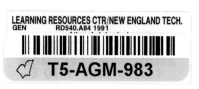

ATLAS OF
ABDOMINAL
SURGERY

Edited by

JOHN W. BRAASCH, M.D., PH.D.

Senior Consultant and Former Chairman
Department of General Surgery
Lahey Clinic Medical Center
Burlington, Massachusetts

Assistant Clinical Professor of Surgery
Harvard Medical School
Boston, Massachusetts

CORNELIUS E. SEDGWICK, M.D.

Department of General Surgery, Emeritus
Lahey Clinic Medical Center
Burlington, Massachusetts

Chairman, Department of Surgery, Emeritus
New England Deaconess Hospital
Boston, Massachusetts

Clinical Professor of Surgery, Emeritus
Harvard Medical School
Boston, Massachusetts

MALCOLM C. VEIDENHEIMER, M.D.

Department of Colon and Rectal Surgery
Former Chairman, Department of General Surgery
Lahey Clinic Medical Center
Burlington, Massachusetts

F. HENRY ELLIS, JR., M.D., PH.D.

Senior Consultant and Former Chairman
Department of Thoracic and Cardiovascular Surgery
Lahey Clinic Medical Center
Burlington, Massachusetts

Chief Emeritus
Division of Thoracic and Cardiovascular Surgery
New England Deaconess Hospital
Boston, Massachusetts

Clinical Professor of Surgery
Harvard Medical School
Boston, Massachusetts

ATLAS OF
ABDOMINAL
SURGERY

1991

W.B. SAUNDERS COMPANY
Harcourt Brace Jovanovich, Inc.

Philadelphia   London   Toronto   Montreal   Sydney   Tokyo

W. B. SAUNDERS COMPANY
Harcourt Brace Jovanovich, Inc.

The Curtis Center
Independence Square West
Philadelphia, PA 19106

Library of Congress Cataloging-in-Publication Data
Atlas of abdominal surgery/edited by John W. Braasch . . . [et al.].
    p.   cm.
ISBN 0–7216–5601–3
    1. Digestive organs—Surgery—Atlases.   I. Braasch, John
        W. (John William)
    [DNLM: 1. Digestive System—surgery—atlases.
WI 17 A874]
RD540.A84   1991
617.5′5—dc20
DNLM/DLC   90–9144

Editor: Edward H. Wickland, Jr.
Developmental Editor: Rosanne Hallowell
Designer: Joan Wendt
Production Manager: Bill Preston
Manuscript Editor: Constance Burton
Illustration Coordinator: Lisa Lambert
Indexer: Kathleen Cole

Atlas of Abdominal Surgery   ISBN 0–7216–5601–3

Last digit is the print number: 9   8   7   6   5   4   3   2   1

The editors wish to dedicate this work to our predecessors on the surgical staff of the Lahey Clinic, to whom we owe a great debt for setting such high standards of surgical practice.

Contributors

JOHN W. BRAASCH, M.D., Ph.D.
Senior Consultant and Former Chairman, Department of General Surgery
Lahey Clinic Medical Center
Burlington, Massachusetts
Assistant Clinical Professor of Surgery
Harvard Medical School
Boston, Massachusetts

JOHN A. COLLER, M.D.
Department of Colon and Rectal Surgery
Lahey Clinic Medical Center
Burlington, Massachusetts
Assistant Clinical Professor of Surgery
Harvard Medical School
Boston, Massachusetts

F. HENRY ELLIS, Jr., M.D., Ph.D.
Senior Consultant, Department of Thoracic and
    Cardiovascular Surgery
Lahey Clinic Medical Center
Chief Emeritus, Division of Thoracic and
    Cardiovascular Surgery
New England Deaconess Hospital
Boston, Massachusetts
Clinical Professor of Surgery
Harvard Medical School
Boston, Massachusetts

ROGER L. JENKINS, M.D.
Director, Division of Hepatobiliary Surgery and
    Liver Transplantation
New England Deaconess Hospital
Boston, Massachusetts
Assistant Clinical Professor of Surgery
Harvard Medical School
Boston, Massachusetts

W. DAVID LEWIS, M.D.
Division of Hepatobiliary Surgery and
    Liver Transplantation
New England Deaconess Hospital–Lahey Clinic
    Medical Center
Boston, Massachusetts

JOHN A. LIBERTINO, M.D.

Staff, Department of Urology
Chairman, Division of Surgery
Lahey Clinic Medical Center
Burlington, Massachusetts
Assistant Clinical Professor of Surgery
Harvard Medical School
Boston, Massachusetts

J. LAWRENCE MUNSON, M.D.

Department of General Surgery
Lahey Clinic Medical Center
Burlington, Massachusetts

C. WRIGHT PINSON, M.D.

Formerly, Fellow in Gastrointestinal Surgery
Lahey Clinic Medical Center
Burlington, Massachusetts
Director, Liver Transplantation Program
Assistant Professor of Surgery and Physiology
Oregon Health Sciences University
Portland, Oregon

STEPHEN G. REMINE, M.D.

Formerly, Department of General Surgery
Lahey Clinic Medical Center
Burlington, Massachusetts
Vice Chairman, Department of Surgery
Associate Professor of Surgery
University of Connecticut Health Center
Farmington, Connecticut

RICARDO L. ROSSI, M.D.

Chairman, Department of General Surgery
Lahey Clinic Medical Center
Burlington, Massachusetts
Assistant Clinical Professor of Surgery
Harvard Medical School
Boston, Massachusetts

JONATHAN M. SACKIER, M.D., F.R.C.S.

Department of Surgery
Cedars-Sinai Medical Center
Los Angeles, California

DAVID J. SCHOETZ, JR., M.D.

Chairman, Department of Colon and Rectal Surgery
Lahey Clinical Medical Center
Burlington, Massachusetts
Assistant Clinical Professor of Surgery
Boston University School of Medicine
Boston, Massachusetts

CORNELIUS E. SEDGWICK, M.D.
Department of General Surgery, Emeritus
Lahey Clinic Medical Center
Burlington, Massachusetts
Chairman, Department of Surgery, Emeritus
New England Deaconess Hospital
Boston, Massachusetts
Clinical Professor of Surgery, Emeritus
Harvard Medical School
Boston, Massachusetts

MALCOLM C. VEIDENHEIMER, M.D.
Department of Colon and Rectal Surgery
Former Chairman, Department of General Surgery
Lahey Clinic Medical Center
Burlington, Massachusetts

Preface

The *Atlas of Abdominal Surgery* outlines for the practicing surgeon the most up-to-date, safe, and effective techniques as used by senior surgeons in the field. The illustrations, created specifically for this volume by the Lahey Clinic's Art Department, are a special strength of this book. Descriptions of the surgical techniques are limited to brief captions in the belief that clear, uncluttered drawings can accomplish more than lengthy narrative. Diagnosis, preoperative preparation, and postoperative care are not discussed. Although these aspects of surgical care are important, this volume concentrates on technique, which, after all, is the art of surgical treatment. A perusal of this volume will enable the surgeon to recognize pitfalls and to concentrate on the essentials of each operation.

In addition to procedures of the gastrointestinal tract, liver, biliary system, pancreas, and spleen, operations for hernias and on the adrenal gland are included. Laparoscopic cholecystectomy is illustrated and described in Chapter 39.

We would like to acknowledge the outstanding work by the members of the Art Department of the Lahey Clinic who created the illustrations for this volume: Paul D. Malone, Francis E. Steckel, Anne S. Greene, and James J. Millerick. We also thank Pauline A. Zorolow of the Editorial Department of the Lahey Clinic for her patient and expert editing of the entire volume, and Elton Watkins, Jr., M.D., for reviewing this work.

Finally, we would like to thank the individual chapter contributors for their descriptions of surgical technique and for their close work with the illustrators, which should ensure that this atlas will be a useful and a beautiful addition to the surgeon's library.

JOHN W. BRAASCH
CORNELIUS E. SEDGWICK
MALCOLM C. VEIDENHEIMER
F. HENRY ELLIS, JR.

Acknowledgments

The contributors acknowledge the vital part played by the members of the Art Department of the Lahey Clinic in the preparation of this volume. The contributing illustrators include Paul D. Malone, Francis E. Steckel, Anne S. Greene, and James J. Millerick. Their work is outstanding.

We also thank Pauline A. Zorolow of the Editorial Department of the Lahey Clinic for her patient and expert editing of the entire volume, and Elton Watkins, Jr., M.D., for reviewing this work.

Contents

Contents

SECTION

1 Gastrointestinal Tract

Esophagogastrectomy for Cancer of the Cardia

1

F. HENRY ELLIS, JR., M.D., PH.D.

▼ IMPORTANT FEATURES
Wide Mobilization of Distal Esophagus and Proximal Stomach
Ligation of Gastric Blood Supply
Division of Stomach Below Growth and Esophagus Above It with
      4-cm Margins or Greater
End-to-Side Esophagogastrostomy

▼ STEPS OR PLANS
Left Thoracotomy
Mobilization of Distal Esophagus
Opening of Diaphragm
Mobilization of Stomach
Division of Stomach
End-to-Side Esophagogastrostomy
Closure of Diaphragm and Chest

1. INCISION

▼

Exposure for esophagogastrectomy for lesions of the esophagogastric junction or of the lower esophagus is best obtained through a left thoracotomy. A thoracoabdominal incision, although providing slightly greater exposure, prolongs the operative procedure unnecessarily and may lead to an unstable costal arch or chondritis or both with a chronically draining sinus.

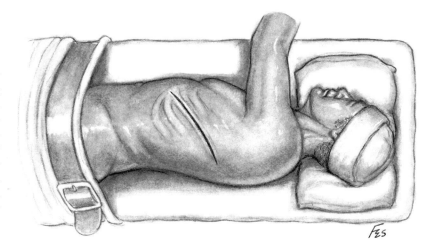

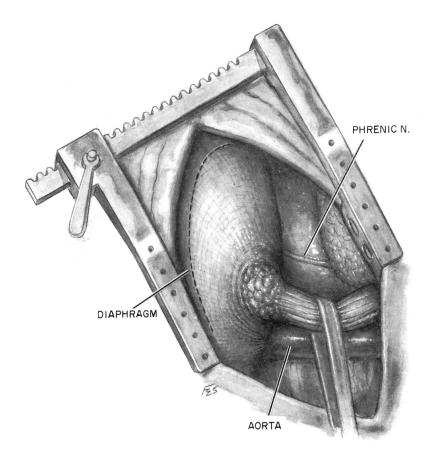

PHRENIC N.

DIAPHRAGM

AORTA

2. ESOPHAGEAL MOBILIZATION

▼

The left thorax is entered through the bed of the nonresected eighth rib, the angle of which may require division to provide better exposure. The mediastinal pleura is opened to permit the esophagus to be mobilized proximal to the growth and encircled with a Penrose drain. *Dashed line* indicates site of incision in the diaphragm.

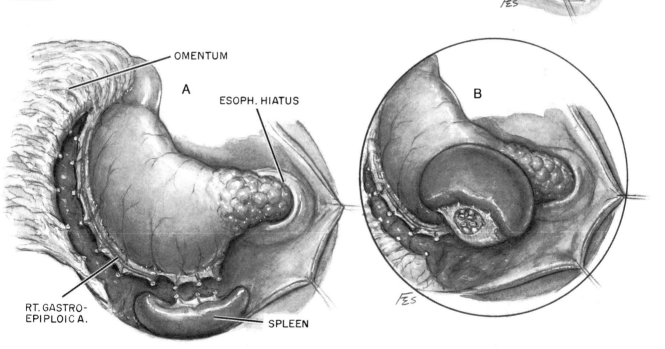

3. DIAPHRAGMATIC INCISION

Although radial incisions in the diaphragm crossing the diaphragmatic crural noose were commonly employed in the past, better exposure of the upper abdomen is obtained through a semilunar incision near the costal arch. This provides a flap of diaphragm that, when elevated and retracted cephalad, provides excellent exposure of the left upper abdomen.

4. INITIAL DISSECTION OF STOMACH

A and B, Mobilization of the stomach is begun by separation of the hiatal attachments of the esophagus and division of the gastrohepatic omentum. Mobilization is continued, as indicated, by division of the short gastric vessels with preservation of the right gastroepiploic artery. When the spleen and tail of the pancreas are involved by the growth, they too can be removed.

5. POSTERIOR GASTRIC DISSECTION

▼

A and *B,* The freed stomach is elevated to expose the posterior vessels (usually two). The posterior gastric artery and recurrent branch of the left inferior phrenic arteries are ligated and divided. The origin of the left gastric artery is exposed. Node-bearing tissue is carefully dissected away from the celiac axis so as to be included in the resected specimen. The left gastric artery is doubly ligated and divided.

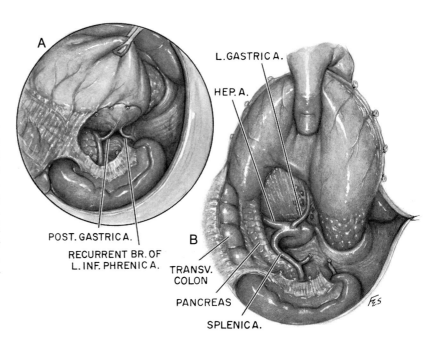

POST. GASTRIC A.

RECURRENT BR. OF
L. INF. PHRENIC A.

L. GASTRIC A.

HEP. A.

TRANSV.
COLON

PANCREAS

SPLENIC A.

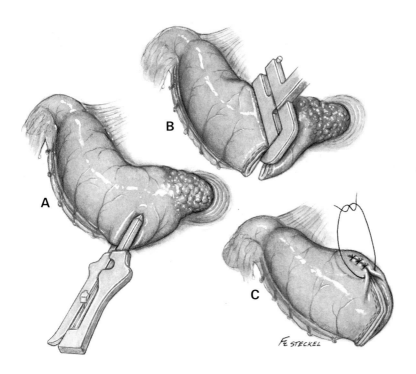

6. DIVISION OF STOMACH

▼

The stomach is divided well below the growth. *A,* A GIA stapling device is placed at right angles to the greater curvature, and the stomach is partially divided. *B,* The lesser curvature point of division is below the point of ligation of the left gastric artery, and a TA-90 stapler is used for this maneuver. *C,* The stapled stomach is then oversewn with nonabsorbable interrupted sutures.

7. ESOPHAGOGASTROSTOMY

▼

After the growth is freed from the surrounding tissues, which may require excision of a part of the diaphragm, the proximal stomach and the growth are passed through the hiatus into the chest after manual widening of the diaphragmatic hiatus. The divided distal stomach is advanced into the chest, and an end-to-side esophagogastrostomy is performed without the use of clamps and without tension. The first layer, illustrated here, is being fashioned with nonabsorbable interrupted sutures.

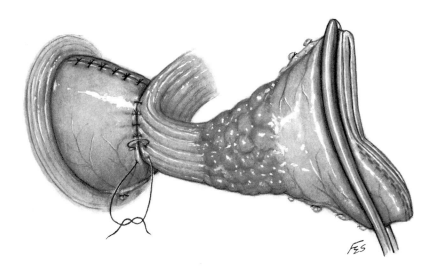

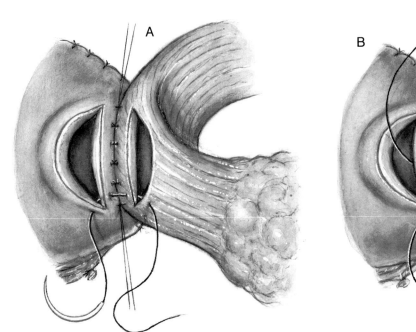
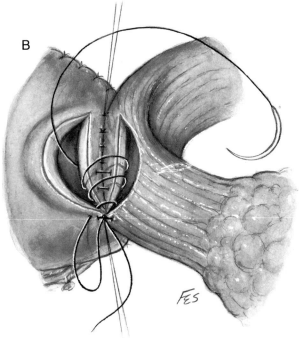

8. ESOPHAGOGASTROSTOMY
(Continued)

▼

A, The esophagus and stomach are opened, and the anastomosis is continued with running fine sutures of chromic catgut. B, The posterior row is completed using through-and-through sutures through the full thickness of the wall of the esophagus and stomach.

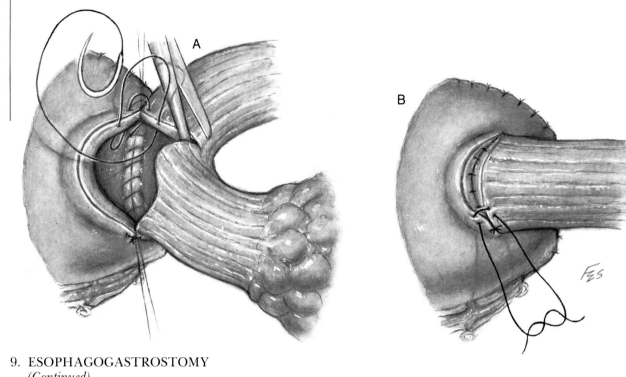

9. ESOPHAGOGASTROSTOMY
(Continued)

A and *B,* The suture is passed to the outside of the bowel before beginning the anterior layer closure. The anterior layer closure is continued, the suture approximating only the mucosa and submucosa. Nonabsorbable interrupted sutures are used for the final seromuscular layer.

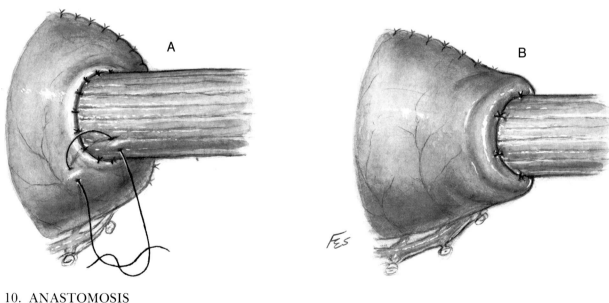

10. ANASTOMOSIS REINFORCEMENT

A, To provide additional safety to the anastomotic site, the anastomosis is "inkwelled" by surrounding it with adjacent fundus using a few nonabsorbable interrupted sutures. *B,* The final appearance of the anastomosis.

11. CLOSURE

After the anastomosis has been completed, the diaphragm is closed with nonabsorbable figure-of-eight sutures. A chest tube is brought out a separate stab wound for postoperative drainage, and the chest is closed in routine fashion.

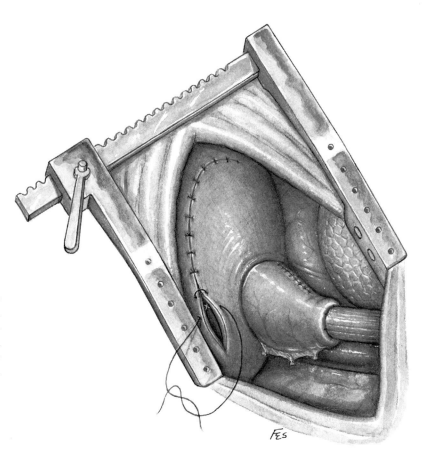

2 Nissen Fundoplication

F. HENRY ELLIS, JR., M.D., PH.D.

▼ IMPORTANT FEATURES
  Mobilization of Distal Esophagus
  Complete Freeing of Gastric Fundus
  Performance of Loose Wrap

▼ STEPS OR PLANS
  Retraction of Left Lobe of Liver
  Mobilization of Esophagus
  Freeing of Gastric Fundus
  Suture Approximation of Diaphragmatic Crura
  Loose Wrap of Distal Esophagus

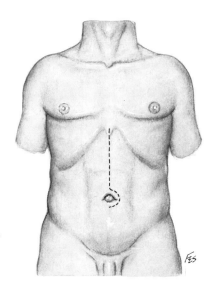

1. INCISION

An upper midline incision is made from the xiphoid to a point just below the umbilicus, skirting this structure on the left. The incision is continued cephalad on the left lateral side of the xiphoid to provide optimal exposure of the esophageal hiatus.

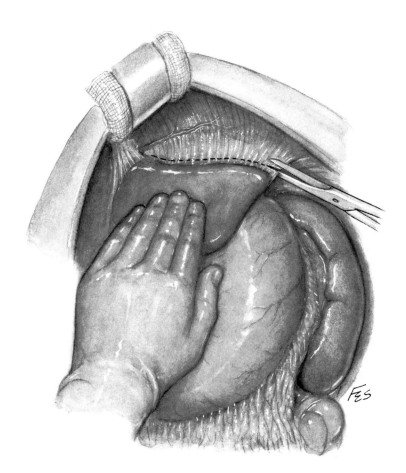

2. MOBILIZATION OF LEFT LOBE OF LIVER

The left lobe of the liver is mobilized by dividing the triangular ligament.

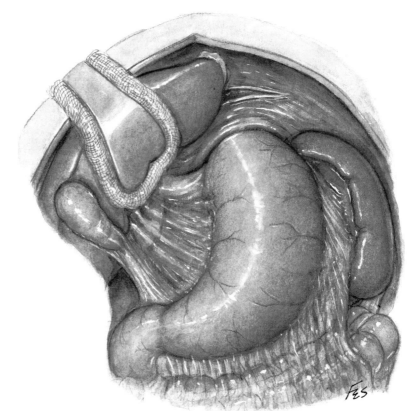

3. EXPOSURE

The liver is retracted using a well-padded liver retractor, thus exposing the region of the esophageal hiatus.

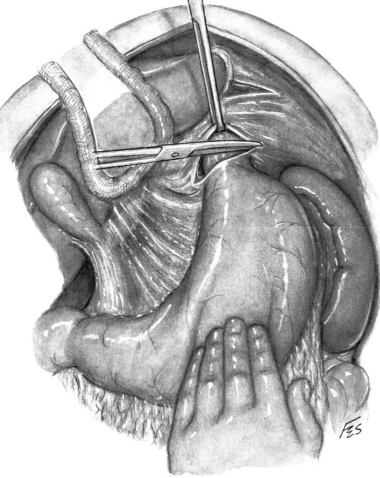

4. SECTION OF PHRENOESOPHAGEAL MEMBRANE

A hernia, if present, is reduced. The phrenoesophageal membrane is incised to expose the anterior aspect of the distal esophagus and permit its accurate mobilization.

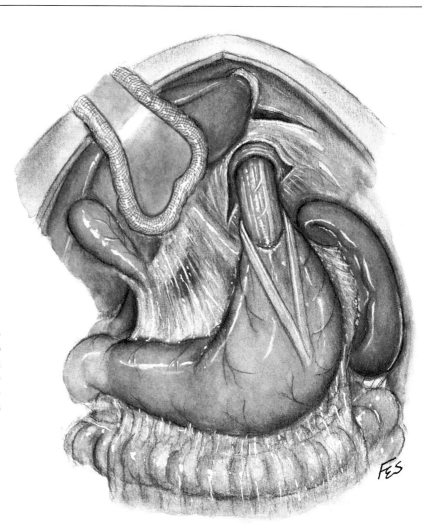

5. MOBILIZATION OF ESOPHAGUS

The esophagus is freed from its hiatal attachments, care being taken to preserve the vagi. It is encircled with a Penrose drain, and esophageal mobilization is continued until approximately 3 to 5 cm of distal esophagus lies free in the abdomen.

6. MOBILIZATION OF GASTRIC FUNDUS

The gastric fundus must be freed completely in preparation for a loose wrap. This part of the procedure is initiated by division of the short gastric vessels and is facilitated by placing a moist pack behind the spleen, thus relieving tension on the short gastric vessels during their control and division. The vessels are successively clamped, divided, and tied starting distally and moving proximally along the greater curvature of the stomach. One or two posterior gastric vessels must also be divided to permit complete mobilization of the gastric fundus.

7. SUTURE OF CRURA

The esophagus is elevated with a special instrument to expose the esophageal hiatus. The hiatus is narrowed by placing two or three nonabsorbable interrupted heavy sutures in the diaphragmatic crura posterior to the esophagus and tying them loosely. This simply prevents migration of the fundoplicated esophagus into the chest; therefore, the degree of narrowing should be slight so as not to compress the esophagus.

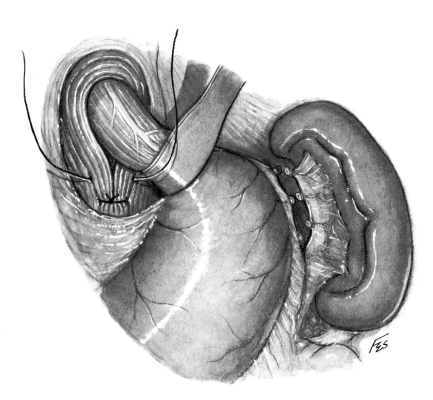

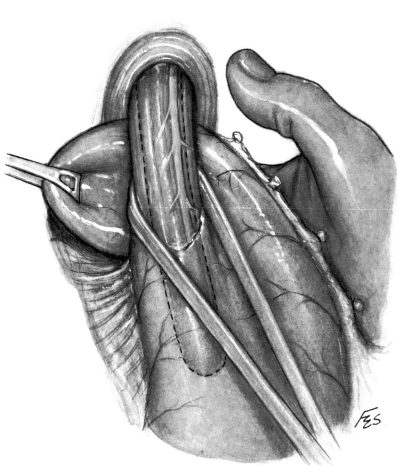

8. WRAP OF GASTRIC FUNDUS

With the operator's right hand, the freed gastric fundus is passed behind the esophagus where it can be grasped with a Babcock clamp to the right of this organ. A large-bore (No. 42 to No. 50 French) Maloney dilator is introduced transorally by the anesthesiologist and passed into the stomach. All subsequent parts of the wrapping procedure are conducted with this in place as a stent to permit performance of a loose wrap.

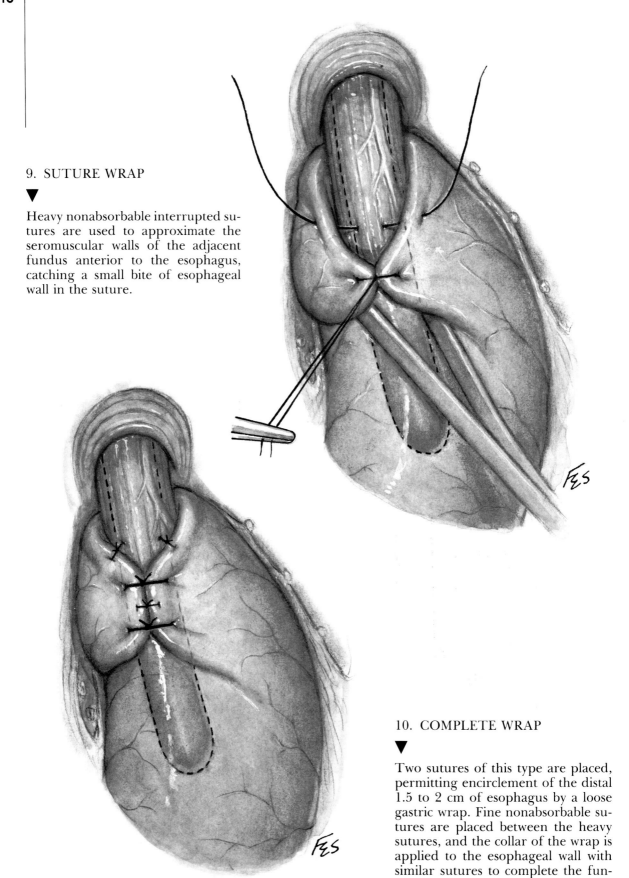

9. SUTURE WRAP

▼

Heavy nonabsorbable interrupted sutures are used to approximate the seromuscular walls of the adjacent fundus anterior to the esophagus, catching a small bite of esophageal wall in the suture.

10. COMPLETE WRAP

▼

Two sutures of this type are placed, permitting encirclement of the distal 1.5 to 2 cm of esophagus by a loose gastric wrap. Fine nonabsorbable sutures are placed between the heavy sutures, and the collar of the wrap is applied to the esophageal wall with similar sutures to complete the fundoplication.

Paraesophageal Hiatus Hernia

3

F. HENRY ELLIS, JR., M.D., PH.D.

▼ IMPORTANT FEATURES
Reduction of Hernia
Excision of Hernia Sac
Approximation of Diaphragmatic Crura Anterior to Esophagus

▼ STEPS OR PLANS
Mobilization of Left Lobe of Liver by Division of Triangular
    Ligament
Manual Reduction of Intrathoracic Stomach and Other Abdominal
    Viscera (If Present) into Abdomen
Excision of Hernia Sac, Protection of Esophagus and Its Normal
    Attachments, and Preservation of Vagi
Traction Elevation of Apex of Esophageal Crura
Approximation of Crura Anterior to Esophagus with Multiple
    Interrupted Sutures of Nonabsorbable Material
Anterior Gastropexy Facilitated by Performance of Stamm
    Gastrostomy

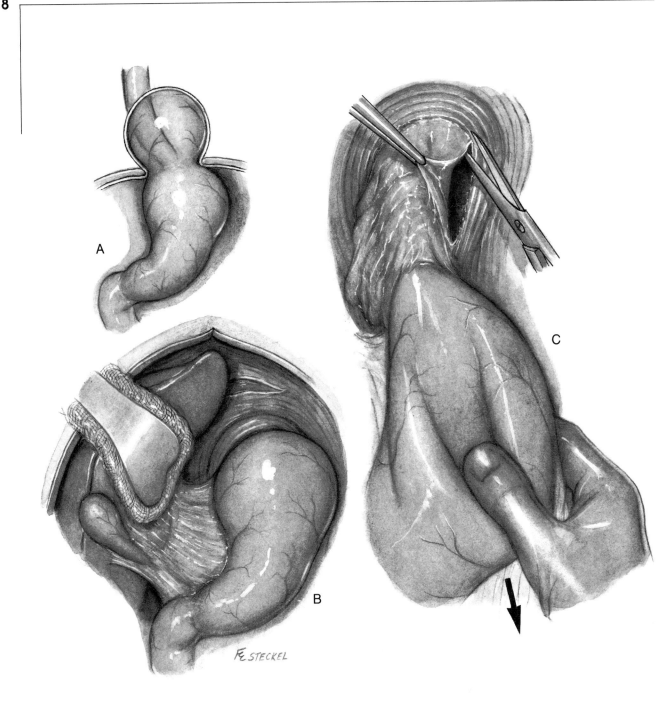

1. EXPOSURE OF HIATUS

▼

A, Semidiagrammatic representation of a true paraesophageal hernia, with the gastric fundus and its peritoneal envelope passing anterior to the esophagus. In advanced cases, greater portions of the stomach migrate into the chest and may rotate counterclockwise. Bowel and spleen also may be found within the hernia sac. *B,* The triangular ligament is divided, permitting mobilization of the left lobe of the liver and visualization of the region of the hiatus. *C,* The redundant peritoneum, which constitutes the hernia sac, is excised, and the edges of the diaphragmatic crura are freshened.

2. ANTERIOR APPROXIMATION OF CRURA

A, The diaphragmatic crus is grasped with a Babcock clamp and elevated toward the ceiling, preserving the normal position and attachments of the esophagus and esophagogastric junction. Heavy nonabsorbable sutures are placed to approximate the crura. *B,* The sutures are placed so that a snug hiatus is achieved but not so tightly as to cause obstruction. An opening two fingerbreadths alongside the esophagus and an indwelling nasogastric tube should provide an opening of adequate size.

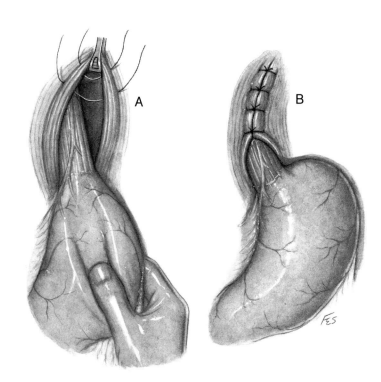

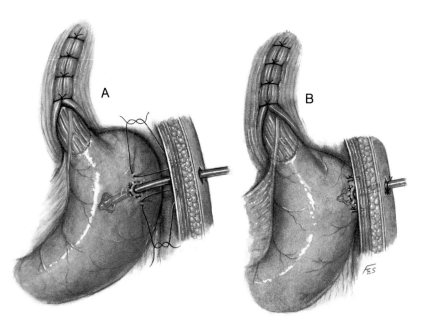

3. GASTROSTOMY AND GASTROPEXY

A, Stamm gastrostomy is performed. A site near the greater curvature of the fundus is selected. *B,* After the gastrostomy has been performed, anterior gastropexy is carried out, approximating the stomach wall to the undersurface of the abdominal wall with absorbable interrupted sutures. This maneuver is performed to minimize gastric dilatation postoperatively and to reduce the possibility of recurrent herniation of the fundus into the chest.

Closure of Perforated Peptic Ulcer

CORNELIUS E. SEDGWICK, M.D.

▼ IMPORTANT FEATURES
All Gastric Ulcers Biopsied
Free Omental Graft for Closure
Minimal Dissection

▼ STEPS OR PLANS
Incision—Upper Right Paramedian or Midline
Irrigation of Abdominal Cavity
Section of Omentum Excised for Graft
Graft Prepared as Solid Tube
Through-and-Through Sutures Placed Around Ulcer
Free Omental Graft Placed Over Ulcer and Secured

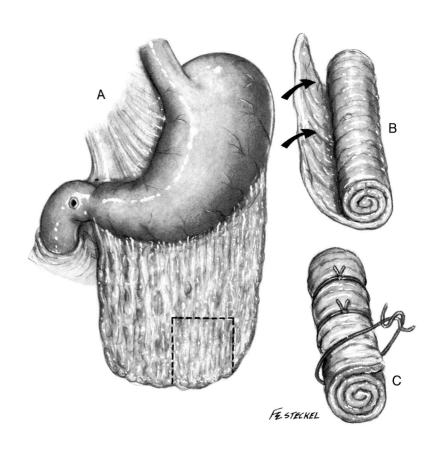

1. PREPARATION FOR CLOSURE

▼

The abdomen is entered through an upper right paramedian or midline incision. All gastric ulcers are biopsied. Minimal abdominal exploration is made for possible multiple perforations. The abdomen is irrigated to flush out foreign material and exudate. *A,* A section of omentum 4 to 5 cm in length is excised. *B* and *C,* The free omentum is fashioned as a solid tube and tied.

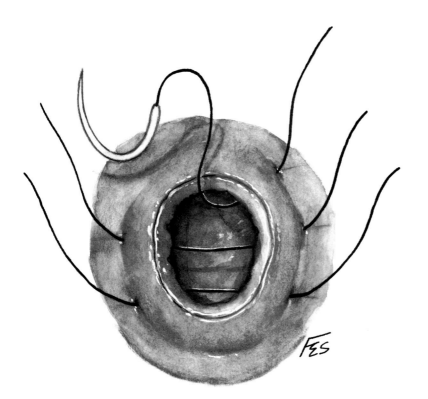

2. SUTURE PLACEMENT

▼

Through-and-through sutures are placed in the duodenum wide of any induration. Care is taken to place the sutures through the duodenum (outside in) and then back (inside out). This prevents inadvertently picking up the mucosa of the opposite duodenal wall.

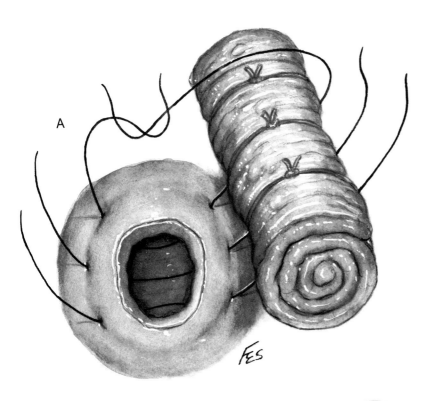

3. CLOSURE PERFORATION

▼

A, The free omental graft is placed over the perforation. *B*, The duodenal sutures are tied without tension.

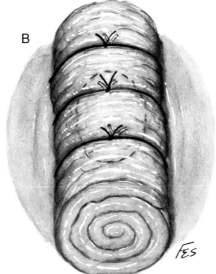

5 Gastrostomy

CORNELIUS E. SEDGWICK, M.D.

▼ IMPORTANT FEATURES

Temporary

> *For Gastric Decompression and Drainage: Gastric Mucosa Inverted to Permit Spontaneous Closure at Later Date*

Permanent

> *For Gastric Feeding: Gastric Wall Everted to Prevent Spontaneous Closure*

▼ STEPS OR PLANS

Temporary

> *Mobilization of Anterior Lower One Third of Stomach*
> *Double Pursestring Suture at Selected Site of Gastrostomy*
> *Incision of Stomach and Insertion of Tube*
> *Closure of Stomach Wall Around Tube (Witzel Procedure)*
> *Tube Exteriorized Through Stab Wound*

Permanent

> *Entire Gastric Wall Tents Through Abdominal Stab Incision*
> *Stomach Opened and Edges Sutured to Skin*

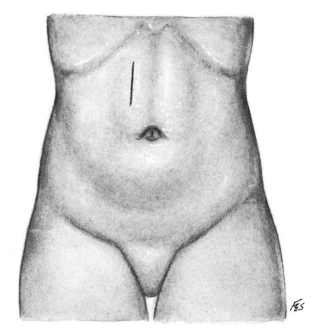

1. INCISION

A right rectus muscle–splitting incision is made above the umbilicus.

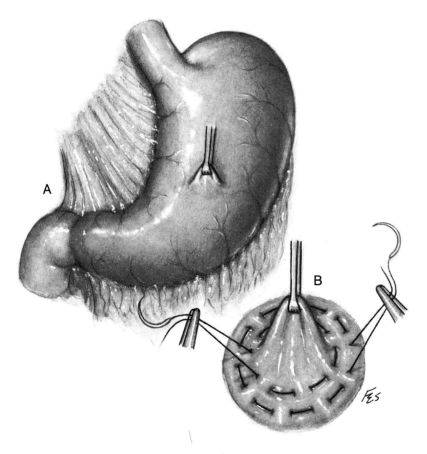

2. PURSESTRING SUTURE PLACED

When the abdomen is entered, the stomach is identified and partially mobilized. *A,* The site of the gastrostomy is determined and grasped with an Allis clamp. *B,* A double pursestring suture is placed around the tented gastric wall.

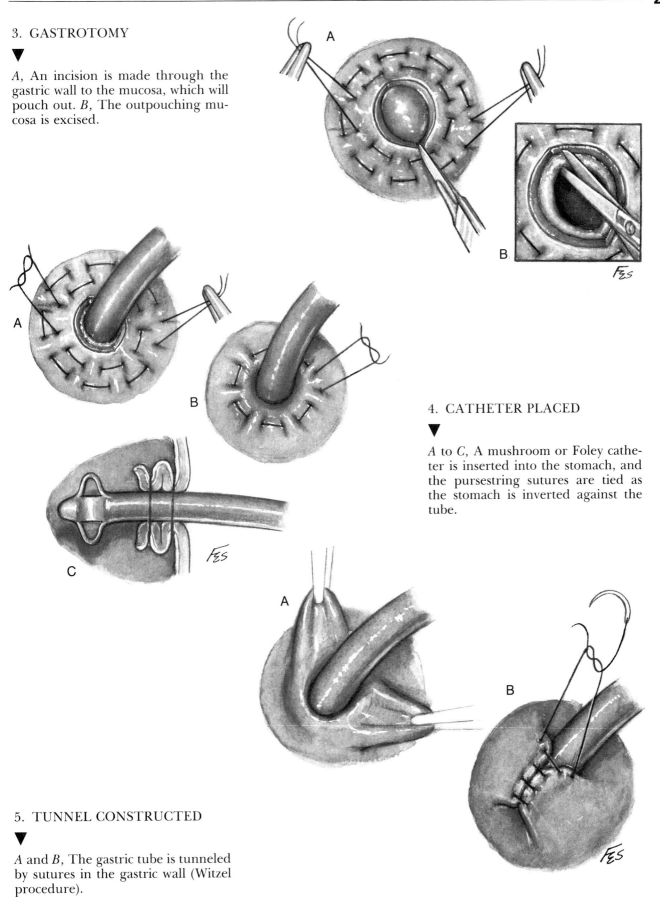

3. GASTROTOMY

▼

A, An incision is made through the gastric wall to the mucosa, which will pouch out. *B,* The outpouching mucosa is excised.

4. CATHETER PLACED

▼

A to *C,* A mushroom or Foley catheter is inserted into the stomach, and the pursestring sutures are tied as the stomach is inverted against the tube.

5. TUNNEL CONSTRUCTED

▼

A and *B,* The gastric tube is tunneled by sutures in the gastric wall (Witzel procedure).

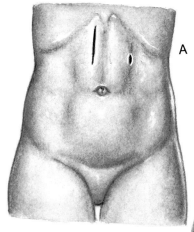

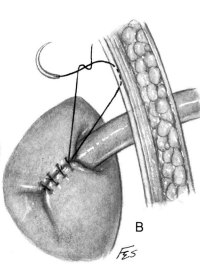

6. STAB WOUND; STOMACH FIXED

▼

A, A stab wound is made in the abdominal wall to the left of the primary incision. *B,* The gastric tube is brought out of the abdomen through the stab wound. The gastric wall is sutured to the peritoneum.

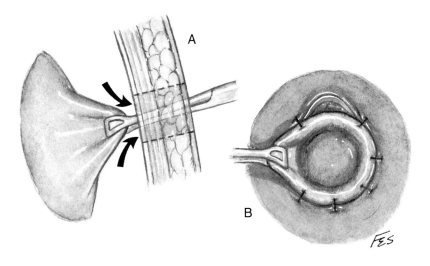

7. PERMANENT GASTROSTOMY

▼

A, A permanent gastrostomy is accomplished by tenting the gastric wall through the abdominal stab incision. *B,* The stomach is incised, and the edges of the stomach are sutured to the skin.

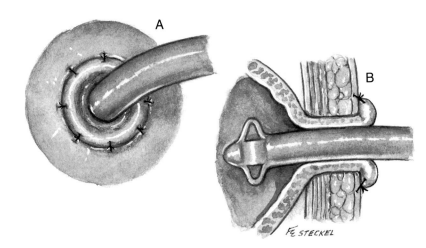

8. TUBE PLACED

▼

A and *B,* The gastric tube is in place with the gastric wall inverted and sutured to the skin.

6 Gastrojejunostomy

CORNELIUS E. SEDGWICK, M.D.

▼ IMPORTANT FEATURES
Stoma Placed on Most Dependent Part of Stomach
Afferent (Proximal) Loop Should Be as Short as Possible but without
    Tension
Jejunal Loop Usually Anterior to Colon Except In Obese Patients
Stoma Placed on Posterior Wall of Stomach
Efferent (Distal) Loop Slightly Lower on Stomach Wall for Better
    Drainage into Distal Jejunum

▼ STEPS OR PLANS
Midline or Upper Left Paramedian Incision
Mobilization of Stomach and Upper Jejunum
Entering Lesser Sac and Mobilization of Greater Curvature of
    Stomach
Free Jejunum from Adhesions Around Ligament of Treitz
Fixation of Jejunal Loop to Posterior Wall of Stomach
Complete Anastomosis
Closure of Lesser Sac

1. LESSER SAC ENTERED

▼

The lesser sac is entered by upward traction on the stomach and downward traction on the colon, permitting the gastrocolic omentum to fall away from the transverse mesocolon. The middle third of the greater curvature of the stomach is freed of the gastrocolic omentum. The posterior wall of the stomach is retracted upward, and the site of the stoma is selected.

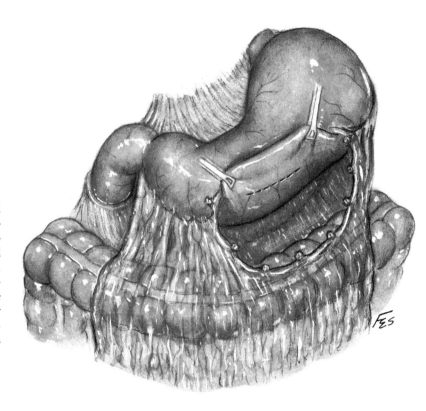

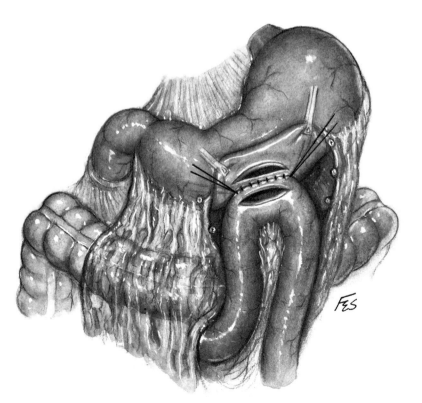

2. ANASTOMOSIS

▼

The proximal jejunum is freed from any adhesions in the region of the ligament of Treitz and is brought up anterior to the colon and fixed to the selected site of the stoma on the posterior wall of the stomach with interrupted mattress sutures. Incisions are made through the walls of the stomach and jejunum.

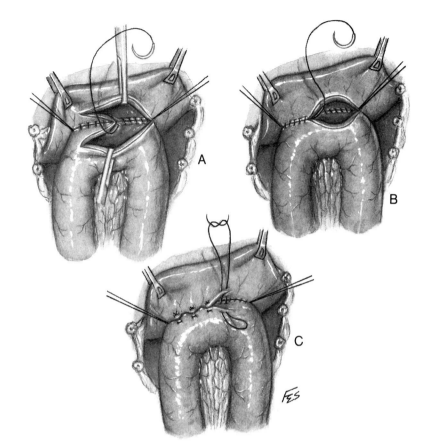

A

B

C

FES

3. ANASTOMOSIS *(Continued)*

▼

A and *B*, A simple running suture through all layers reinforces the posterior layer and is continued as a running Connell inverting suture closing the anterior layer. *C*, Interrupted mattress sutures on the anterior walls complete the anastomosis.

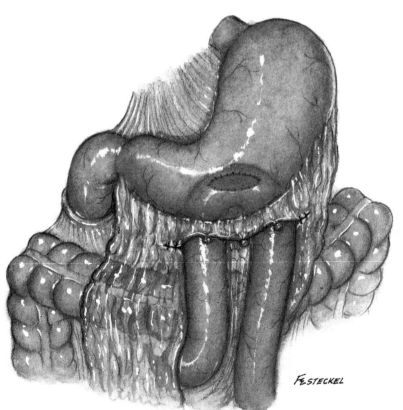

FESTECKEL

4. LESSER SAC CLOSED

▼

The open edges of the gastrocolic omentum are sutured to the loops of the jejunum to close the lesser sac. The stoma lies comfortably on the most dependent area of the posterior wall of the stomach.

7 | Gastrectomy

CORNELIUS E. SEDGWICK, M.D.

▼ IMPORTANT FEATURES

Mobilization of Stomach and First Portion of Duodenum (or Lower
Esophagus)
Extragastric Ligation of Blood Supply
Resection of Stomach and First Portion of Duodenum (or Lower
Esophagus)
Reestablish Continuity of Upper Gastrointestinal Tract

▼ STEPS OR PLANS

Identification and Partial Mobilization of First Portion of Duodenum
Entering Lesser Sac
Mobilization of Greater Curvature of Stomach (High)
Complete Mobilization of Greater Curvature of Stomach and
Ligation of Right Gastroepiploic Vessels
Complete Mobilization of Distal Stomach and First Portion of
Duodenum and Ligation of Right Gastric Vessel
Division of Duodenum
Closure of Duodenum
Ligation of Left Gastric Vessel
Division of Stomach
Closure of Lesser Curvature Side of Stomach
Gastrojejunostomy—Billroth II
Gastroduodenostomy—Billroth I
Esophagojejunostomy—Total Gastrectomy
Enteroenterostomy

1. ANATOMY

Blood supply of the stomach with usual extent of resection for peptic ulceration. Subtotal gastrectomy involves mobilization of the stomach, extragastric ligation of the blood supply, excision of the desired gastric and duodenal mass, and reestablishment of continuity of the upper gastrointestinal tract by gastroduodenal anastomosis (Billroth I) or gastrojejunostomy (Billroth II).

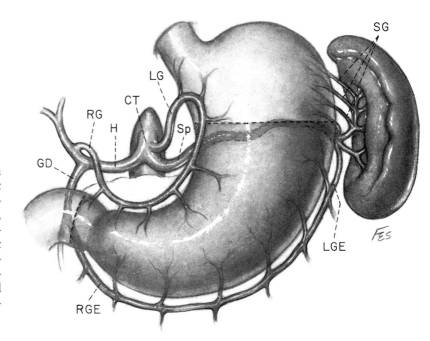

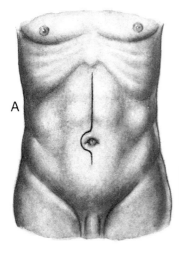

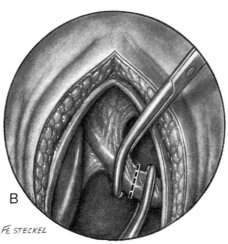

2. INCISION

A, Long vertical midline incision extends from xiphoid around and below the umbilicus. This gives adequate exposure of both the duodenum and the high lesser gastric vessels. B, After the abdominal cavity has been entered, the round ligament is divided to mobilize partially the left lobe of the liver. This allows better exposure of the proximal stomach and the left gastric artery and vein.

3. IDENTIFICATION AND PARTIAL MOBILIZATION OF FIRST PORTION OF DUODENUM DISTAL TO PATHOLOGY

▼

The first portion of the duodenum may be closely adherent to the gallbladder, colon, omentum, and mesentery. The duodenum is separated from these structures to establish normal relationships. The pathology is visualized. Distal to the site of disease and at a level where the duodenum appears normal, incisions are made both above and below close to the margins of the duodenum. This allows normal duodenum to bulge from its attachments and to act as a target area for later mobilization and section of the duodenum.

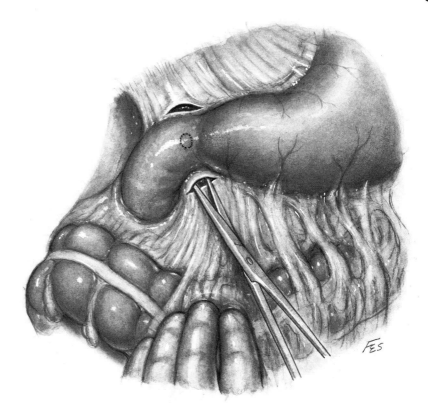

4. ENTERING LESSER SAC

▼

The lesser sac is entered left of the midpoint. Entering the lesser sac to the right is difficult, particularly in ulcer disease, as the gastrocolic omentum may be fused by inflammatory adhesions to the mesocolon, and at this site the colic vessels may be injured. The lesser sac is entered by upward traction on the stomach and downward traction on the transverse colon. This puts the gastrocolic omentum on the stretch and allows it to fall away from the transverse mesocolon.

5. MOBILIZATION OF GREATER CURVATURE OF STOMACH

▼

With continued upward traction on the stomach and downward traction on the transverse colon, putting the gastric omentum on the stretch, mobilization of the greater curvature of the stomach to the left is accomplished by dividing the short gastric vessels. It makes no difference whether these vessels are divided and ligated close to the stomach or outside the arcuate of the epiploic vessels. Ligation of the high short gastric vessel allows better mobilization of the stomach. Careful traction avoids injury to the spleen.

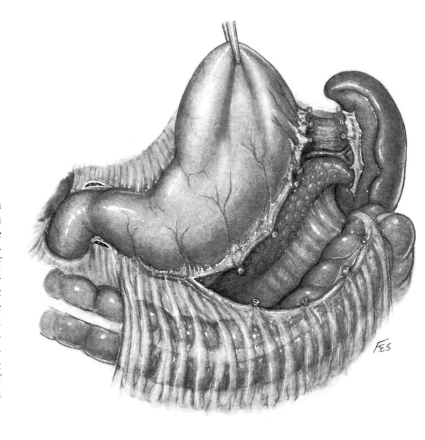

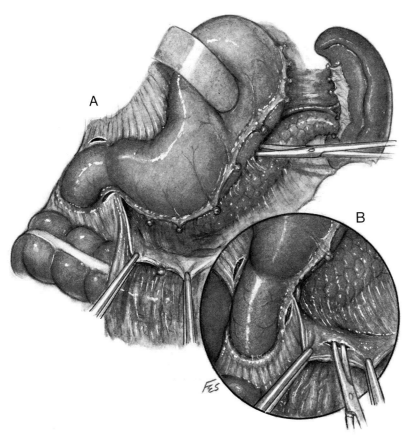

6. COMPLETE MOBILIZATION OF GREATER CURVATURE OF STOMACH AND LIGATION OF RIGHT GASTROEPIPLOIC VESSELS

▼

A, With the left half of the greater curvature freed, the stomach is retracted upward, anterior, and to the left. Frequently, adhesions have formed between the posterior wall of the stomach and the reflection of the peritoneum over the pancreas. These are avascular and are divided to mobilize the posterior wall of the stomach from the pancreas.

B, Attention is then turned to the right side of the greater curvature. Again, downward traction on the transverse colon allows dissection in an avascular plane, separating the gastric omentum from the transverse mesocolon. Care must be taken not to injure the right colic artery, which may be pulled into a posterior duo-

Continued

Figure 6 *Continued*
denal ulcer. The remaining vessels along the greater curvature are divided. The neck of the pancreas is visualized, and the gastroduodenal artery crossing the pancreas is identified.

7. LIGATION OF RIGHT GASTROEPIPLOIC VESSEL

▼

The gastroepiploic artery is identified near its origin from the gastroduodenal artery. The stomach is retracted at right angles to the abdomen. The original target area beyond the ulcer is visualized. The remaining tissue together with the right gastroepiploic artery is divided close to its origin, completing the mobilization of the greater curvature of the stomach and first portion of the duodenum distal to the ulcer.

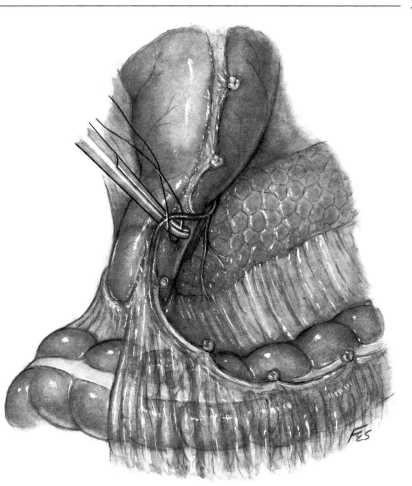

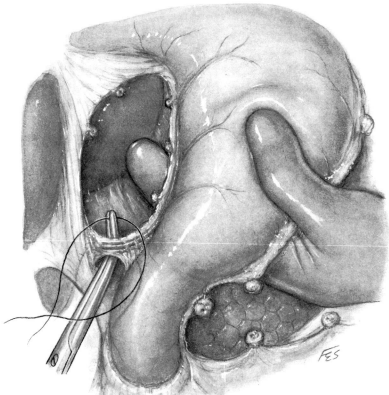

8. COMPLETE MOBILIZATION OF DISTAL STOMACH AND FIRST PORTION OF DUODENUM; LIGATION OF RIGHT GASTRIC VESSELS

▼

An avascular area in the gastrohepatic omentum is identified and entered. The vessels along the lesser curvature are divided distal to the left gastric vessels. An avascular plane is developed so that the caudal lobe of the liver is visualized. This will give better visualization of the left gastric vessels later in the procedure. As dissection proceeds distally along the lesser curvature, the right gastric vessels are identified and ligated close to the duodenum. If an anterosuperior duodenal or pyloric ulcer is encountered, extreme care must be used to avoid injury to the common bile duct.

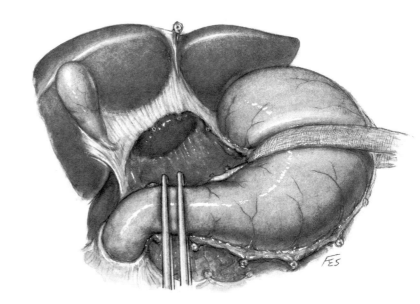

9. DIVISION OF DUODENUM

Traction is applied to the stomach. Kocher clamps are applied across the duodenum just distal to the ulcer and pylorus. The duodenum is transected between the clamps. The transected duodenum is covered with a pad and placed upward and to the left, allowing exposure for duodenal closure.

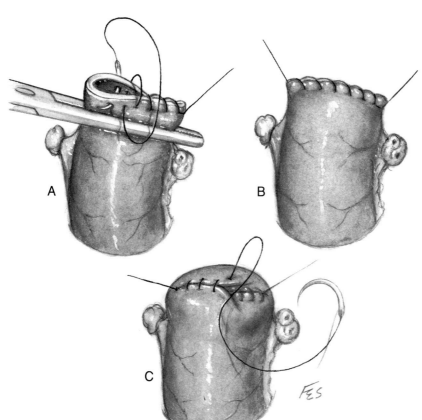

10. CLOSURE OF DUODENAL STUMP (ROUTINE)

Closure of the duodenum depends on pathologic findings. *A*, When adequate duodenum is available, the cuff of the duodenum above the clamp may be closed with a running absorbable suture. *B* and *C*, The clamp is removed, and the closed cuff is inverted with a running Connell absorbable suture.

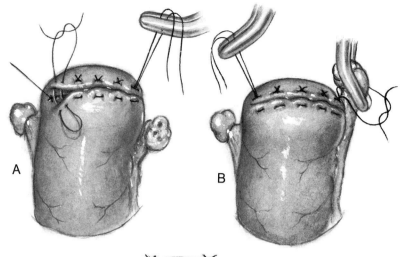

11. CLOSURE OF DUODENAL STUMP (ROUTINE, *Continued*)

▼

A to C, A layer of interrupted mattress silk sutures completes the closure. The angles of the closure are reinforced by tying in the stumps of the right gastric vessels above and the gastroepiploic vessels below. This also further secures these vessels.

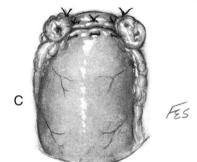

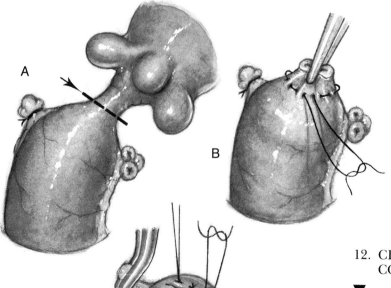

12. CLOSURE FOR CONSTRICTED DUODENUM

▼

Ulcerations may present with a constricted duodenum and pseudopolyposis above. *A* and *B,* This may be managed by division of the constricted area and by inversion and closure with a pursestring suture. *C,* The inverted stump is then reinforced with interrupted silk mattress sutures.

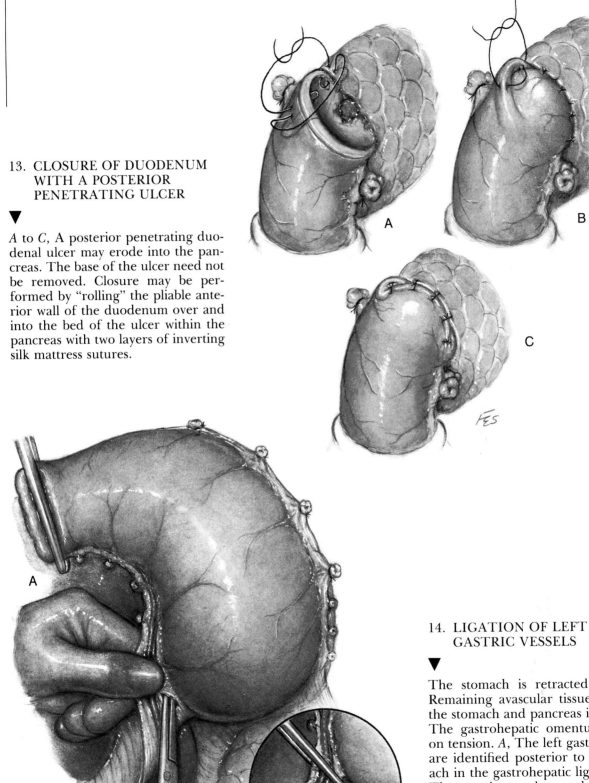

13. CLOSURE OF DUODENUM WITH A POSTERIOR PENETRATING ULCER

▼

A to *C,* A posterior penetrating duodenal ulcer may erode into the pancreas. The base of the ulcer need not be removed. Closure may be performed by "rolling" the pliable anterior wall of the duodenum over and into the bed of the ulcer within the pancreas with two layers of inverting silk mattress sutures.

14. LIGATION OF LEFT GASTRIC VESSELS

▼

The stomach is retracted upward. Remaining avascular tissue between the stomach and pancreas is divided. The gastrohepatic omentum is put on tension. *A,* The left gastric vessels are identified posterior to the stomach in the gastrohepatic ligament. *B,* The gastric vessels are clamped, ligated, and divided. The lesser curvature is cleared of any remaining tissue, which completes the extragastric devascularization and mobilization of the stomach.

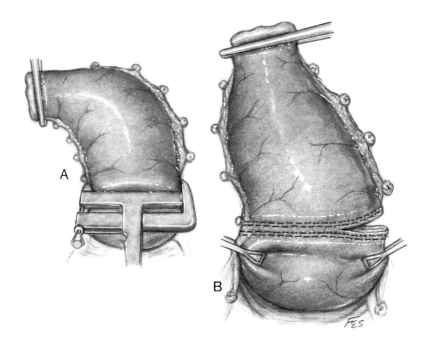

15. DIVISION OF STOMACH

A and *B*, With the stomach on upward traction, two rows of staples are applied. The stomach is divided between the rows of staples with the electrocautery. This ensures minimal bleeding.

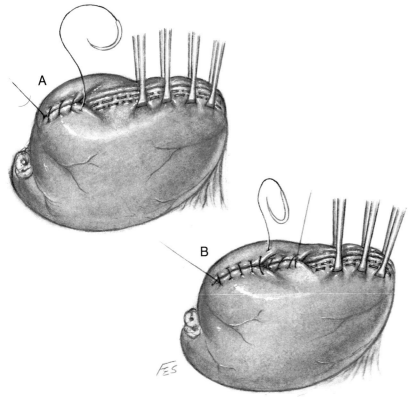

16. CLOSURE OF LESSER CURVATURE SIDE OF STOMACH

A and *B*, The stomach is retracted with Allis clamps. The lesser curvature side of the divided stomach is closed in three layers. A running absorbable suture is placed over the staples for hemostasis. A second running inverting Connell suture inverts the closed stomach and staples. A third layer of inverted silk mattress sutures is placed (see Fig. 17*A*). Each suture is held with a separate clamp.

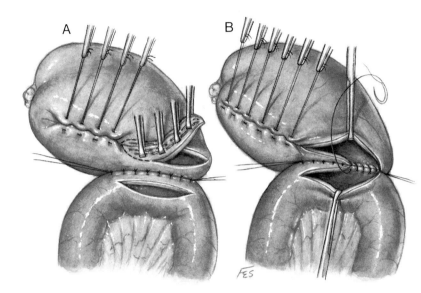

17. GASTROJEJUNOSTOMY—BILLROTH II

▼

Usually a short loop of jejunum (15 cm) from the ligament of Treitz is brought over the transverse colon for anastomosis. Occasionally to obtain a short loop, particularly in the patient with a large fatty omentum and transverse mesocolon, it may be necessary to bring the jejunal loop through an opening in the transverse mesocolon. We prefer an antiperistaltic gastrojejunostomy with the afferent (proximal) loop of jejunum sutured to the greater curvature side of the stomach. The posterior layer of sutures is placed between the stomach and jejunum. An appropriate incision, slightly larger than the diameter of the small bowel, is made through the jejunal wall. *A,* The staples are removed from the gastric margin. *B,* A simple running absorbable suture reinforces the posterior layer.

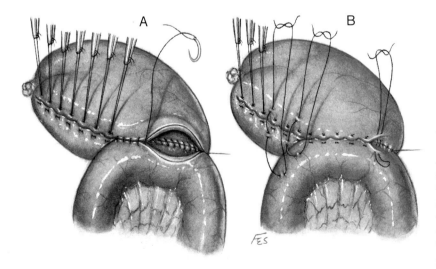

18. CLOSURE OF ANASTOMOSIS

▼

A and *B,* The posterior running absorbable suture is continued anteriorly as a running Connell inverting suture to close the anastomosis. Interrupted nonabsorbable sutures are used for the second layer of closure. The lesser curvature of the anastomosis is buttressed with two or three pursestring sutures between the jejunum and posterior and anterior walls of the stomach.

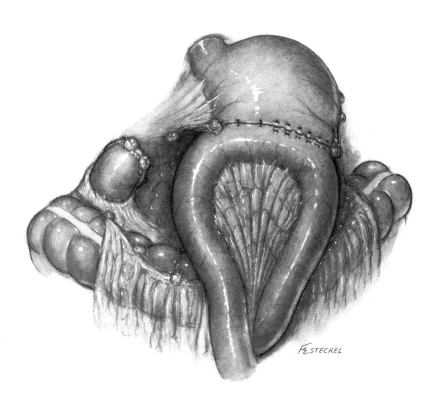

19. COMPLETED OPERATION

The stump of the left gastric vessel is tied to the lesser curvature angle of the anastomosis. Illustration shows the completed procedure. The duodenal stump is closed. A small gastric remnant is left with an anticolic-antiperistaltic gastrojejunostomy.

20. GASTRODUODENOSTOMY— BILLROTH I

The initial steps for a Billroth I subtotal gastrectomy are the same as for a Billroth II subtotal gastrectomy (see Figs. 2 to 16). The duodenum is brought up to the greater curvature side of the stomach. A posterior layer of nonabsorbable mattress sutures approximates the stomach and duodenum. The staples on the closed gastric remnant are removed.

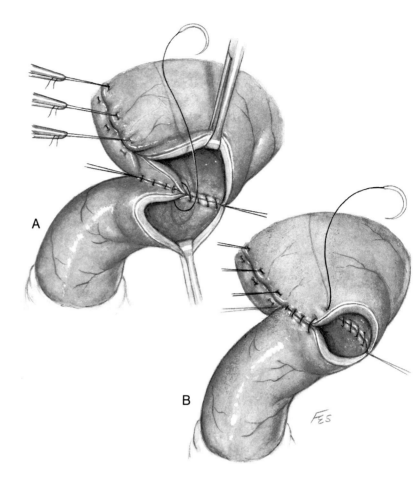

21. GASTRODUODENOSTOMY

▼

A and *B*, The posterior layer is reinforced with a running absorbable suture, which is continued anteriorly as a running inverting Connell suture as a first layer to close the anastomosis.

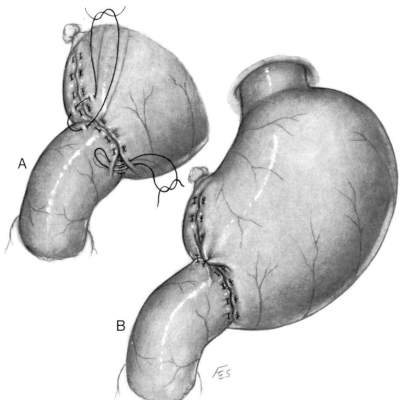

22. COMPLETION OF GASTRODUODENOSTOMY

▼

A and *B*, A layer of interrupted nonabsorbable mattress sutures completes the anastomosis. The lesser curvature angle of the anastomosis is reinforced with a pursestring suture between the duodenum and posterior and anterior walls.

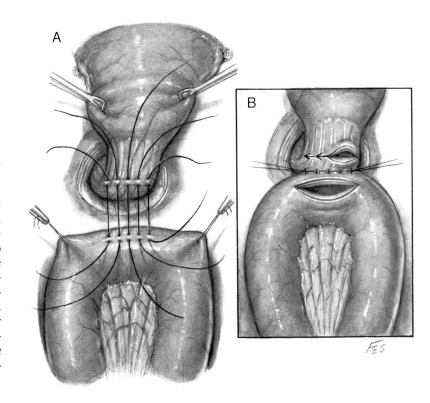

23. TOTAL GASTRECTOMY—ESOPHAGOJEJUNOSTOMY

▼

The initial steps in performing total gastrectomy are the same as for subtotal gastrectomy (see Figs. 2 to 14). After the left gastric vessels are dissected, the remainder of the stomach is mobilized by dividing the remaining high short gastric vessel. A loop of jejunum is brought adjacent to the lower esophagus. *A,* A layer of posterior mattress sutures is placed between the esophagus and jejunum. An opening, the size of the diameter of the jejunum, is made in the jejunum. *B,* A small opening is made at the lateral angle of the anastomosis.

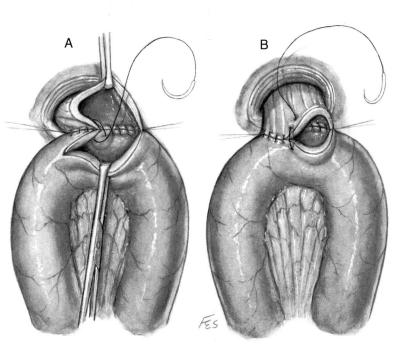

24. ESOPHAGOJEJUNOSTOMY

▼

A, A running posterior absorbable suture is started to reinforce the posterior layer. As one continues with this suture, additional esophagus is incised. By not completely incising the esophagus, the mobilized stomach is used to retract the site of anastomosis for better visualization. *B,* The esophagus is completely divided at the medial angle of the anastomosis, and the posterior suture is continued anteriorly as a running inverting Connell suture.

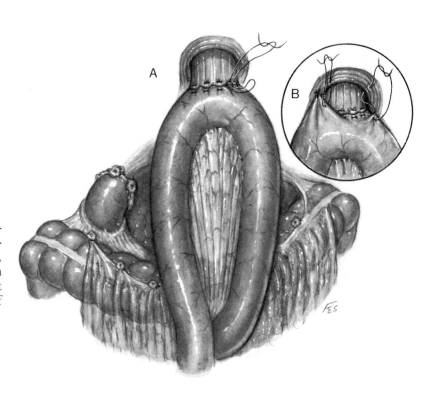

25. ESOPHAGOJEJUNOSTOMY

▼

A, Inverting interrupted mattress sutures are placed to complete the anterior layer of the anastomosis. *B,* The peritoneum over the diaphragm is sutured to the jejunum to support the anastomosis and seal the line of the anastomosis.

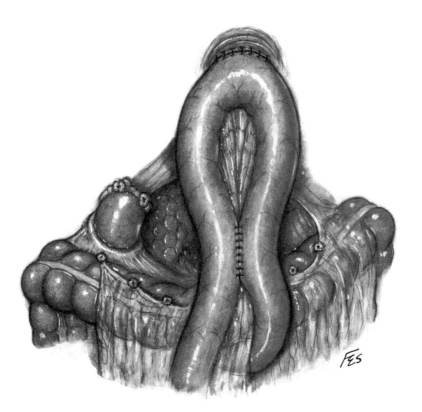

26. ENTEROENTEROSTOMY

Truncal Vagotomy and Heineke-Mikulicz Pyloroplasty Including Selective Vagotomy

8

JOHN W. BRAASCH, M.D.

▼ IMPORTANT FEATURES

Mobilization of Distal Esophagus and Vagus Trunks
Appropriate Selection of Vagus Nerves
Dissection for Additional Vagal Fibers
Mobilization of Pylorus, Longitudinal Incision, and Transverse
   Closure

▼ STEPS OR PLANS

Finger Mobilization of Lower Posterior Esophagus
Posterior Vagus Trunk Projected Anteriorly
Clip Posterior Trunk and Section
Incise Anterior Peritoneum of Lower Esophagus
Dissect Anterior Trunk, Section Appropriately
Dissect Periesophageal Tissues for Small Branches of Vagus Nerve
Preparation of Pylorus
Longitudinal Incision
Transverse Closure

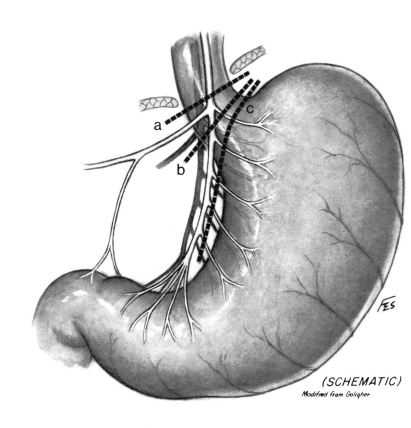

(SCHEMATIC)
Modified from Goligher

1. VAGAL GASTRIC ANATOMY

The course of the vagal trunks and their branches is shown. With section at level *a*, the entire vagus trunk is severed. With section at level *b*, the branch anterior to the hepatobiliary system and the branch from the posterior trunk to the celiac ganglia are preserved. With section at level *c*, a parietal cell or highly selective or proximal gastric vagotomy is accomplished.

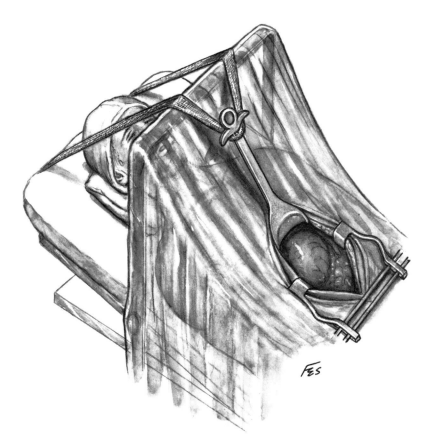

2. PROXIMAL STOMACH EXPOSED

Exposure for transabdominal vagotomy is illustrated with the use of the Balfour retractor and the third blade of the Balfour retractor for sternal elevation. Alternatively, the Bookwalter retractor serves the purpose. Mobilization and retraction of the left lateral segment of the liver are not necessary. The left lobe may simply be elevated with a retractor, giving access to the esophagogastric junction.

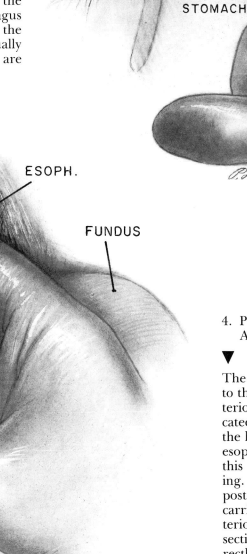

ANT. VAGUS N.

LEVIN TUBE
IN ESOPHAGUS

FUNDUS

STOMACH

CRURA

ESOPH.

POST.
VAGUS N.

FUNDUS

3. BLUNT POSTERIOR DISSECTION

▼

The groove at the angle of His is indicated by the placement of the surgeon's right index finger. Blunt dissection in this area enables the finger to be placed posterior to the lower intra-abdominal esophagus and to the posterior trunk of the vagus nerve. This dissection is usually bloodless when the proper planes are used.

4. POSTERIOR VAGUS ACCESSED

▼

The finger has been placed posterior to the lower esophagus, and the posterior vagus trunk has been dislocated to the right where a window on the lesser curvature side of the distal esophagus can be made to visualize this trunk for clipping and sectioning. Careful palpation of all tissues posterior to the esophagus must be carried out to avoid missing any posterior trunks. The back of the dissecting index finger must pass directly on the anterior surface of the crura and the abdominal aorta.

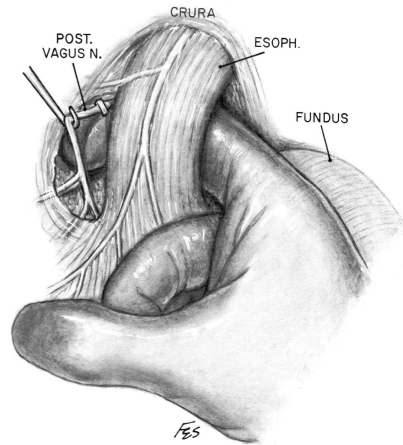

CRURA

POST.
VAGUS N.

ESOPH.

FUNDUS

FES

5. POSTERIOR VAGUS SECTIONED

After the posterior vagus nerve has been secured with the nerve hook, clips can be placed at either extremity and a middle segment excised for histologic study.

6. ANTERIOR VAGUS DISSECTED

Attention is then directed to the anterior esophagus. A rubber sling is passed around the esophagus for traction. As shown, the peritoneum over the anterior surface of the distal esophagus is opened with the point of the scissors. With suitable traction on the stomach, the anterior nerve can be felt as a bowstring.

7. ANTERIOR VAGUS SECTIONED

This nerve is elevated with a nerve hook and clipped, and a segment is removed for histologic study. All tissue around the esophagus is dissected down to the muscle plane, and this level is inspected for the presence of other vagus nerve trunks, which are found in many patients. With mobility obtained in this way, the abdominal esophagus should lengthen appreciably, and inspection for extra vagus trunks should be easy. When selective vagotomy is preferred because of the possible deleterious effect of diarrhea or in (for instance) Crohn's disease of the small bowel, care is taken to preserve the branches of the anterior and posterior vagus nerves to the hepatobiliary system and to the celiac ganglia.

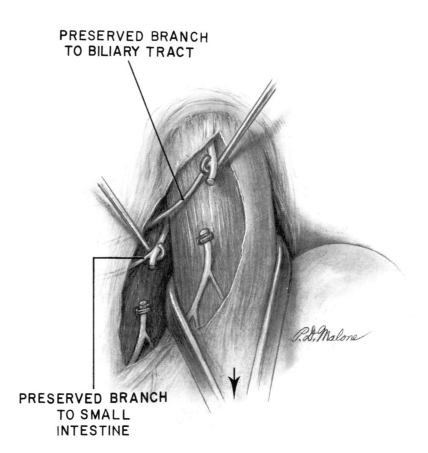

PRESERVED BRANCH
TO BILIARY TRACT

PRESERVED BRANCH
TO SMALL
INTESTINE

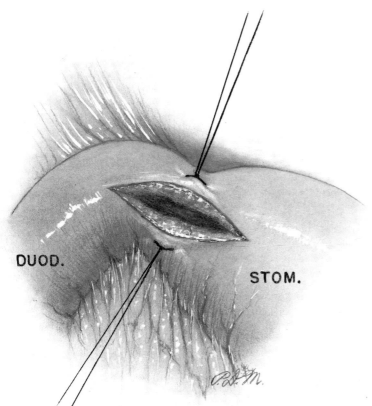

DUOD.

STOM.

8. PYLOROPLASTY–PYLORUS INCISED

Heineke-Mikulicz pyloroplasty is preferred and initiated with a longitudinal incision centered over the pyloric muscle as illustrated. This incision should extend for 2 cm on either side of the pylorus.

9. HORIZONTAL CLOSURE

Partial closure of the vertical incision in a horizontal direction is shown, using a single-layer interrupted suture technique in which the serosal surfaces of the stomach and duodenum are carefully apposed. These sutures are placed first at the lateral extremities of the closure to ensure an even contour.

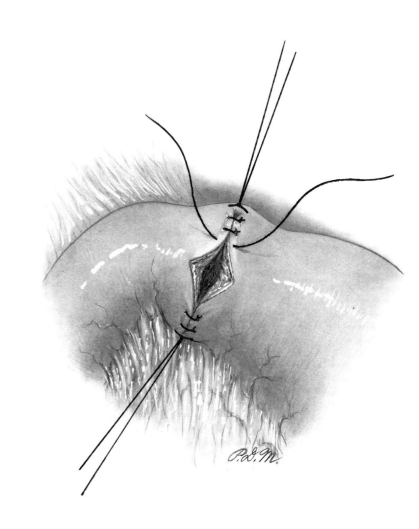

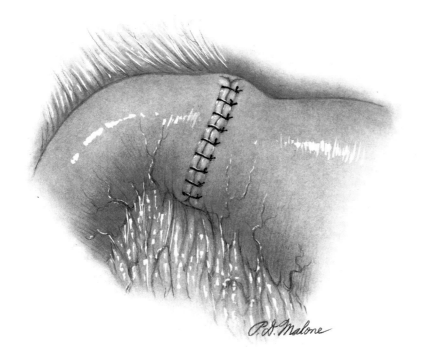

10. PYLOROPLASTY COMPLETED

The completed Heineke-Mikulicz pyloroplasty gives an adequate lumen through this area.

Parietal Cell Vagotomy (Highly Selective Vagotomy)

9

RICARDO L. ROSSI, M.D.

▼ IMPORTANT FEATURES

Lyse Adhesions of Omentum to Spleen at Exploration to Avoid
Splenic Tear

Traction of Stomach to Left; Gastrohepatic Ligament to Right

Avoid Excessive Traction on Short Gastric Vessels to Prevent Splenic
Tear

Dissection of Gastrohepatic Ligament Close to Stomach to Preserve
Anterior and Posterior Nerves of Latarjet

Avoid Injury to Gastric Wall

Dissect Distal Esophagus for 5 to 7 cm

Distal Extent of Dissection to Left of Crow's Foot at About 7 cm
from Pylorus

Best Results In Intractable Duodenal Ulcer; Less Effective for Gastric
Ulcer

▼ STEPS OR PLANS

Midline Vertical Incision

Abdominal Exploration and Lysis of Adhesions to Spleen

Optimal Exposure Using Self-Retaining Retractors

Exposure of Nerve of Latarjet, Stomach, Duodenum, Distal
Esophagus

Assessment of Distal Extent of Denervation

Division of Anterior Leaf of Gastrohepatic Ligament Close to
Stomach

Division of Posterior Leaf of Gastrohepatic Ligament

Dissection of Distal Esophagus and Esophagogastric Area

Assessment of Proximal Extent of Denervation

Evaluation of Completed Denervation

Assess Hemostasis, Rule Out Splenic Tears, Close Wound

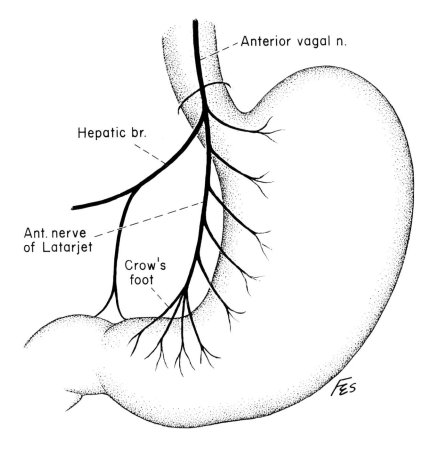

1. ANATOMY OF VAGUS NERVES

▼

The left (anterior) vagus nerve continues in the anterior leaf of the lesser omentum parallel to the lesser curvature of the stomach about 1 to 2 cm from it, forming the anterior nerve of Latarjet. It reaches the pyloric antral area where it fans out into branches forming the crow's foot. The anterior vagus nerve supplies the hepatic branch to the gallbladder and biliary tree.

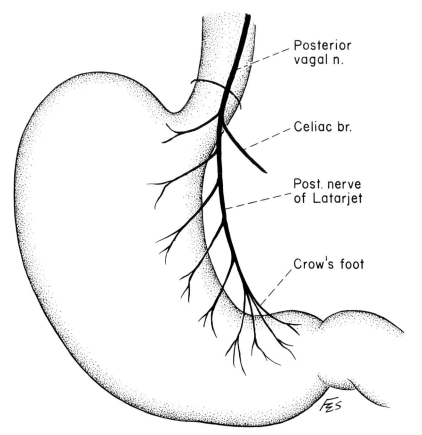

2. ANATOMY OF VAGUS NERVES *(Continued)*

▼

The right (posterior) vagus nerve continues in the posterior leaf of the lesser omentum, forming the posterior nerve of Latarjet, which has a similar position to that of the anterior nerve. Early in its course, a branch to the celiac plexus supplies vagal fibers to the bowel and other abdominal viscera.

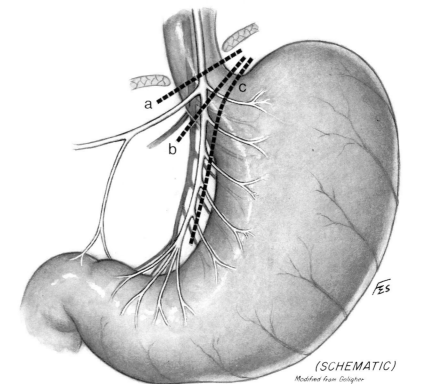

(SCHEMATIC)

Modified from Goligher

3. TYPES OF VAGOTOMY

▼

a, Truncal vagotomy: Vagal denervation of all abdominal viscera. *b,* Selective vagotomy: Vagal denervation of the stomach but preservation of innervation to other abdominal viscera. *c,* Parietal cell vagotomy: Vagal denervation of the acid-producing stomach with preservation of vagal innervation to the antrum, the pylorus, and other abdominal viscera.

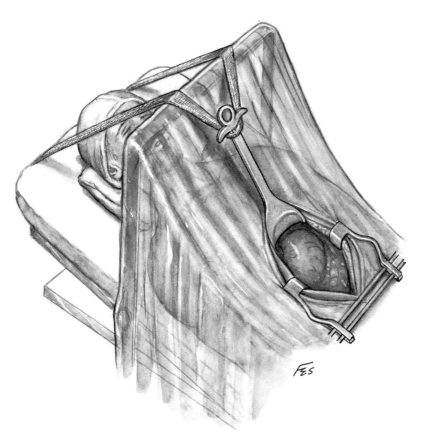

4. EXPOSURE

▼

A midline incision extends from along the xiphoid process to the umbilicus. The falciform ligament is divided and ligated and the abdomen explored. Omental adhesions to the spleen are lysed. The bladder blade of a Balfour retractor is placed substernally and tied over the ether screen of the anesthesiologist with a sterile, double-folded strip of cloth or gauze. A regular Balfour retractor is placed in the lower half of the incision. Alternatively, mechanical devices attached to the operating table achieve excellent exposure. The operating table is placed in the reverse Trendelenburg position of approximately 15 to 20 degrees.

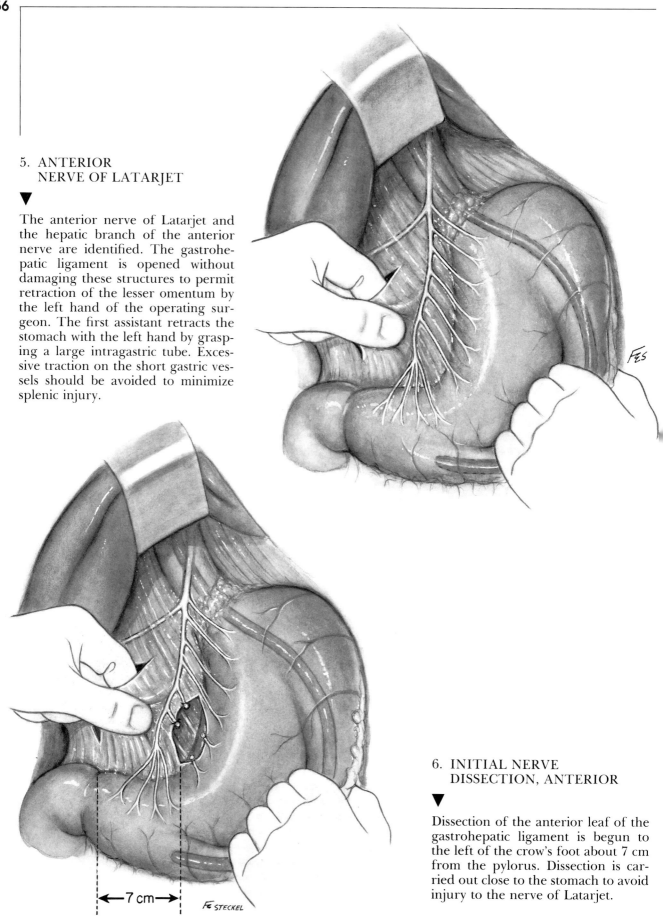

5. ANTERIOR NERVE OF LATARJET

▼

The anterior nerve of Latarjet and the hepatic branch of the anterior nerve are identified. The gastrohepatic ligament is opened without damaging these structures to permit retraction of the lesser omentum by the left hand of the operating surgeon. The first assistant retracts the stomach with the left hand by grasping a large intragastric tube. Excessive traction on the short gastric vessels should be avoided to minimize splenic injury.

←—7 cm—→

6. INITIAL NERVE DISSECTION, ANTERIOR

▼

Dissection of the anterior leaf of the gastrohepatic ligament is begun to the left of the crow's foot about 7 cm from the pylorus. Dissection is carried out close to the stomach to avoid injury to the nerve of Latarjet.

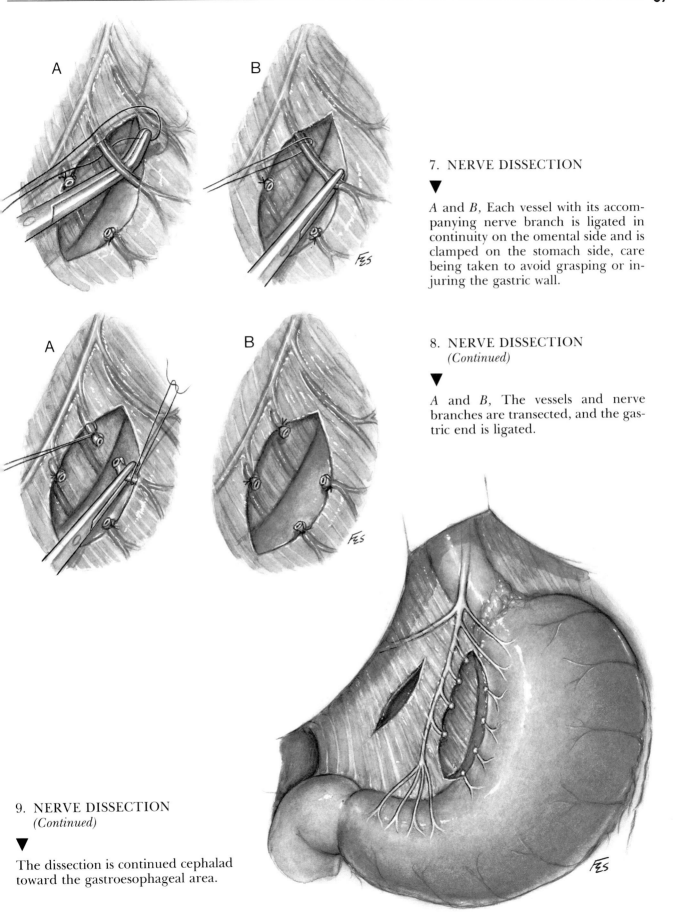

7. NERVE DISSECTION

▼

A and *B,* Each vessel with its accompanying nerve branch is ligated in continuity on the omental side and is clamped on the stomach side, care being taken to avoid grasping or injuring the gastric wall.

8. NERVE DISSECTION
(Continued)

▼

A and *B,* The vessels and nerve branches are transected, and the gastric end is ligated.

9. NERVE DISSECTION
(Continued)

▼

The dissection is continued cephalad toward the gastroesophageal area.

10. POSTERIOR DISSECTION

▼

When dissection permits easy visibility of the posterior leaf of the gastrohepatic ligament, its vessels can be clamped and transected using the same precautions as with the anterior leaf. The lesser sac is entered. A Penrose drain aids in retraction of the gastrohepatic ligament to the right for better exposure of its vessels and nerve fibers. Alternatively, the surgeon can achieve this exposure by placing the left hand in the rent between the stomach wall and the gastrohepatic ligament. The dissection is continued to the angle of His. A fat pad overlying the gastroesophageal area indicates the line of dissection.

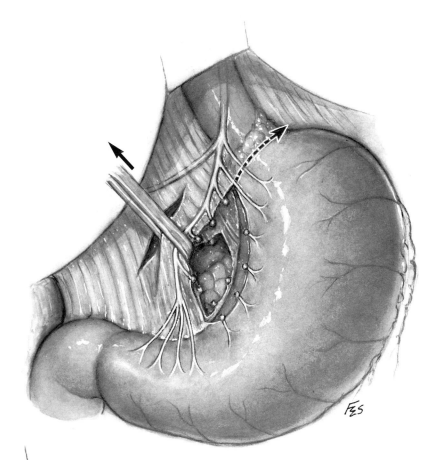

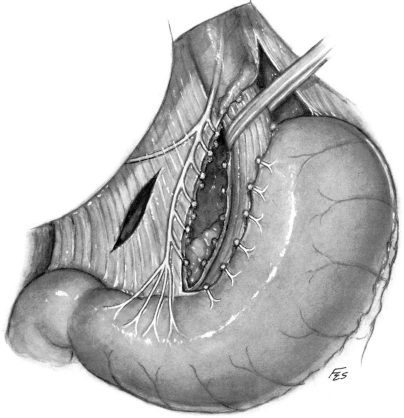

11. ESOPHAGOGASTRIC DISSECTION

▼

Dissection of the lower esophagus is begun and extended to the first short gastric vessel. The lesser omentum is always retracted to the right to avoid injury to the main vagal trunks.

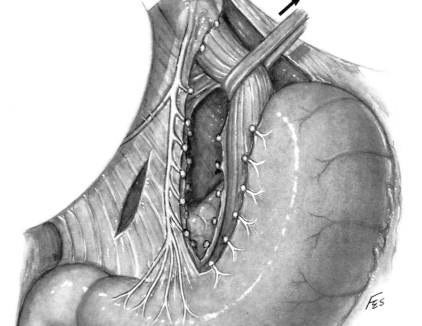

12. ESOPHAGEAL DISSECTION

The distal esophagus is retracted anteriorly and to the left with a Penrose drain, and any nerve branches to the posterior wall of the esophagus or gastric fundus are divided.

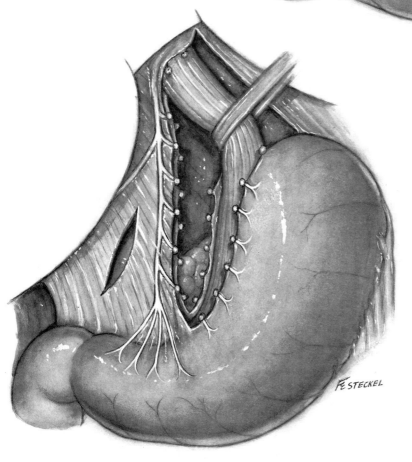

13. ESOPHAGEAL DISSECTION
(Continued)

The esophagus is dissected for a length of 5 to 7 cm, isolating it completely from vagal branches. Hemostasis is ensured, and the extent of vagal denervation is reassessed.

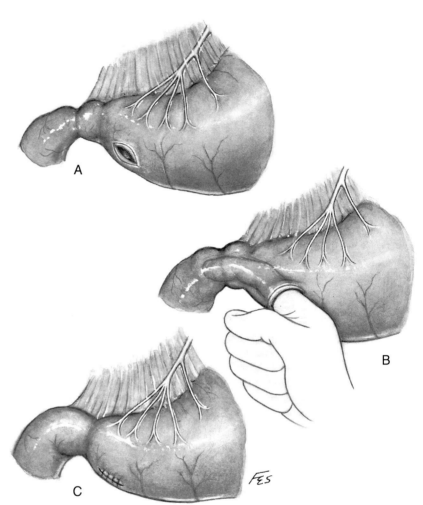

14. DUODENAL DILATATION

▼

Surgical dilatation can be used for patients with pyloroduodenal stenosis from peptic ulcer disease. Because of frequent unsatisfactory functional results as expressed by the Visick criteria, in most cases we prefer gastric resection, pyloroplasty, or gastrojejunostomy. *A,* A small gastrostomy is performed close to the pylorus and to the greater curvature of the stomach to avoid antral denervation. *B,* The pyloroduodenal area is assessed by palpation. Gentle finger dilatation is performed, usually passing the proximal interphalangeal joint through the area of stenosis. The pyloroduodenal area is inspected for possible perforations. *C,* The gastrostomy is closed.

10 | Stapling Techniques

STEPHEN G. ReMINE, M.D.

▼ IMPORTANT FEATURES
Staple Design—Apposition and Maintenance of Blood Supply
Side-to-Side and End-to-End Enteroenterostomy Variations
Precautions and Pitfalls
Permanent Tube Gastrostomy
Alternative Methods Using EEA Stapler

▼ STEPS OR PLANS
Staple Design
Side-to-Side Enteroenterostomy
Setup, Placement of GIA Stapler, and Closure
End-to-End Enteroenterostomy
Small Bowel and Colon
Functional End-to-End Enteroenterostomy
Small Bowel and Colon
Pitfalls to Avoid
Permanent Tube Gastrostomy
Alternative Uses for EEA Stapler
Antegrade and Retrograde Anastomosis

1. PRINCIPLES OF STAPLING

▼

Standard staple loads are usually 3.5 mm in height and when fired compress to 1.5 mm. The main goal with staples, as with sutures, is apposition of tissue. However, tissue thickness varies, and hemostasis may not always be achieved. For some tissue

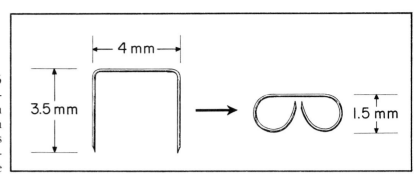

that is edematous or thicker than usual, 4.5-mm loads are available. Judgment in the appropriate use of staples is as important as with other techniques. Because stapling techniques have made some aspects of bowel surgery quicker and simpler, their limitations and proper use are important to understand. The four main principles that should always be applied when using staples are to check for hemostasis, avoid crossing staple lines when possible, avoid devascularizing tissue, and reinforce with sutures areas of stress, corners of anastomosis, and areas of possible tissue compromise to avoid delayed perforation.

A

B

2. SIDE-TO-SIDE ENTEROENTEROSTOMY

▼

A, With use of the antimesenteric border of two loops of bowel apposed with several silk stay sutures, small enterotomies (3 to 4 mm) are made with a knife or cutting electrocautery. The enterotomies should not be too large because they can be stretched easily to accommodate the stapler. Allis clamps are used to hold the lateral margin of the enterotomy. B, A GIA stapler can now be placed through the enterotomy and advanced along the antimesenteric border. Clamping the GIA stapler sets its position. Avoid gathering too much tissue. The GIA stapler is designed to give a smooth 5-cm double-edged staple line. Advancing the blade forward implants the staples and cuts between the two rows simultaneously. C, Final closure of the
Continued

C

Figure 2 *Continued*

enterotomy is accomplished by lifting the lateral margins and placing a TA-55 stapler across transversely. A third Allis clamp may be placed combining the medial edge of both enterotomies. This facilitates final closure. Secure the end of the staple line by tying down the end stay suture.

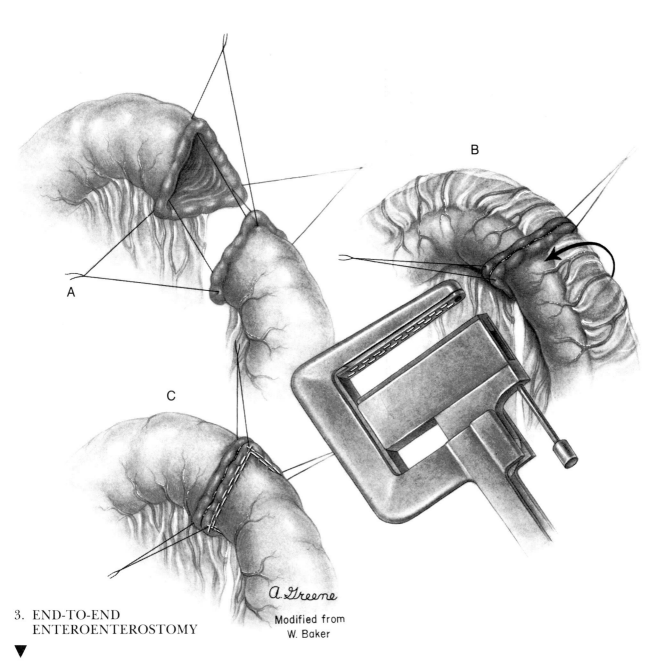

a. Greene

Modified from
W. Baker

3. END-TO-END ENTEROENTEROSTOMY

▼

A, Placement of stay sutures in three corners is seen. The lumen of the bowel must be large enough to avoid a compromised lumen when the anastomosis is complete. *B,* Application of the TA-55 stapler between two stay sutures completes one of the three sides. Care must be taken not to injure the mesenteric vessels and possibly compromise anastomotic healing. *C,* The completed anastomosis is seen. Note the crossed staple lines at the apex of each side. These can be reinforced with several inverting silk sutures for security.

4. COLOCOLOSTOMY

▼

A, A technique similar to that for the small bowel can be used for the colon. Because of the larger lumen of the colon, the first row is placed as an inverting staple line, thus avoiding much dissection along the mesocolon and inadvertent vascular injury. *B,* With use of the silk stay sutures to hold up the margins, the final two sides of the triangular anastomosis can be completed. Again, because of overlapping suture lines, additional inverting stay sutures may be needed to secure the corners.

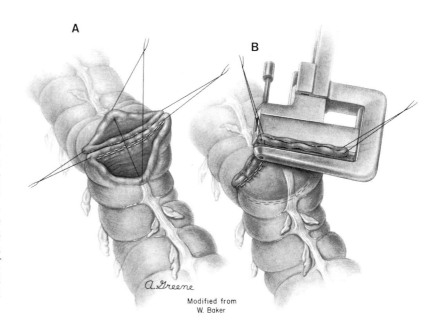

Modified from
W. Baker

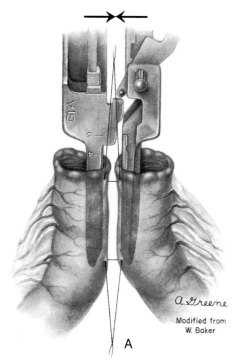

Modified from
W. Baker

A

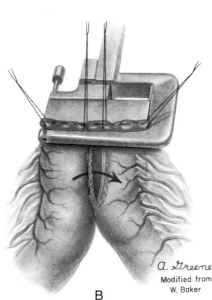

Modified from
W. Baker

B

5. MODIFIED END-TO-END ENTEROENTEROSTOMY

▼

A, After the antimesenteric border of two limbs of small bowel have been secured with stay sutures, a GIA stapler can be placed and fired along the antimesenteric margin. *B,* To complete the anastomosis, a TA-55 stapler can be placed across the ends, being sure that the mucosa is completely everted. Areas where staple lines may cross and the apex of the GIA staple line are reinforced.

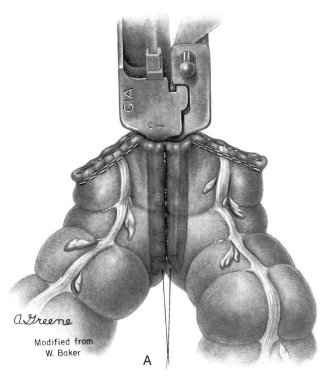

Modified from
W. Baker

A

6. MODIFIED END-TO-END COLOCOLOSTOMY

A, After the colon has been transected with a GIA stapler, the antimesocolonic borders are approximated with stay sutures. Small stab wounds are made, permitting placement of the GIA stapler. An alternative method is to leave the antimesocolonic margin unstapled. However, the benefit of having the bowel sealed while the surgical field is being prepared should be considered when additional work needs to be completed before finishing the anastomosis. After the GIA stapler has been fired, the inner lumen is inspected for bleeding. *B*, To com-

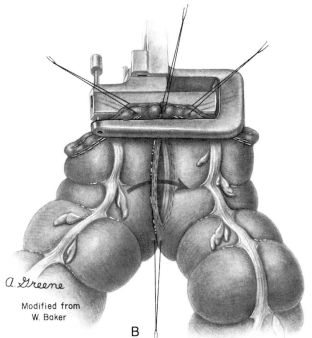

Modified from
W. Baker

B

plete the anastomosis, a TA-55 stapler can be applied. The three areas where multiple staple lines cross are areas of potential weakness and may need to be reinforced with inverting sutures. The anastomosis is tested for patency and continence.

7. PITFALLS

Although stapler techniques in surgery are relatively straightforward, care must be taken to apply them properly and safely. Awareness of a few basic principles will help avoid problems. Staples are designed for uniform apposition. Because of differences in tissue thickness, hemostasis may not always be obtained or staples may not be completely set. In addition, inappropriately placed staples may cause vascular compromise. A good example of a problem to avoid is shown with a side-to-side enteroenterostomy. *A*, After the side-to-side closure of the stoma has been completed with a GIA stapler, avoid setting up final closure in this alignment. *B*, Offsetting the edges of the new stoma before final staple closure avoids stapling across two staple rows twice. Because staples do not take into account differences in quality of tissue, good surgical judgment should always be applied. Appropriateness of staples should be considered when prior radiation exposure, chemotherapy, collagen disorders, and chronic steroid use are factors.

8. GASTROSTOMY

A, A permanent tube gastrostomy can be made with a GIA stapler when it is applied to the lesser curvature side of the distal body of the stomach. *B*, The base of the tube can then be inverted approximately 1 cm and sutured in place, thus creating some continence and avoiding skin erosion from gastric effluent. *C*, Staple lines are reinforced, and the tube is brought out through the abdominal wall. The stomach is secured to the abdominal wall. Finally, the stoma is matured, resulting in a mucosa-lined continent permanent tube gastrostomy.

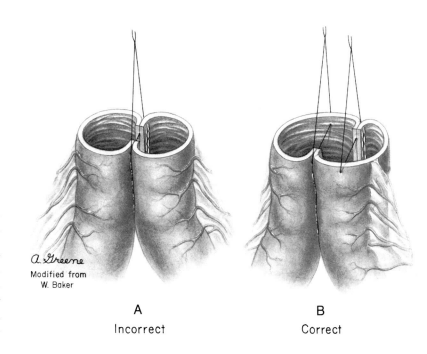

a. Greene
Modified from
W. Baker

A
Incorrect

B
Correct

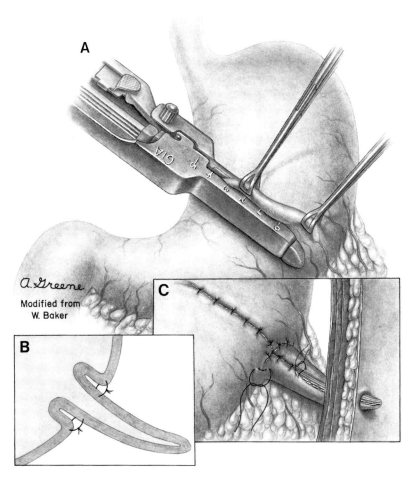

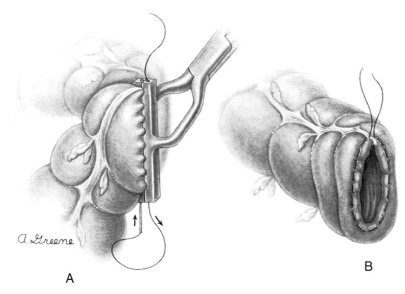

A

B

9. PURSESTRING SUTURE FOR EEA USE

▼

A, Before the bowel is transected, a pursestring suture is applied using the angled bowel clamp of the EEA stapler. *B,* This results in a complete pursestring suture with minimal additional tissue. A hand-sutured pursestring or a circumferential whipstitch suture can accomplish the same thing. However, care must be taken not to incorporate too much tissue, causing incomplete apposition of the anvil.

10. ANTEGRADE EEA USE FOR COLON ANASTOMOSES

▼

A, The standard retrograde insertion of the EEA stapler is detailed in Chapter 20. *B,* An alternative to retrograde placement of the EEA stapler is antegrade insertion. The rectum can be everted if necessary for lower placement of the anastomosis. This method requires another staple line to close the insertion site. When the antegrade method is used for a low rectal anastomosis, the curved EEA stapler will facilitate the procedure.

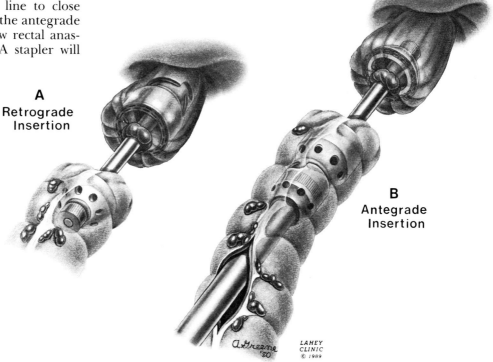

A
Retrograde
Insertion

B
Antegrade
Insertion

LAHEY
CLINIC
© 1989

11. OTHER EEA USES

▼

The techniques used in EEA coloco-lostomy can be applied to many areas of the bowel, such as in esophagogas-tric or esophagocolonic interposition. *A*, The EEA stapler is advanced through a small stab wound along the antimesocolonic border of the bowel. The anvil is secured in posi-tion, and a pursestring suture is placed around the proximal and dis-tal bowel lumens. *B*, The EEA stapler is tightened completely and fired. After the entire stapler has been withdrawn, check to be sure that two complete doughnuts of tissue have been excised around the pursestring sutures. When these are not com-plete, an incomplete staple line is

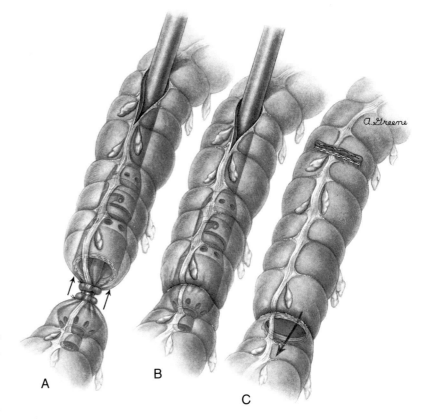

possible, and the anastomosis should be examined carefully and re-inforced. *C*, Patency of the anasto-mosis should be assessed. The anas-tomosis is completed by transverse closure of the colotomy with a TA-55 stapler.

Gastric Partitioning or Gastric Bypass

11

RICARDO L. ROSSI, M.D.
JOHN W. BRAASCH, M.D.

▼ IMPORTANT FEATURES
Adequate Exposure Through Midline Incision
Mobilization of Proximal Stomach
Double Set of Staples Applied Across Upper Stomach
Gap In All Rows In Gastric Partitioning
Proximal Pouch 50 to 60 ml Capacity
Roux-en-Y Loop Jejunum Brought Up for Anastomosis to Proximal
Stomach In Gastric Bypass
Small (1 cm) Stoma Between Pouch and Distal Stomach or Jejunum

▼ STEPS OR PLANS
Detach Upper Greater Curvature of Stomach from Short Gastric
Vessels
Dissect Posterior Surface of Proximal Stomach from
Retroperitoneum
Determine Position for Line of Clips So That Proximal Pouch Is 50
to 60 ml Capacity
Place TA-90 Stapler Across Upper Stomach; Two Applications for
Quadruple Line of Clips
In Gastric Bypass
Bring Roux-en-Y Loop Up for Anastomosis to Proximal Pouch
In Gastric Partitioning
*Remove Three Clips from Upper Row and Two Clips from Bottom
Row, Leaving Gap at Junction of Middle and Lateral Thirds of
Stomach or on Greater Curvature*
Opening In Rows of Clips Admits No. 32 French Dilator
*Nonabsorbable Circular Suture Placed In Gastric Wall Around
Dilator to Maintain Proper Gap*

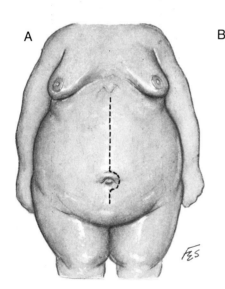

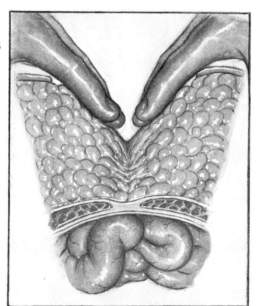

1. EXPOSURE

▼

A, Midline incision extends from the xiphoid process to below the umbilicus. B, After the skin incision has been made, the midline is dissected bluntly by lateral traction, which permits identification of the rectus fascia at the midline. An incision is then made between the rectus muscles into the abdomen. After the abdominal exploration has been completed, adhesions from the omentum to the spleen are lysed to avoid capsular tears of the spleen during traction on the omentum. A Bookwalter self-retaining retractor is useful for adequate exposure for the subsequent steps.

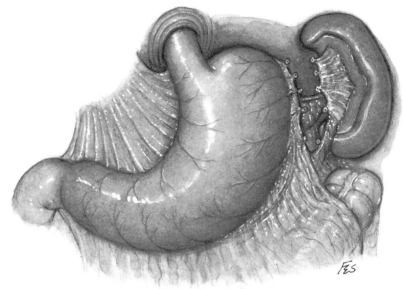

2. MOBILIZATION OF GASTRIC FUNDUS

The short gastric vessels are clamped, severed, and ligated to free the upper part of the greater curvature of the stomach.

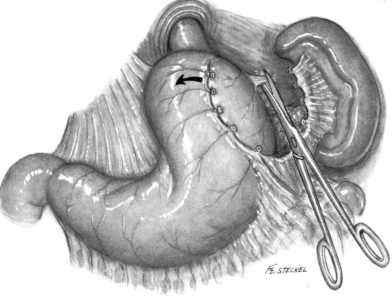

3. POSTERIOR MOBILIZATION

The posterior portion of the upper stomach is freed and devascularized from its retroperitoneal blood supply.

4. PLACEMENT OF STAPLER

A rent is made in the gastrohepatic ligament by dissection at the gastric wall so that one arterial branch of the left gastric artery is preserved to the proximal stomach. A catheter is passed through the rent in the gastrohepatic ligament and drawn behind the stomach, emerging from the greater curvature side of the stomach, which has been mobilized. The TA-90 stapler is inserted into the open end of the catheter, and traction on the catheter permits the stapler to be placed in position for application of a double row of staples across the proximal stomach. For gastric partitioning, two or three staples in each row need to be removed from the cartridge before loading the TA-90 instrument.

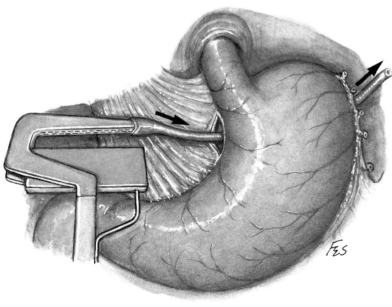

5. POUCH VOLUME MEASURED

▼

After the stapler has been positioned to achieve a proximal pouch with a volume of 50 to 60 ml, the TA-90 stapler is tightened to occlude the stomach at that point; the volume of the pouch is tested by injecting a catheter passed down the esophagus into the upper part of the stomach. A Penrose drain placed around the esophagus can be used to prevent reflux into the esophagus while injecting saline solution into the pouch.

6. STAPLER FIRED

▼

A, The final position of the TA-90 stapler is determined, and the staples are fired. *B*, The TA-90 stapler is replaced and fired again within 5 mm of the previous double stapled line.

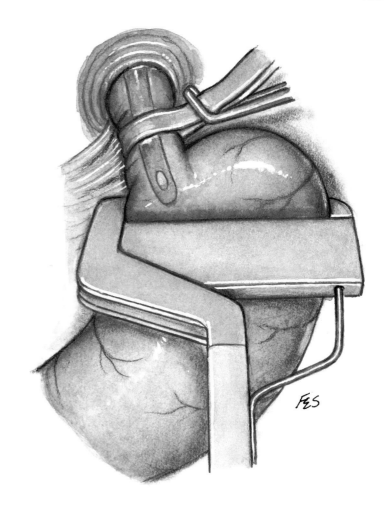

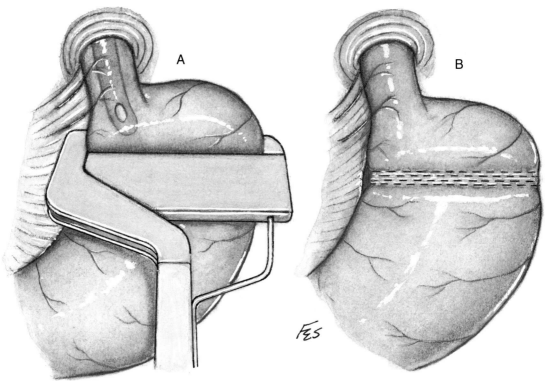

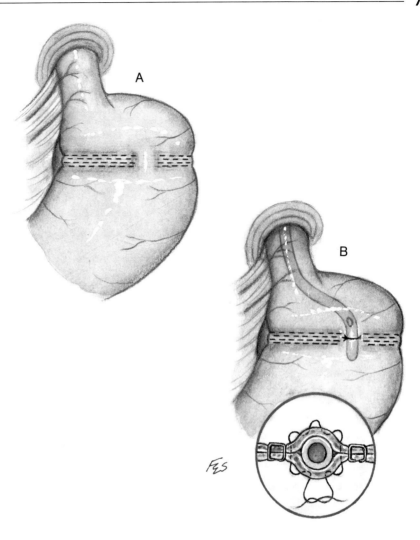

7. CREATION OF GAP IN STAPLE LINE FOR PARTITIONING

▼

A, In gastric partitioning, in each double row of clips, three clips are removed from the upper row and two clips are removed from the lower row so that a gap is produced through the rows of clips at about the junction of the middle and lateral thirds of the stomach or at the greater curvature. When the gap is on the greater curvature side of the stomach with recreation of the normal angle of His in the postoperative period, angulation of the gap may occur. This decreases the diameter of the passageway, and obstruction may occur. *B*, A No. 32 French dilator is passed into the stomach and through the gap in the stapled lines. *Inset*, The opening is maintained by placing a nonabsorbable circular suture around the dilator.

8. BYPASS

▼

In gastric bypass, a Roux-en-Y loop at least 40 cm long is brought through the mesocolon. A 10-mm side-to-side gastrojejunostomy is made with two layers of interrupted sutures. This anastomosis can be positioned to the anterior *(A)* or posterior *(B)* wall of the stomach close to the greater curvature. The gastrotomy incision should be made not less than 2 cm from the stapled line. After the posterior aspect of the anastomosis has been completed, a nasogastric tube may be passed into the jejunum, leaving side holes in the stomach and jejunum. This type of tube is also used in the gastric partitioning operation. The rent in the mesocolon is closed.

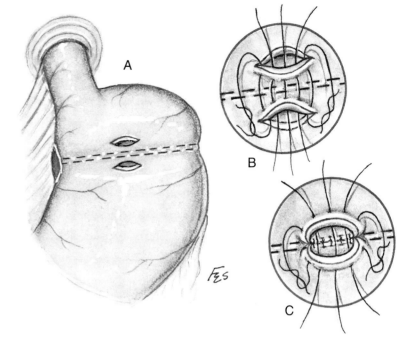

9. GASTRIC OBSTRUCTION RELIEVED

▼

A to C, When gastric obstruction occurs after gastric partitioning, gastric continuity can be restored by making an anastomosis between the proximal and distal pouches of the stomach. This anastomosis should have a lumen approximately 1 cm in diameter and can be constructed with interrupted sutures joining incisions above and below the stapled line.

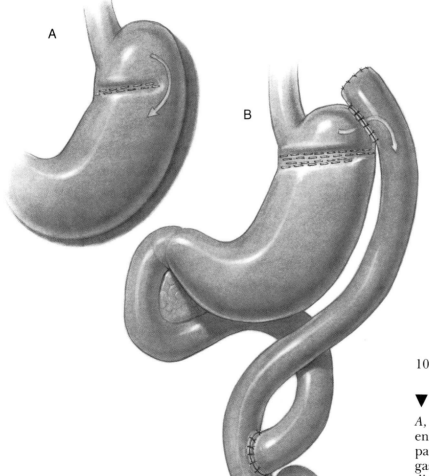

10. STAPLE LINE DISRUPTION REPAIRED

▼

A, With disruption of staple line or enlargement of the stoma, gastric partitioning should be converted to gastric bypass (B) by placing an additional double staple line across the upper stomach and bringing a Roux-en-Y loop of jejunum up for anastomosis to the proximal pouch.

12

Vertical Banded Gastroplasty

STEPHEN G. ReMINE, M.D.

▼ IMPORTANT FEATURES
Creation of Proximal Volume-Limiting Gastric Pouch
Creation of Small Aperture Banded Stoma

▼ STEPS OR PLANS
Setup
Placement of Anteroposterior Gastrotomy
Precautions in EEA Stapler Placement
Creation of Lesser Curvature Pouch
Method of Rechecking Reservoir Volume
Completion of Vertical Banding

▼ SPECIAL PRECAUTIONS
The Smaller the Pouch, the More Extreme the Weight Loss
Band Should Not Be Sutured to Stomach
Gastroplasty Stoma Should Not Be Too Small

1. MOBILIZATION OF ESOPHAGUS AND STOMACH

Through an upper midline incision and the use of fixed lateral retractors, the stomach and diaphragm are easily visualized. The esophagogastric junction is mobilized, and a 0.5-inch Penrose drain is placed around the esophagus. The upper aspect of the greater curvature is freed up by ligating the two most superior short gastric vessels. For best visualization, approximately 3 inches of upper greater curvature must be freed up. The lesser sac is entered along the lesser curvature, and the serosal surface is dissected free approximately midway between the esophagogastric junction and the terminal branches of the nerve of Latarjet.

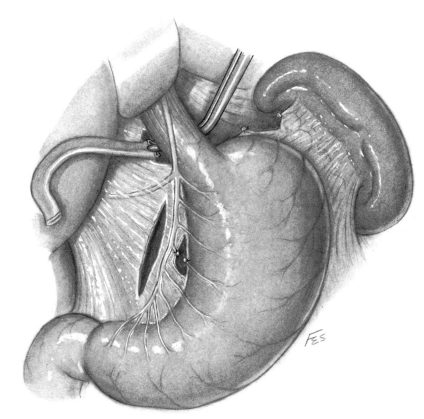

2. EEA STAPLER PLACED

A No. 15 French Silastic suction drain is attached to the bare end of an EEA stapler without the anvil portion of the cartridge. A 24-mm EEA cartridge is used. A trocar introducer is attached to the other end of the suction catheter. The tip of the trocar is bent in a gentle, 45-degree angle curve to facilitate placement in the tight subhepatic space. The trocar is passed through the stomach from anterior to posterior, exiting out the lesser sac. The point most appropriate to pass the trocar is approximately 8.5 cm from the greater curvature and 2.5 cm from the lesser curvature. Another way to check this site is to place a No. 32 French esophageal dilator into the stomach along the lesser curvature and place the EEA stapler lateral to this site.

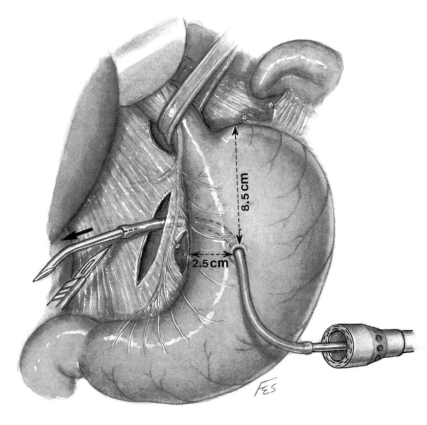

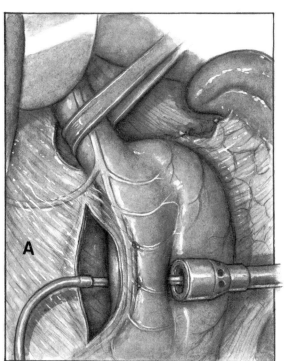

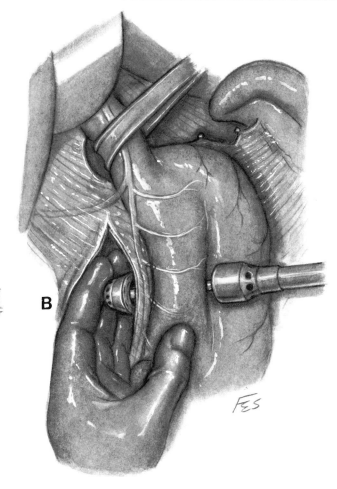

3. ROUND DEFECT CREATED IN GASTRIC WALLS

▼

A and *B,* Care must be taken to avoid inadvertent injury to the pancreas, liver, or vagal nerves. Curving the tip of the trocar facilitates placement of the stapler. When the handle of the stapler is in place, it is rotated to permit good visualization of the posterior aspect of the stomach. All soft tissue, particularly if it might include the posterior vagus nerve, must be cleared from around the stylet of the stapler before placing the anvil in position. The anvil is attached, and the stapler is fired.

4. LESSER CURVATURE POUCH CREATED

▼

A and *B,* The EEA staple line is reinforced with interrupted figure-of-eight or simple 3-0 silk sutures. At this point, a TA-90 stapler is used to create a lesser curvature pouch. A standard 3.5-mm load is usually used. Two staple loads are placed several millimeters apart. The size of the pouch (shown in Fig. 5) is estimated before firing the staples in place.

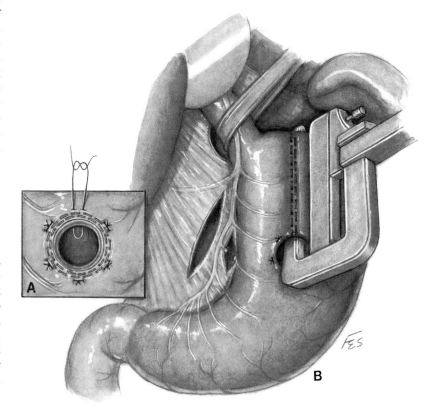

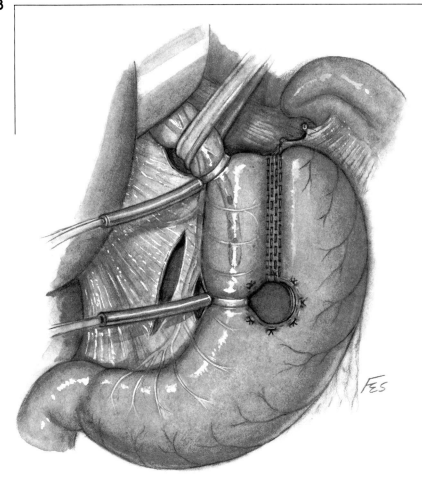

5. LESSER CURVATURE POUCH CREATED (Continued)

▼

After the stapler has been tightened into position and before it is fired, a nasogastric tube is placed into the proximal stomach. Proximal and distal pouch orifices are occluded, and 30 to 45 ml of saline solution is placed down the nasogastric tube. The pouch should distend but not be under any undue pressure, and no saline solution should return when the pressure is let up on the plunger of the syringe. Too large a pouch will result in less than desired weight loss, and too small a pouch may lead to excessive weight loss and severe nutritional problems. After the pouch has been created, the volume should be checked again for reassurance.

6. BAND POUCH OUTLET

▼

A strip of Marlex mesh or Gore-Tex patch, 7 by 1.5 cm, is placed around the outlet of the pouch. A point 5.5 cm from one of the ends is premarked as the point where the band will be sutured to itself with four to six interrupted sutures of 3-0 polypropylene (Prolene). The band is placed with a No. 32 French esophageal dilator in position to ensure that the outflow aperture of the pouch will be 1.2 cm in diameter. Excess stomach wall gathered during banding will result in a smaller lumen than expected and outflow obstruction. When the band is greater than 1.5 cm in width, the result will be partial outflow obstruction, much the same as when a Nissen fundoplication wrap is too long. When the band is not sutured to the serosa of the stomach, the chance of foreign body reaction and migration is theoretically less.

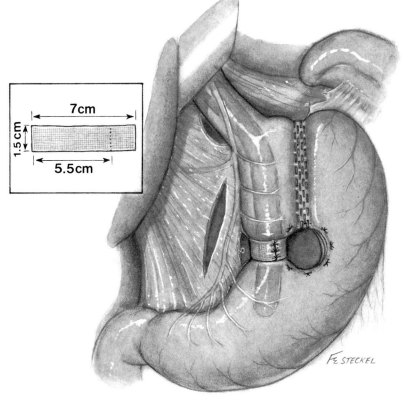

13 | Local Resection of the Duodenum

JOHN W. BRAASCH, M.D.

▼ IMPORTANT FEATURES
    Exposure and Mobilization of Duodenum
    Resection of Portion of Duodenum
    Reconstruction of Gastrointestinal Tract

▼ STEPS OR PLANS
    Wide Kocher Maneuver to Elevate Second and Third Portions of
        Duodenum
    Anterior Exposure of Second and Third Portions of Duodenum by
        Elevating Right Colon and Small Bowel Mesentery
    Isolation and Resection of Duodenal Segment
    End-to-End Anastomosis of Duodenum

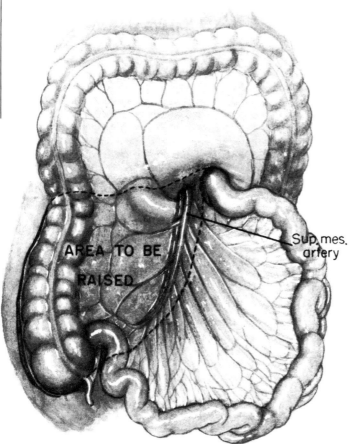

1. AREA TO BE MOBILIZED

The area of the right colon and mesentery to be raised to expose the retroperitoneal duodenum is shown.

2. MOBILIZATION OF RIGHT COLON

Initial dissection of the cecum, which is extended upward to mobilize the entire right colon, is shown. This dissection is extended medially to mobilize the mesentery of the small intestine.

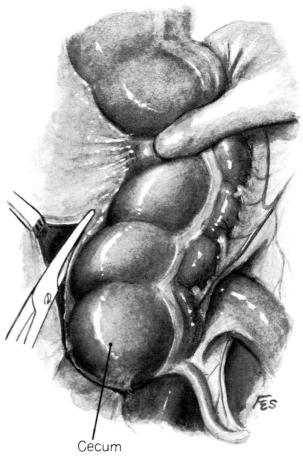

Cecum

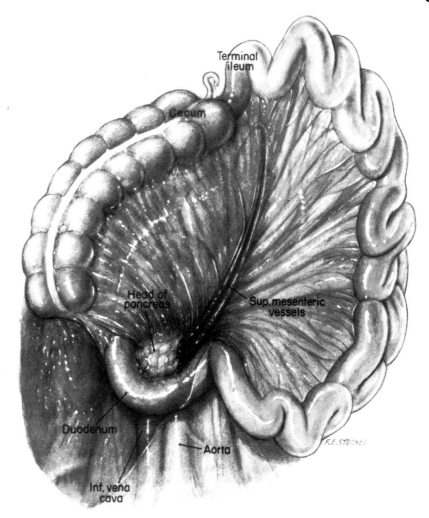

3. MESENTERY ELEVATED

▼

The entire right colon and small bowel mesentery are elevated, exposing the second, third, and fourth portions of the duodenum.

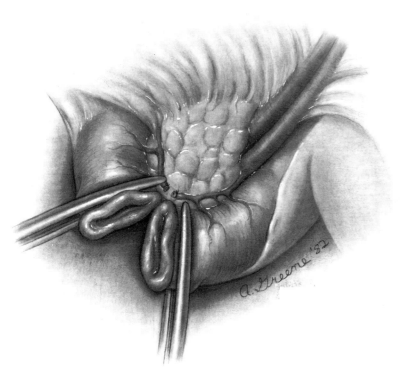

4. DUODENAL SEGMENT RESECTED

After an extensive Kocher maneuver has been completed, resection of a segment of the duodenum can be accomplished. Control of luminal contents can be with occluding clamps or with staples. Preservation of the ampulla of Vater is, of course, important.

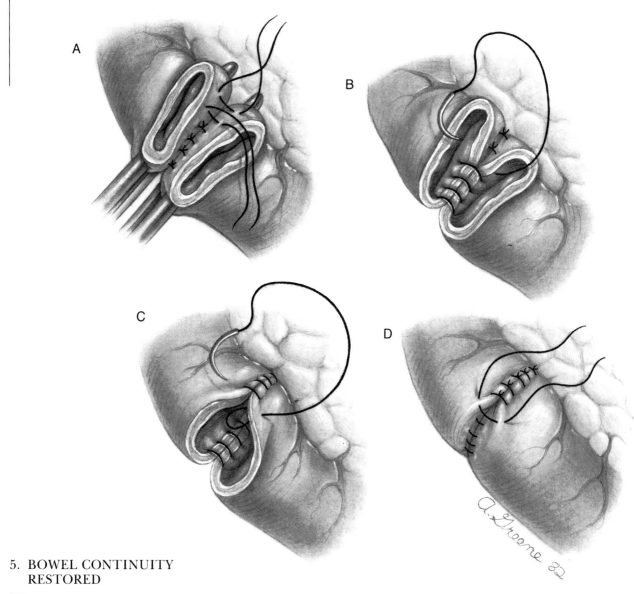

5. BOWEL CONTINUITY RESTORED

▼

When extensive resection of the duodenum is required, end-to-end anastomosis is impossible; a Roux-en-Y loop of jejunum must be brought up for anastomosis to the proximal duodenum and the distal duodenojejunum closed.

A, After local resection of the duodenum, reconstruction of the duodenum is with posterior permanent interrupted Lembert sutures. *B* and *C,* The inner layer of sutures of chromic catgut is placed in a running locking suture posteriorly and in a running Connell suture anteriorly. *D,* External seromuscular Lembert sutures are placed anteriorly as before.

14 Enteroenterostomy (Small Bowel Bypass)

RICARDO L. ROSSI, M.D.

▼ IMPORTANT FEATURES
Type of Disease (Tumor, Radiation) and Its Location Determine Site
of Anastomosis
Preserve as Much Functional Bowel as Is Safely Possible
Adequate Blood Supply
Rule Out Distal Obstruction
Minimize Contamination
Precise Suturing to Avoid Narrowing Lumen and to Achieve
Watertight Anastomosis
No Tension on Suture Line

▼ STEPS OR PLANS
Abdominal Exploration
Assess Type and Extent of Disease
Determine Site of Anastomosis
Wound Packing and Exposure
Outer Posterior Suture Line
Enterotomies
Inner Posterior Suture Line
Anterior Suture Lines

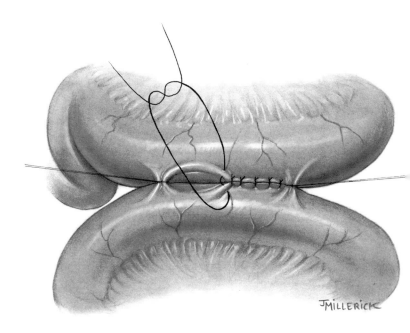

1. POSTERIOR SUTURES

Interrupted seromuscular Lembert sutures of 3-0 silk are placed just posterior to the antimesenteric bowel wall approximating both bowel loops.

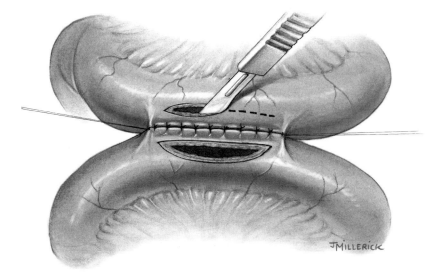

2. ADJACENT ENTEROTOMIES

The bowel is opened. Incisions are made close to the suture line and in the antimesenteric border of each bowel loop. They are made with a scalpel and completed with scissors or electrocautery. Hemostasis of the walls of the enterotomies is achieved.

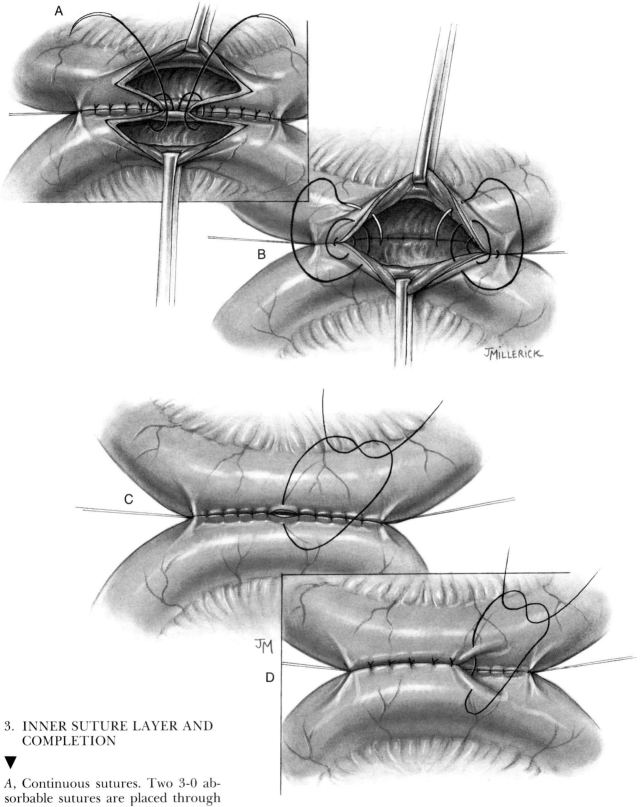

3. INNER SUTURE LAYER AND COMPLETION

▼

A, Continuous sutures. Two 3-0 absorbable sutures are placed through the full thickness of the bowel wall in the midline. B, Each suture is tied, run to the corners, and continued in the anterior wall in a through-and-through fashion, C, The sutures are tied in the midline anteriorly. D, Interrupted seromuscular sutures complete the anterior outer layer of the anastomosis.

15 | Small Bowel Resection

RICARDO L. ROSSI, M.D.

▼ IMPORTANT FEATURES
Nature and Extent of Disease Influence Decision for Resection,
    Extent and Type of Anastomosis, and Need for Other Surgical
    Maneuvers
Adequate Blood Supply
Precise Suturing to Avoid Narrowing and for Watertight
    Anastomosis
Suture Line without Tension
Minimize Contamination
Accurate Hemostasis of Mesentery
Mesenteric Rent Closed
Patency of Distal Bowel Assessed

▼ STEPS OR PLANS
Abdominal Exploration
Assess Type and Extent of Disease
Determine Amount of Bowel and Mesentery to Be Resected
Prepare Mesenteric Border of Bowel
Prepare Mesentery for Transection
Transection and Ligation of Mesentery
Bowel Transection
Techniques of Anastomosis
Anastomosis In Special Circumstances
Close Rent In Mesentery

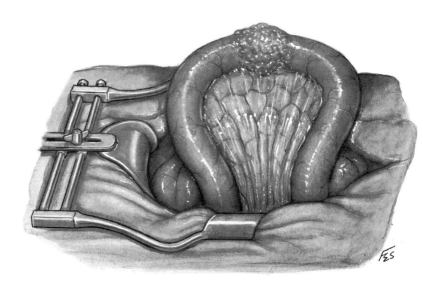

1. EXPOSURE

▼

The abdomen is explored, the disease process assessed, and the length of bowel and amount of mesentery to be removed determined. In general, a limited segment of mesentery is removed for benign disease, whereas more extensive resections (approaching the base of the mesentery) are preferred for a malignant process when it is believed that this procedure could be curative. The bowel to be resected is exteriorized, the wound is protected with drapes or plastic sheeting, and the rest of the abdomen is packed to decrease contamination. A self-retaining retractor aids the exposure.

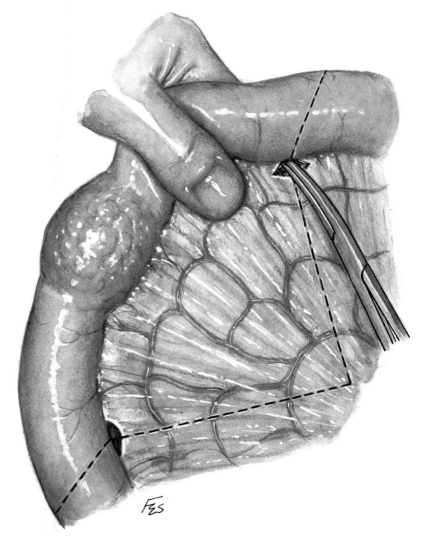

2. MESENTERIC DISSECTION

▼

In preparation of the mesenteric border of the bowel at the resection line, a small curved hemostat is used to make an opening in an avascular portion of the mesentery adjacent to the bowel.

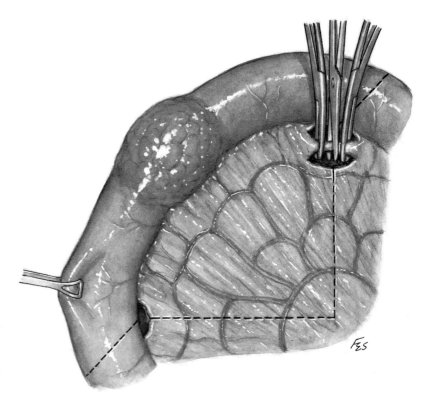

3. MESENTERIC DISSECTION
(Continued)

▼

Enough mesenteric border of bowel is freed to permit an accurate anastomosis, but excessive devascularization should be avoided. A segment of mesentery is divided between curved hemostats for this purpose. A similar technique has been used in the second site of resection.

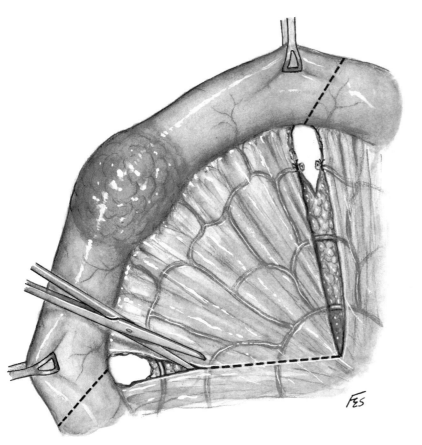

4. MESENTERIC DISSECTION
(Continued)

▼

The visceral peritoneum of the mesentery is incised with scissors following the estimated lines of transection. For traction, Babcock clamps are placed on the side of the bowel to be resected.

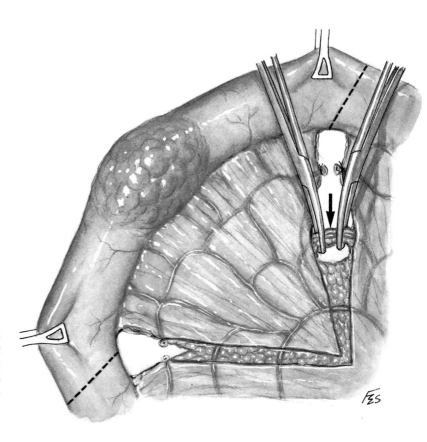

5. MESENTERIC DISSECTION
(Continued)

The mesentery is serially clamped with curved hemostats. The tissue between the clamp is divided with scissors and ligated. Suture ligation is preferred in thick or inflamed mesentery.

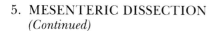

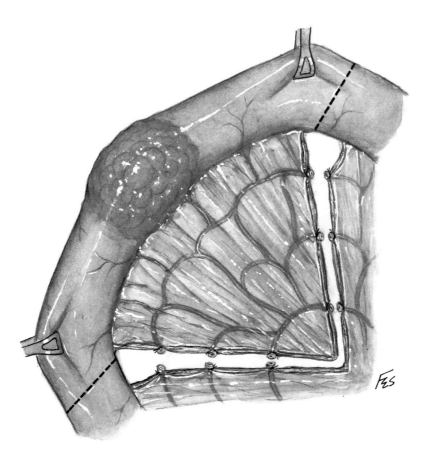

6. MESENTERIC DISSECTION COMPLETED

The mesentery has been divided completely. Hemostasis is reassessed.

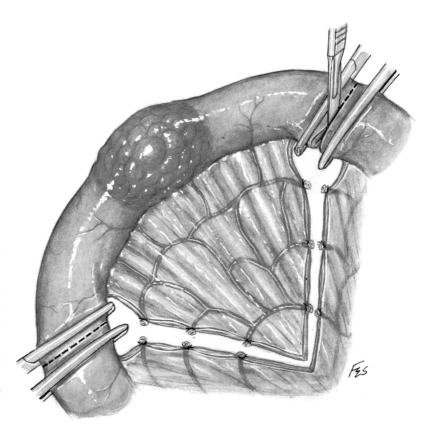

7. BOWEL CLAMPS PLACED

Drapes and packing are readjusted or changed if necessary. The bowel is clamped at an angle to excise more bowel in the antimesenteric border to optimize the blood supply. Kocher (Ochsner) clamps are used on the resected side and noncrushing clamps on the anastomotic side. The tip of the clamp points to the mesenteric side of the bowel. Enough freed bowel has to be left on the anastomotic side of the noncrushing clamp to enable later resection of tissue within the clamp.

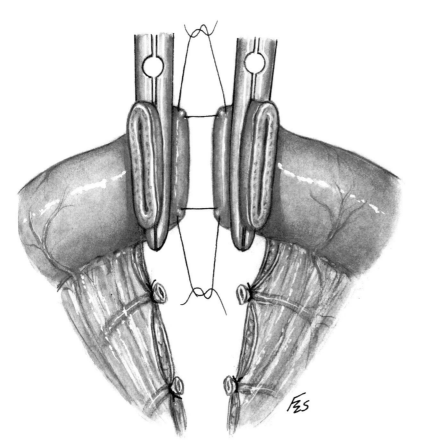

8. POSTERIOR ANASTOMOSIS

The bowel is approximated, and a posterior row of interrupted Lembert sutures of 3-0 silk is placed for end-to-end anastomosis.

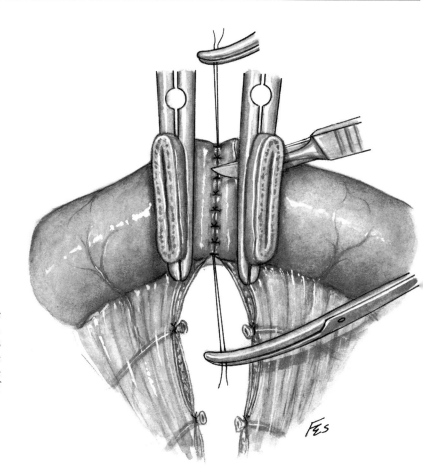

9. POSTERIOR ANASTOMOSIS
(Continued)

The sutures are tied and cut. The end (corner) sutures are clamped. The tissue included in the clamp is excised with a knife blade in close contact with the undersurface of the clamp. Hemostasis of the edges of the bowel is obtained.

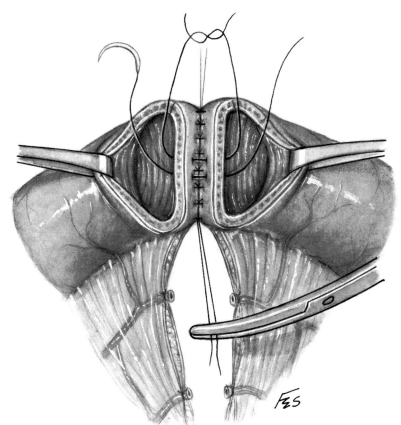

10. INTERNAL SUTURE LAYER

The free edges of the anterior bowel wall are retracted with Allis clamps. Hemostasis is achieved. The internal layer (second layer) is started in the midline of the posterior wall using absorbable 3-0 sutures. This can be accomplished with interrupted sutures or with running sutures.

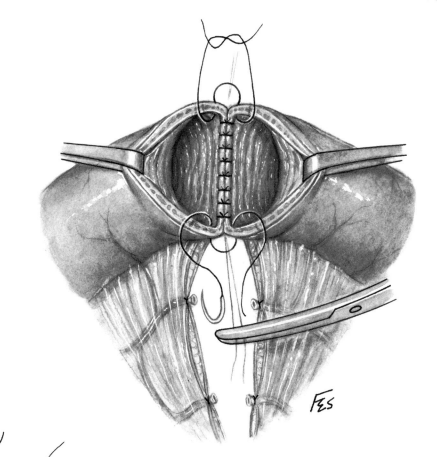

11. ANASTOMOSIS

▼

When interrupted or separated sutures are used, they are placed posteriorly, advancing toward the corners and ending anteriorly in the midline. Accurate closure of the corners is mandatory. The sutures are placed so that they can be tied within the lumen and invert the mucosa.

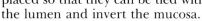

12. ANASTOMOSIS *(Continued)*

▼

An exception to this is that the final two or three sutures are placed anteriorly in the midline. Interrupted through-and-through sutures take more seromuscular tissue than mucosa and permit more accurate closure.

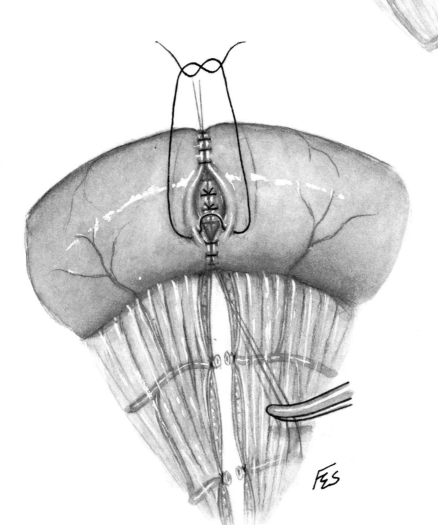

13. ANASTOMOSIS (Continued)

▼

When running sutures are used, two sutures are tied posteriorly in the midline. The suture is continued through and through in the posterior layer and corners. The sutures can be continued in the anterior wall in a similar fashion to achieve inversion. An alternative procedure is to proceed with a Connell stitch.

14. COMPLETION OF ANTERIOR LAYER

▼

After the inner layer has been completed, the anterior wall is reinforced with interrupted Lembert sutures of 3-0 silk.

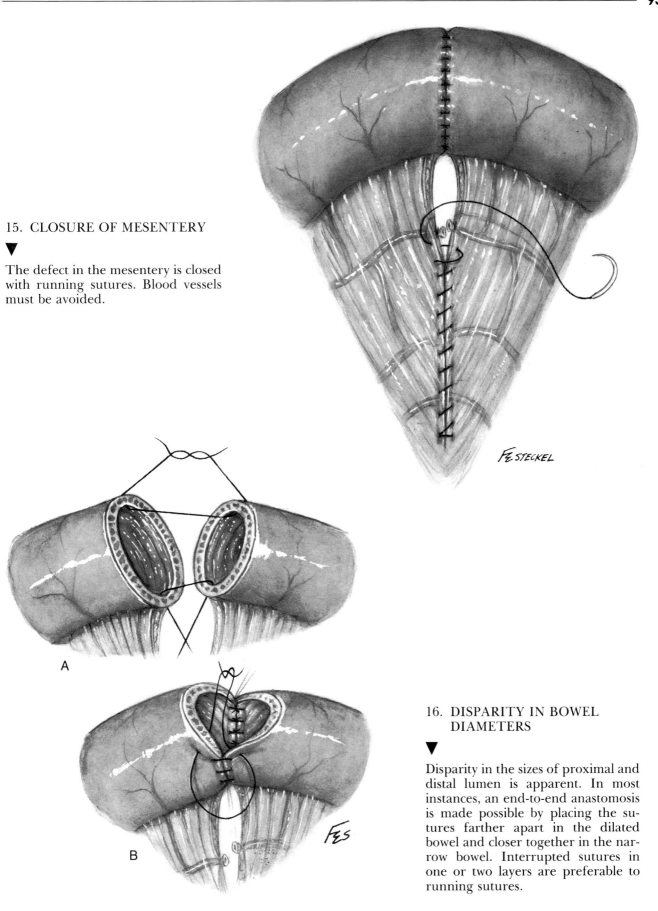

15. CLOSURE OF MESENTERY

▼

The defect in the mesentery is closed with running sutures. Blood vessels must be avoided.

A

B

16. DISPARITY IN BOWEL DIAMETERS

▼

Disparity in the sizes of proximal and distal lumen is apparent. In most instances, an end-to-end anastomosis is made possible by placing the sutures farther apart in the dilated bowel and closer together in the narrow bowel. Interrupted sutures in one or two layers are preferable to running sutures.

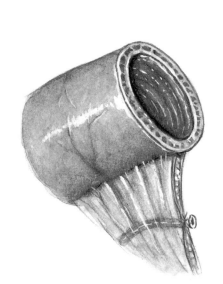
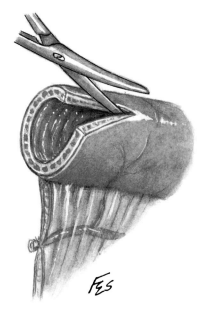

17. DISPARITY IN LUMENS

▼

Alternatively, the antimesenteric border of the narrow bowel is incised, enlarging its opening. An end-to-end anastomosis is then performed.

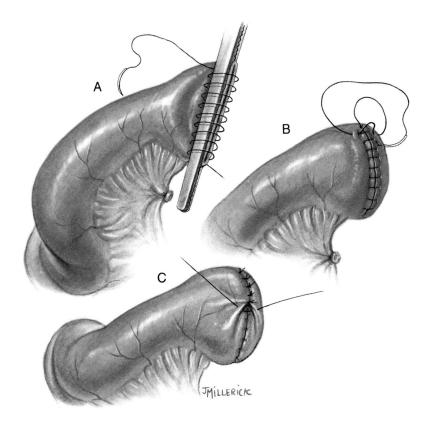

18. SIDE-TO-SIDE ANASTOMOSIS

▼

A side-to-side anastomosis can also be performed. *A,* The distal ends of both dilated and nondilated loops are closed in two layers. A running catgut suture is passed through and looped over the noncrushing clamp. The clamp is then removed, and both ends of the suture are stretched to tighten the closure. *B,* The same suture is brought backward to invert the previous suture line, using seromuscular stitches. Both ends of the suture are then tied. *C,* The closure is reinforced with an interrupted inverting layer of sutures of 3-0 silk.

19. INITIAL SUTURES

The bowel loops are approximated by placing the posterior interrupted 3-0 silk suture line. The sutures are placed just posterior to the antimesenteric border so that the opening in the bowel can be fashioned just at the antimesenteric border. The bowel is incised close to the suture line. To avoid the blind loop syndrome, no excess bowel should be left between the anastomosis and the closed end of the bowel loop.

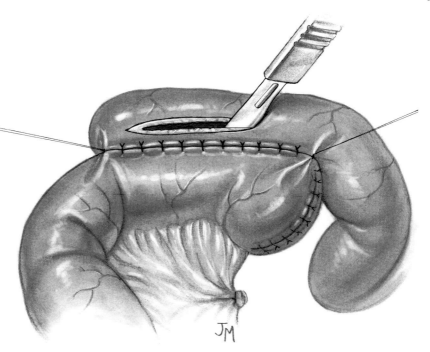

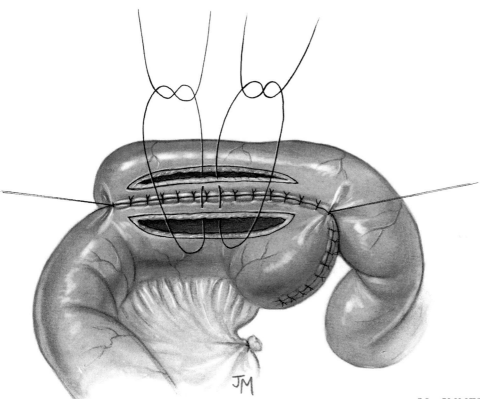

20. INNER LAYER

The inner layer is closed with interrupted sutures.

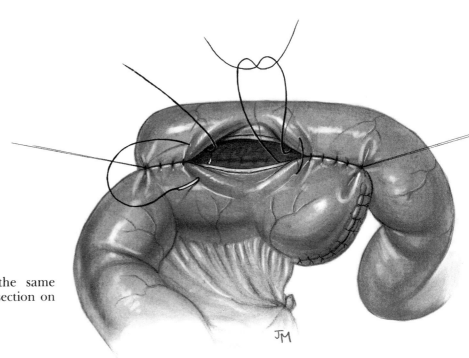

21. RUNNING SUTURE

▼

Running sutures follow the same principles outlined in the section on end-to-end anastomosis.

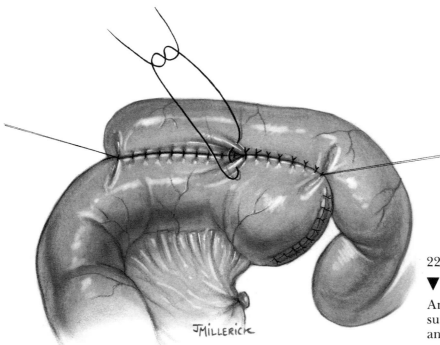

22. ANTERIOR LAYER

▼

An anterior layer of seromuscular sutures of 3-0 silk completes this anastomosis.

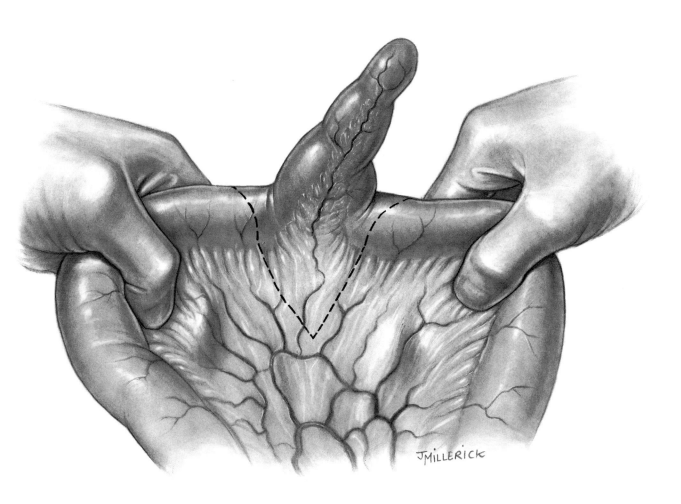

23. EXCISION OF MECKEL'S DIVERTICULUM

For excision of a Meckel's diverticulum that is acutely inflamed or causing gastrointestinal bleeding, we favor segmental small bowel resection.

16 Appendectomy

MALCOLM C. VEIDENHEIMER, M.D.

▼ IMPORTANT FEATURES
Site of Incision
Muscle-Splitting Incision
Control Mesoappendix and Appendiceal Base
Care of Appendiceal Stump

▼ STEPS OR PLANS
Incision Over Appendix
Muscle-Splitting Entry into Abdomen
Deliverance of Appendix into Wound
Control Mesoappendix
Control Appendiceal Stump
Sealing Appendiceal Stump by Mesoappendix
Careful Approximation of Abdominal Wall Musculature

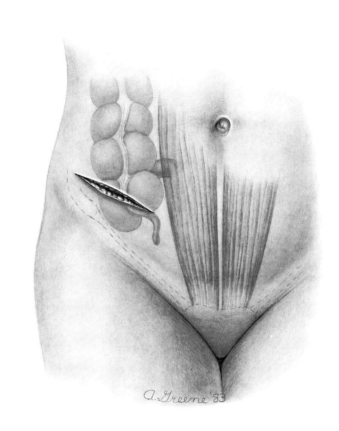

1. INCISION FOR ACCURATE DIAGNOSIS

▼

The abdomen is entered through an oblique right lower quadrant incision centered over the external oblique muscle and sited lateral to the lateral border of the rectus abdominis muscle.

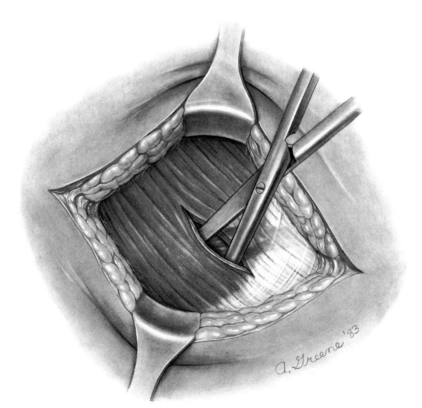

2. INCISION (*Continued*)

▼

The fibers of the external oblique muscle are split in the direction of their fibers, exposing the underlying internal oblique muscle.

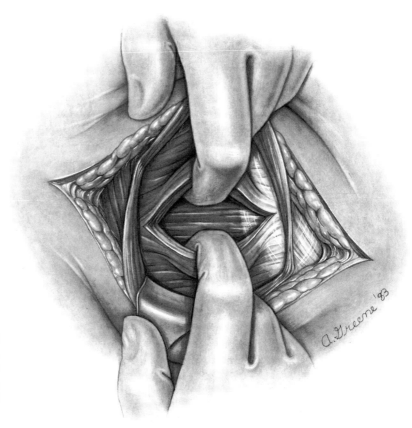

3. INCISION *(Continued)*

The internal oblique muscle is opened in the direction of its fibers, permitting a transverse window onto the transversus abdominis muscle, which is similarly separated in the direction of its fibers.

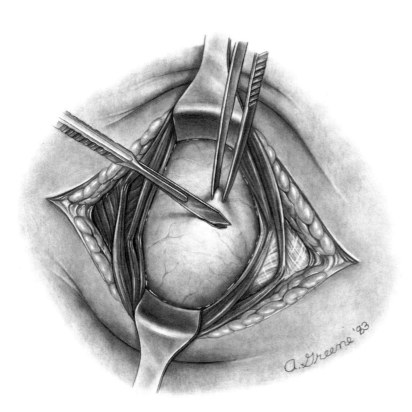

4. INCISION *(Continued)*

The peritoneum is entered.

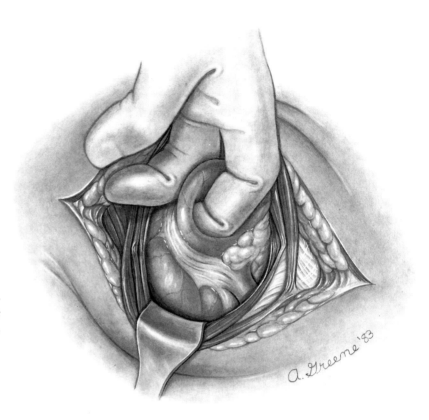

5. APPENDIX VISUALIZED

The cecum is visualized, and by rolling the cecum into the wound, the appendix is mobilized, visualized, and delivered into the wound.

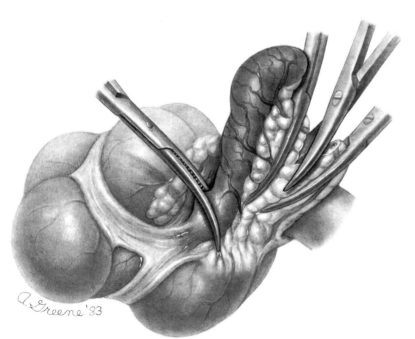

6. MESOAPPENDIX SEVERED

The mesoappendix is grasped between Kelly clamps and divided with scissors. The base of the appendix is controlled by a Kelly clamp applied across the appendix.

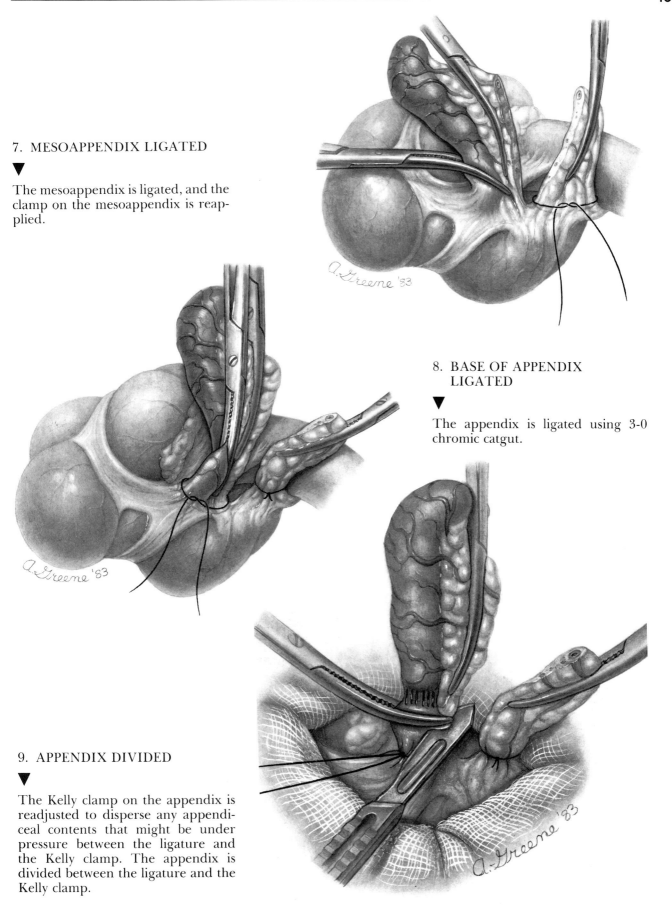

7. MESOAPPENDIX LIGATED

▼

The mesoappendix is ligated, and the clamp on the mesoappendix is reapplied.

8. BASE OF APPENDIX LIGATED

▼

The appendix is ligated using 3-0 chromic catgut.

9. APPENDIX DIVIDED

▼

The Kelly clamp on the appendix is readjusted to disperse any appendiceal contents that might be under pressure between the ligature and the Kelly clamp. The appendix is divided between the ligature and the Kelly clamp.

10. TREATMENT OF APPENDICEAL STUMP

The mesoappendix is tied down over the appendiceal stump. The appendiceal stump may be pretreated with phenol and alcohol or may receive no such antiseptic application.

11. APPENDECTOMY COMPLETED

▼

The completed appendectomy is visualized with the mesoappendix sealing off the appendiceal stump from the general abdominal cavity.

12. INCISIONAL CLOSURE

▼

The abdomen is closed in layers using either continuous or interrupted sutures on the peritoneum and interrupted sutures on the transversus abdominis and internal oblique muscles.

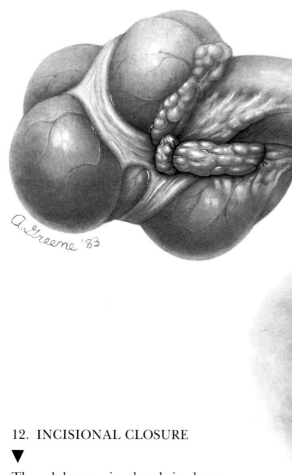

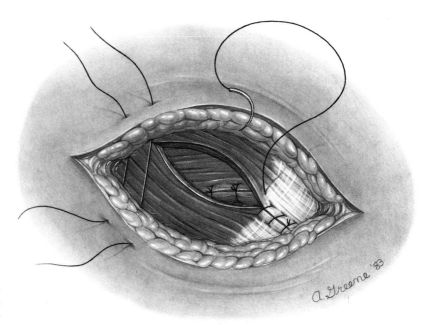

13. CLOSURE (Continued)

▼

The external oblique muscle and its aponeurosis are closed with a running catgut suture, and the skin may be closed using subcuticular or interrupted nylon sutures. A drain may be placed within the wound when the appendix is badly infected.

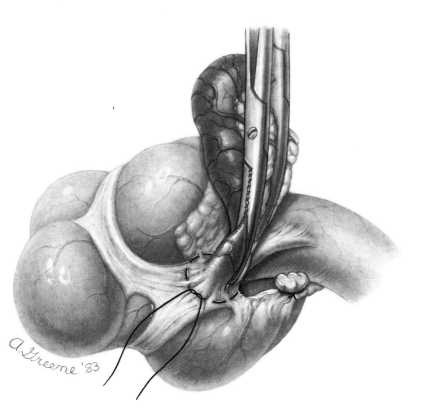

14. PURSESTRING SUTURE MANAGEMENT OF APPENDICEAL STUMP

▼

An alternative to the handling of the appendiceal stump as previously described is the inversion of the stump using a pursestring suture, which is placed before the appendix is ligated.

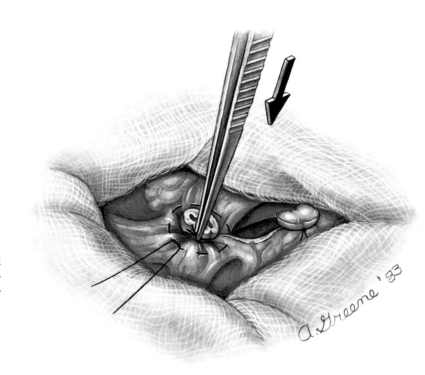

15. STUMP INVAGINATED

The appendix has been ligated and is now divided. The stump is invaginated into the cecum, and the purse-string suture is tightened.

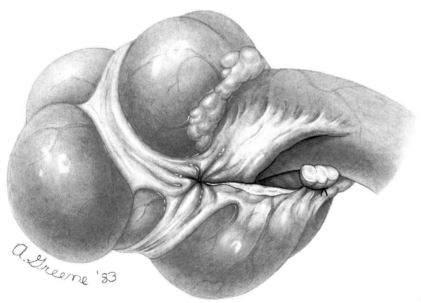

16. COMPLETED APPENDECTOMY

The completed appendectomy with the inverted stump is demonstrated.

17 Loop Ileostomy

MALCOLM C. VEIDENHEIMER, M.D.

▼ IMPORTANT FEATURES
Proper Preoperative Marking
Transrectus Position
Rotation Stoma with Afferent Limb Positioned Inferiorly
Primary Maturation of Stoma

▼ STEPS OR PLANS
Skin Ellipse Excised at Appropriate Site
Loop of Ileum Mobilized without Tension
Bowel Rotated with Afferent Limb Situated Inferiorly
Transverse Incision on Efferent Limb Close to Abdominal Skin
Eversion of Mucous Membrane
Primary Maturation with Eversion Proximal Limb of Ileostomy

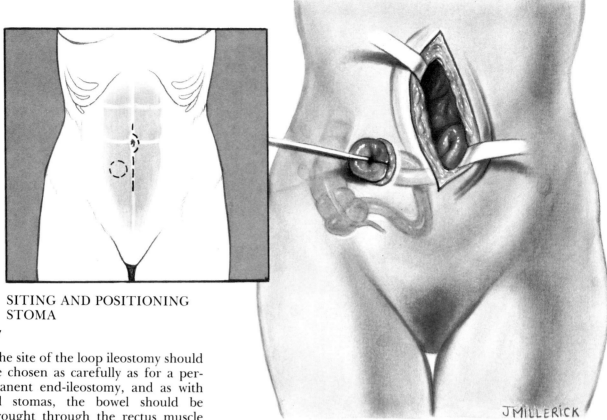

1. SITING AND POSITIONING STOMA

The site of the loop ileostomy should be chosen as carefully as for a permanent end-ileostomy, and as with all stomas, the bowel should be brought through the rectus muscle rather than lateral to the rectus sheath. As the bowel is brought through the abdominal wall, it is rotated so that the afferent limb of the bowel lies inferior to the efferent limb of the bowel. The bowel is not fixed to the abdominal wall.

2. ENTEROTOMY

The bowel is opened transversely with the electrocautery, care being taken to locate the incision close to the upper skin edge as close as possible to the point where the efferent limb of ileum passes back into the abdominal wall. A little more than one half of the circumference of the ileum is divided with the electrocautery. The bowel is supported on the abdominal wall by a plastic rod inserted through the mesentery of the ileum close to the mesenteric border of the intestine.

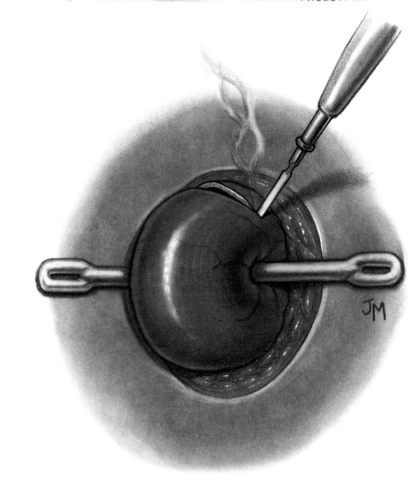

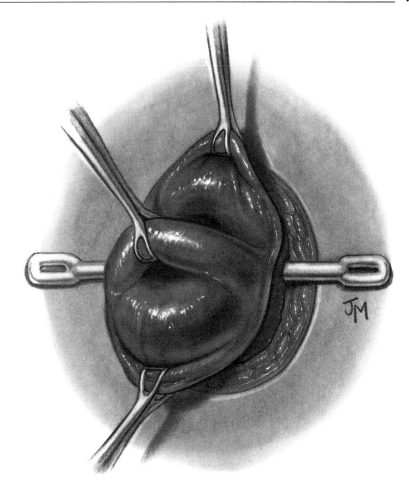

3. PROXIMAL LIMB EVERTED

The cut edges of the ileum are grasped with Babcock clamps, and the proximal limb of the ileum is everted as a protruding spout by Babcock clamps, which have been insinuated up the proximal lumen to grasp the bowel wall and cause its extrusion as traction is applied.

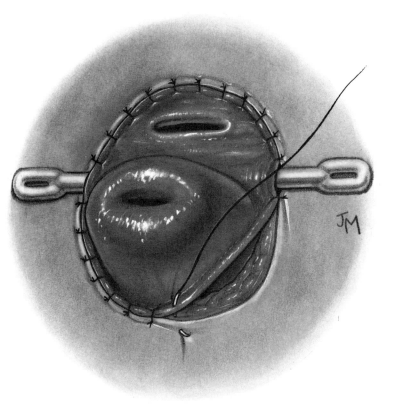

4. FIXATION TO SKIN

The bowel is sewed primarily to the skin by sutures passed through the full thickness of the ileum and either sutured in a subcuticular fashion to the skin or as full-thickness bites into the skin. The suture material is 4-0 chromic catgut. An ileostomy appliance is applied in the operating room.

18 Loop Colostomy

MALCOLM C. VEIDENHEIMER, M.D.

▼ IMPORTANT FEATURES
Proper Choice for Stoma Site
Transrectus Position of Stoma
Long Antimesocolonic Colotomy
Primary Maturation of Colostomy

▼ STEPS OR PLANS
Separate Incision for Stoma
Transrectus Position of Stoma
Support of Stoma on Abdominal Wall without Tension
Long Antimesocolonic Colotomy
Primary Maturation of Stoma with Prominent Posterior Wall Spur

BASIC INFORMATION

▼

The usual loop colostomy is performed in the transverse colon. For left colon lesions, we prefer to make the colostomy in the left transverse colon close to the splenic flexure so that no redundancy occurs between the colostomy and the splenic flexure. This minimizes the risk of prolapse of the distal limb of the colostomy should the loop colostomy have to remain in place for more than a few weeks. As in the case of all abdominal stomas, the stoma is placed through the body of the rectus muscle and is situated in an incision that is separate from the major laparotomy incision.

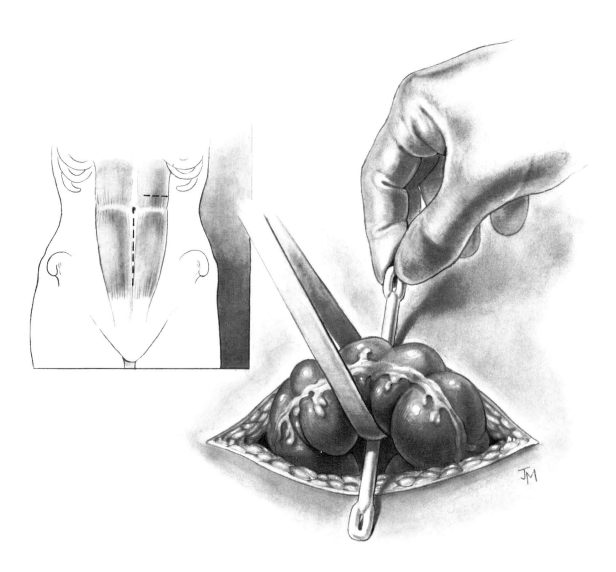

1. EXTERIORIZATION

▼

The bowel is brought through the incision and supported on the abdominal wall by means of a plastic rod.

2. COLOTOMY

The colon is opened longitudinally at a site equidistant between the attachments of the mesocolon on each side, and the incision made with the electrocautery knife should be long enough to permit a good spur of posterior wall to evert. Such an incision should, therefore, be close to 3 inches in length.

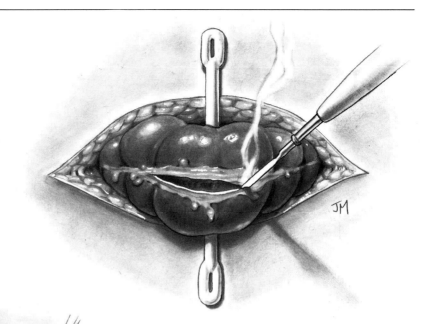

3. SPUR DEVELOPED

The cut edges of the bowel are grasped with Babcock clamps to demonstrate the full development of the spur of the posterior wall of the colon.

4. MATURATION

Primary maturation of the stoma with interrupted sutures of 4-0 chromic catgut is achieved. An appliance is placed on the stoma in the operating room. The supporting rod is left in place for one week.

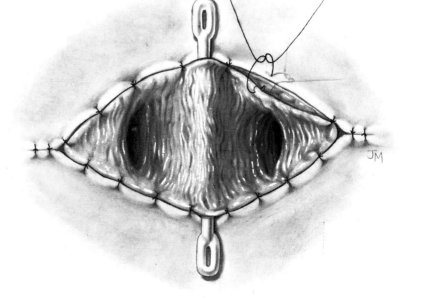

19 Abdominoperineal Resection

MALCOLM C. VEIDENHEIMER, M.D.

▼ IMPORTANT FEATURES
Positioning Patient In Stirrups
Mobilization of Rectum
Preservation of Ureters
Wide Excision Through Perineal Wound

▼ STEPS OR PLANS
Midline Incision
Colostomy Site Marked Preoperatively
Ligation of Sigmoidal Branches of Inferior Mesenteric Artery
Identification and Preservation of Ureters
Identification and Preservation of Seminal Vesicles and Vaginal Wall
Mobilization from Presacral Space
Ligation of Lateral Ligaments
Identification of Urethra Distal to Prostate
Fashioning Colostomy with Maturation
Perineal Dissection into Ischiorectal Fossa
Division of Levator Muscles
Excision of Rectum
Closure of Perineal Wound

1. POSITIONING ON TABLE

The patient is positioned with the legs in stirrups. Partial flexion of the thighs permits ready access to the abdomen by the abdominal team of operators, but the use of stirrups permits access to the perineum by the perineal operators. A moderate degree of Trendelenburg tilt aids in the dissection.

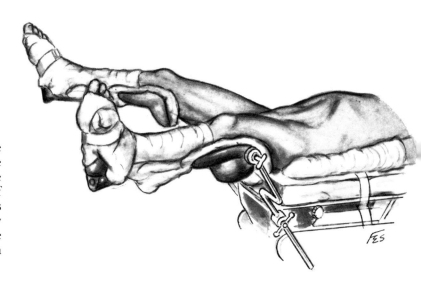

2. INCISION AND SITING COLOSTOMY

The location of the incision is important not only in consideration of access to the abdominal contents but also in consideration of deformity of the abdominal wall and the relationship of such deformity to the placement of an abdominal stoma. Because of the importance of such a consideration, all of our incisions are made in the midline so that neither the right nor the left half of the abdomen has scarring that might interfere with the selection of a site for a stoma.

The colostomy, ideally, should be situated over the rectus muscle and beneath the beltline at a distance from the iliac crest, umbilicus, and rib margin that will permit easy application of an appliance. Paracolostomy herniation is less likely to occur when the stoma is placed through the rectus muscle than when it is in a pararectal situation or more laterally in the oblique musculature of the abdominal wall.

3. BLOOD SUPPLY OF RECTUM

▼

The operation of abdominoperineal excision evolves around control of the three major areas of blood supply to the rectosigmoid and rectum. These are the sigmoidal and superior rectal branches of the inferior mesenteric artery; the middle rectal arteries, which pass through the lateral ligaments of the rectum; and the inferior rectal vessels, which are found in the ischiorectal fossa. We do not believe in ligation of the inferior mesenteric artery at its origin because nodal involvement at that level is found only in patients with incurable rectal carcinoma. We therefore ligate distal to the main inferior mesenteric trunk and thus ensure a more viable blood supply to the colostomy.

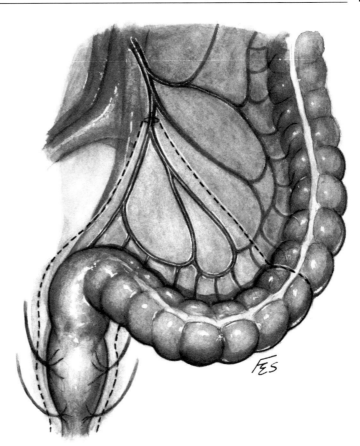

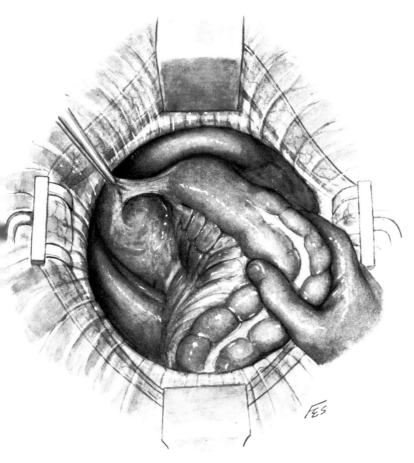

4. INITIAL DISSECTION

▼

After insertion of a self-retaining Balfour retractor and a plastic wound protector, the abdomen is explored for evidence of spread of the primary disease. Mobilization of the sigmoid and rectosigmoid colon begins in the left paracolic gutter to obtain sufficient mobility to bring the bowel to the abdominal wall at the level of the proposed colostomy.

5. LEFT PARASIGMOID AREA INCISED AND DISSECTED

The peritoneum on the left aspect of the sigmoid and rectosigmoid is incised with scissors. The site of this incision is guided by the location of the branches of the inferior mesenteric artery mentioned in Figure 2. The left ureter must be observed and protected during the course of this dissection. All patients should have preoperative excretory urography to determine the course and number of ureters present from each kidney. Dissection of the peritoneum is continued anteriorly to the base of the bladder.

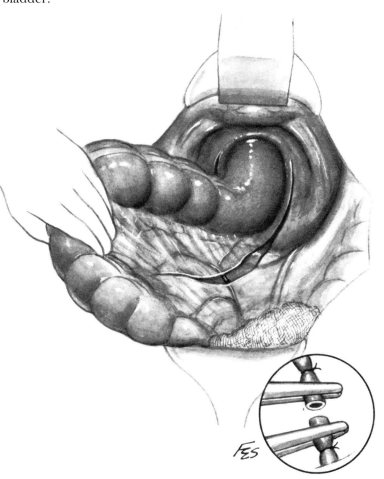

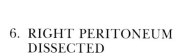

6. RIGHT PERITONEUM DISSECTED

▼

The peritoneal incision on the right side of the sigmoid and rectosigmoid is made in a similar fashion. Again, the ureter is preserved. A gauze pad protects the small bowel from the operative field. The vasculature is ligated between clamps.

7. ANTERIOR AND POSTERIOR DISSECTION

▼

The peritoneal incisions have been joined across the base of the bladder anteriorly just anterior to the bottom of the rectovesical pouch, and the retrorectal presacral space is entered in front of the sacral promontory by inserting dissecting scissors into this region while maintaining gentle anterior traction on the rectosigmoid. The loose areolar tissue in the presacral space is relatively avascular and usually readily entered.

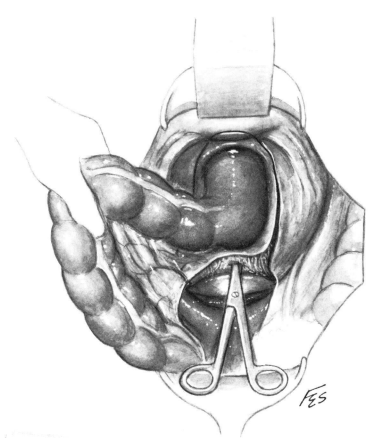

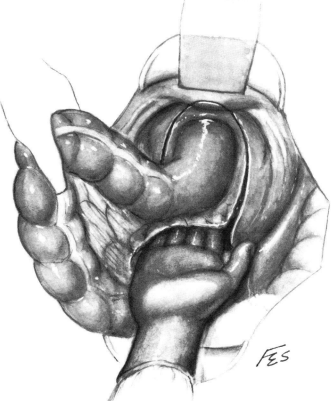

8. PRESACRAL DISSECTION

▼

When the presacral space has been demonstrated with sharp dissection, the operator's right hand is inserted into the region, and the presacral dissection is carried out by means of blunt finger dissection and gentle anterior displacement of the rectum.

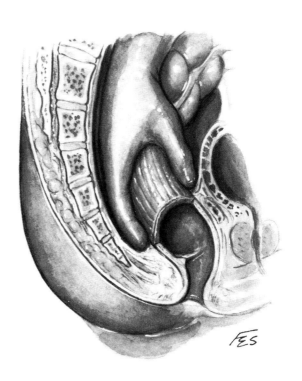

9. COCCYGEAL TIP DISSECTION

The rectum is freed from the presacral fascia distally to the level of the tip of the coccyx. The dissection is performed in a plane anterior to the presacral fascia, and thus damage to the presacral veins is avoided. Occasionally, branches of the middle sacral artery require ligation.

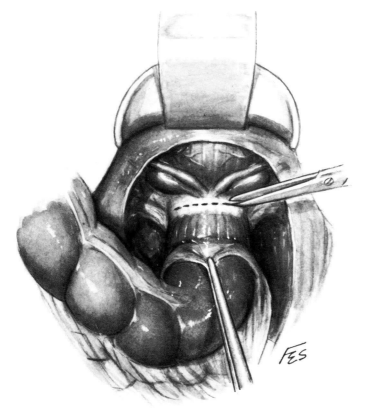

10. ANTERIOR RECTUM MOBILIZATION

The anterior dissection, aided by retraction on the bowel, is now carried to a deeper plane. The posterior wall of the bladder and the seminal vesicles are demonstrated by a combination of sharp and blunt dissection. Denonvilliers' fascia must be incised by sharp dissection, as depicted here, to mobilize the rectum farther from the prostate and seminal vesicles.

11. ANTERIOR DISSECTION TO PROSTATIC APEX

▼

When this layer has been incised, the bladder, prostate, and seminal vesicles may be swept away from the rectum by finger and scissors dissection, displaying the now bared longitudinal muscle wall of the anterior rectal surface. By means of retraction of the bladder and prostatic area and countertraction on the rectum, the dissection is carried distally until the apex of the prostate and the urethra with its contained catheter can be palpated.

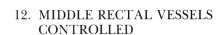

12. MIDDLE RECTAL VESSELS CONTROLLED

▼

Attention is now turned to the middle rectal vasculature. By means of a corkscrew motion with the index finger passed along the right and then the left lateral borders of the rectum, the lateral ligament with its contained middle rectal vessels is isolated from the surrounding fascial structures, clamped, cut, and ligated. On conclusion of this step of the procedure, the rectum is completely isolated anteriorly, laterally, and posteriorly. A few strands of remaining fascia may require division with scissors, but no important vascular control is needed to complete the abdominal dissection.

13. COLOSTOMY SITE PREPARATION

The site of the colostomy is now prepared by grasping the skin in a Kocher clamp and excising a circular segment of skin, the diameter of which should approximate the diameter of the sigmoid colon to be used for the sigmoid colostomy. The subcutaneous fatty tissue is retracted, and the anterior sheath of the rectus muscle is incised in a cruciate fashion. The rectus muscle fibers are split in a longitudinal direction, and the peritoneal cavity is entered with scissors. The colostomy aperture in the peritoneum, muscle, and skin must be of a size to admit two fingers.

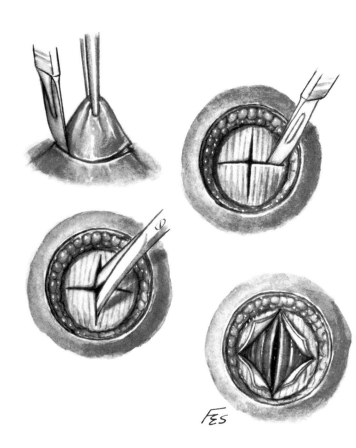

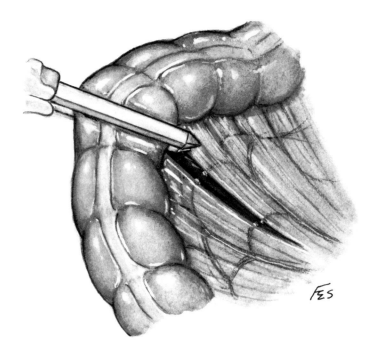

14. COLOSTOMY

A GIA stapler is passed across the sigmoid colon at the site of the proposed division of the bowel.

15. COLOSTOMY (Continued)

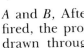

A and *B*, After the stapler has been fired, the proximal sigmoid colon is drawn through the colostomy incision to lie without tension on the abdominal wall. Before maturation of the colostomy, the staple line is excised with the electrocautery knife. The upper closed end of the rectum has been sealed by the staple line.

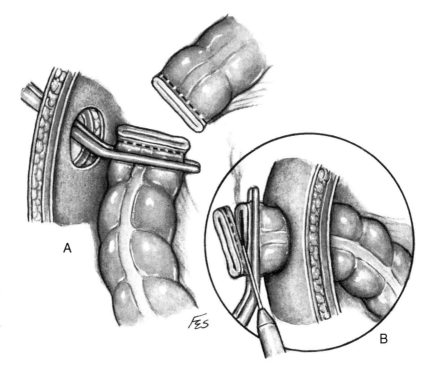

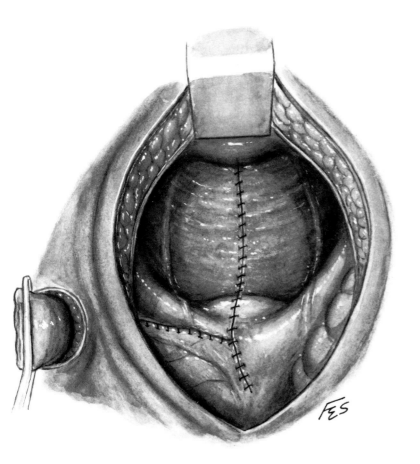

16. PELVIC PERITONEUM CLOSURE

The rectum is buried in the pelvic cavity, and by finger dissection the peritoneum on either lateral wall is mobilized to a degree that will permit closure with sutures of continuous chromic catgut. We do not close the lateral gutter in relation to the afferent limb of the colostomy.

17. CLOSURE OF INCISION AND MATURATION OF COLOSTOMY

The colostomy is completed by immediate mucocutaneous suture using about eight sutures of 4-0 chromic catgut. A disposable colostomy bag is applied to the colostomy in the operating room. Note the clothesline drain: a series of 0.5-cm Penrose drains suspended from a silk suture. These drains, 3 to 5 cm in length, are inserted between each skin stitch and removed on the fourth postoperative day. We believe copious irrigation of the wound before skin closure and use of the clothesline drain diminish the incidence of wound infection.

SYNCHRONOUS TECHNIQUE

The peritoneal dissection is started when the operability of the lesion has been ascertained by the abdominal surgeon. Thus, the dissection can be performed synchronously from both the abdominal and perineal routes. When two teams are not available to perform the abdominoperineal excision, the abdominal dissection, as depicted in Figures 1 to 17, can be performed first and the perineal dissection performed as a separate operative approach after the colostomy has been fashioned and the abdominal incision has been closed. However, both the abdominal and the perineal dissections are facilitated by use of the synchronous technique.

18. PERINEAL INCISION

A pursestring suture of heavy catgut is placed around the anal verge to close the anus. A rectangular incision is made surrounding the area of the anus, including a generous margin of perianal skin and extending from the tip of the coccyx posteriorly to the bulb of the urethra anteriorly. The edges of the skin are grasped by Lahey double-hook clamps, and the perianal skin is grasped anteriorly and posteriorly with Kocher forceps.

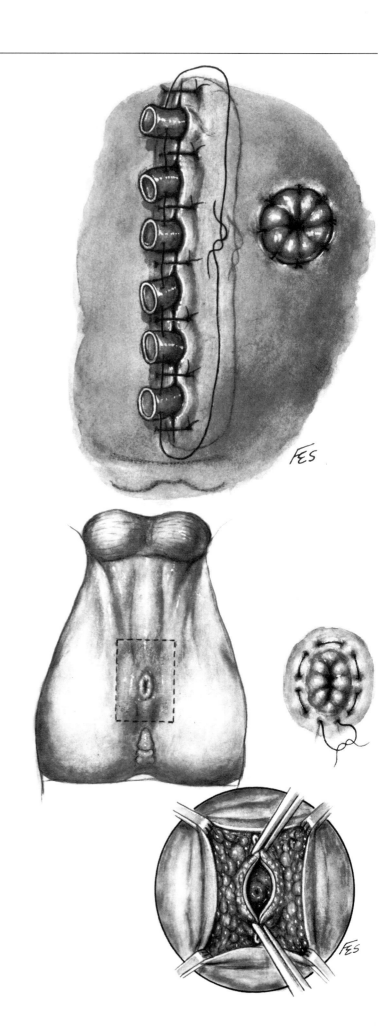

19. LATERAL DISSECTION

The dissection begins laterally. Blunt scissors are used to divide the perianal fat and to enter the ischiorectal fossa. Usually two distinct vascular bundles lie anteriorly and posteriorly deep in the ischiorectal fat. These inferior rectal vessels require ligation.

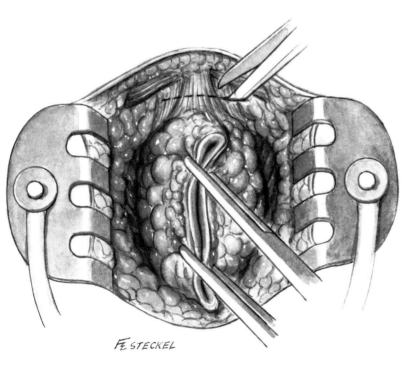

20. ANTERIOR DISSECTION DEEPENED

When the ischiorectal fossa has been entered bilaterally and posteriorly to the level of the tip of the coccyx, the anterior dissection is deepened in a plane at the posterior border of the deep transverse perineal muscle.

21. PRESACRAL SPACE
ENTERED

▼

A self-retaining retractor facilitates the dissection. The presacral space is entered by inserting scissors into this plane at the level of the coccygeal tip. These scissors should be inserted in a truly anterior direction so that they penetrate the presacral fascia and do not strip this fascia from the front of the sacrum. Thus, hemorrhage from the presacral veins is avoided. At this juncture, the abdominal and perineal dissections meet, and the rectum and anus will be free in the midline posteriorly.

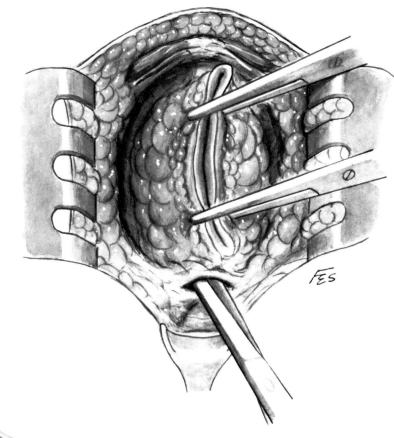

22. LEVATOR MUSCLES
DIVIDED

▼

A finger inserted through the pre coccygeal incision will enter the a ready dissected pelvic space. This fin ger is swept across the superio aspect of the levator muscles on th left and right side of the pelvis, an the levator muscles are divided alon their pelvic wall attachment with scis sors. This plane is usually avascular

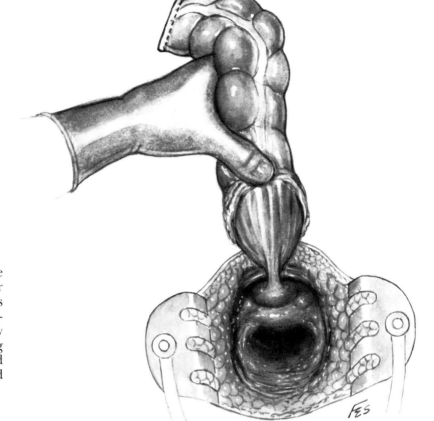

23. ANTERIOR URETHRAL ATTACHMENTS DIVIDED

▼

The rectum is delivered from the pelvis, and by traction in an anterior direction, the remaining attachments of the rectourethral muscle and fascia in the region of the urethra may be divided with safety. The palpating finger should readily ascertain and protect the urethra with its contained catheter.

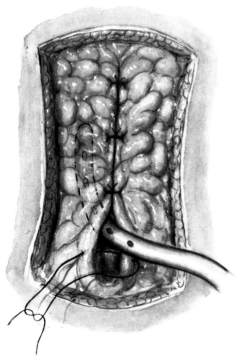

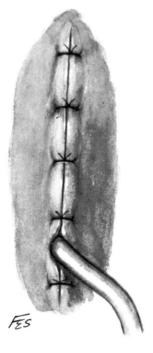

24. IRRIGATION, DRAINAGE, AND CLOSURE OF PERINEUM

▼

The perineal wound is copiously irrigated and closed using interrupted sutures of chromic catgut in the ischiorectal fat. A suction sump drain is placed into the pelvic cavity and brought out through the posterior aspect of the perineal wound. The perineal wound is closed with interrupted sutures of silk.

20 Low Anterior Resection with Hand-Sutured Anastomosis

MALCOLM C. VEIDENHEIMER, M.D.

▼ IMPORTANT FEATURES
Wide Dissection within Pelvis
Adequate Margin Distal to Tumor
Preservation of Ureters
Anastomosis Under Direct Vision

▼ STEPS OR PLANS
Assessment of Tumor
Identification of Ureters
Incision of Mesosigmoid and Peritoneum of Pelvis
Mobilization from Presacral Space
Preservation of Anterior Structures
Ligation of Blood Vessels
Division of Bowel Between Clamps
Two-Layer Anastomosis Under Direct Vision
Drainage of Extraperitoneal Anastomosis

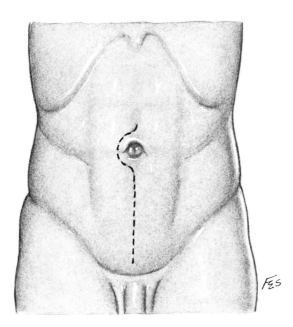

1. PREPARATION FOR EXPLORATION

▼

As with all patients having rectal operations, preoperative excretory urography has been performed. Not only does this study delineate any abnormalities of the genitourinary system that may be a result of the disease for which the operation is to be performed but it also demonstrates any anatomic variation, such as a single kidney or a double ureter. Patients with low-lying tumors are operated on in stirrups in case the anterior resection cannot be completed and an abdominoperineal resection is required. The incision is a midline incision carried to the right of the umbilicus; it leaves the left side of the abdomen free of scarring should a decision be made to perform colostomy as part of the operative procedure. When the abdomen is opened, a Balfour retractor is inserted, and a wound protector is also used.

2. EXTENT OF RESECTION

▼

A thorough exploration of the abdomen is performed. Attention is then given to the rectal area to determine the extent of any potential spread of the tumor into the perirectal tissues and into the structures within the pelvis. Nodes along the superior rectal vessels and in the preaortic region are examined. As the anterior resection for rectal carcinoma is performed, a wide margin of pelvic structures is removed posteriorly, laterally, and to some degree, anteriorly. The dissection should not funnel into the rectum as the pelvis is entered. The planned excision should include ligation of the sigmoidal and superior rectal branches of the inferior mesenteric artery as depicted. The distal margin of rectal excision should include a cuff of normal rectum at least 2 to 3 cm distal to the tumor.

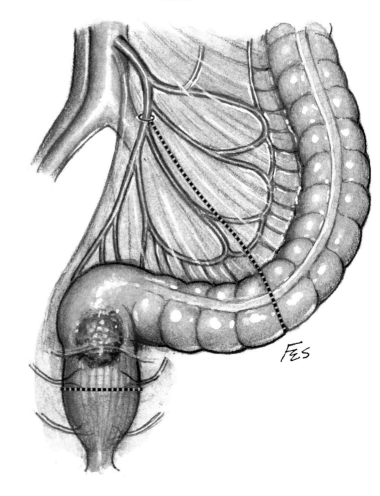

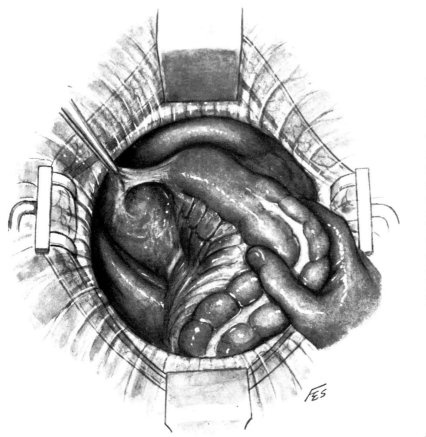

3. INITIAL LATERAL DISSECTION

▼

The patient in this illustration is positioned with the feet superior and the head inferior. The peritoneum along the left side of the sigmoid colon is freed of any adhesions to mobilize the distal sigmoid colon. The right ureter should be visible through the posterolateral parietal peritoneum. The left ureter is usually visualized only after the left posterolateral parietal peritoneum has been incised.

4. FURTHER LATERAL DISSECTIONS

▼

Incisions along each side of the posterolateral parietal peritoneum are carried distally to the base of the bladder. Both ureters must be identified and preserved.

5. SIGMOIDAL AND RECTAL VESSELS LIGATED

▼

After the right lateral parietal peritoneum has been incised, the bowel is further mobilized by ligating the vascular pedicles of the sigmoidal and superior rectal arteries and veins. We have not found any curative value from ligation of the inferior mesenteric artery at the level of the aorta.

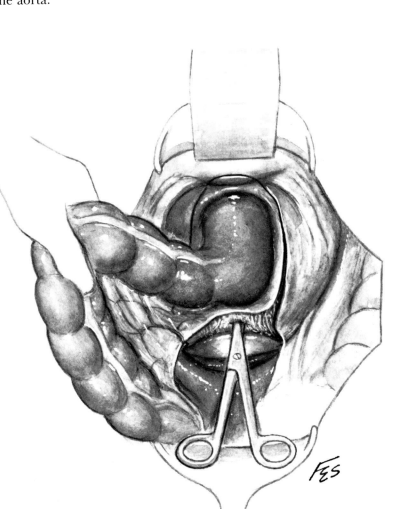

6. INITIAL MOBILIZATION OF RECTUM

▼

The parietal peritoneum is incised across the base of the bladder in men and along the posterior aspect of the vagina in women. With traction on the sigmoid colon, the loose areolar fascia of the presacral space is penetrated with sharp dissection by scissors.

7. FURTHER MOBILIZATION OF RECTUM

▼

The presacral dissection is further enlarged by finger and hand dissection to mobilize the rectum from the presacral space. The tissues on each lateral aspect of the rectum are avascular and permit blunt finger dissection in a wide fashion along the lateral walls of the pelvis bilaterally.

8. POSTERIOR DISSECTION TO COCCYX

▼

The dissection posteriorly extends to the level of the tip of the coccyx. Care must be taken not to enter the presacral fascia because that action would expose the presacral veins and create the potential for serious bleeding. The rectum should be mobilized at least 5 cm distal to the lower border of the tumor to encompass any potential lymphatic and venous spread of tumor.

9. VESICLES AND PROSTATE SEPARATED

▼

Denonvilliers' fascia is incised anteriorly by sharp dissection to separate the plane of the prostate and seminal vesicles anteriorly from the muscle of the anterior wall of the rectum posteriorly.

10. FURTHER ANTERIOR DISSECTION

▼

Sharp and blunt dissection frees these structures from the anterior rectal wall and permits more distal mobilization of the rectum anteriorly. In women, this dissection is somewhat easier, and the vagina is separated from the front of the rectum by this same technique.

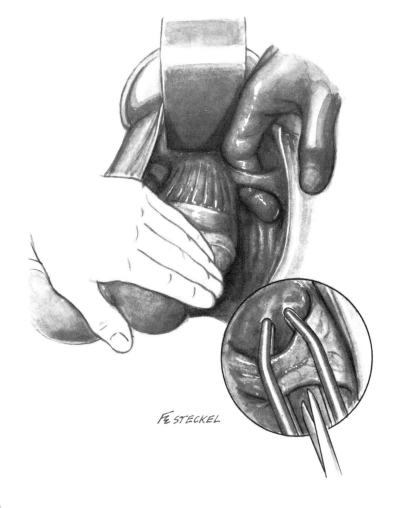

11. MIDDLE RECTAL VESSELS LIGATED

▼

With traction on the rectum and with a corkscrew motion of the operator's index finger, the right and left lateral ligaments of the rectum can be identified, clamped, and cut. The middle rectal vessels lie within these structures and are thus readily ligated.

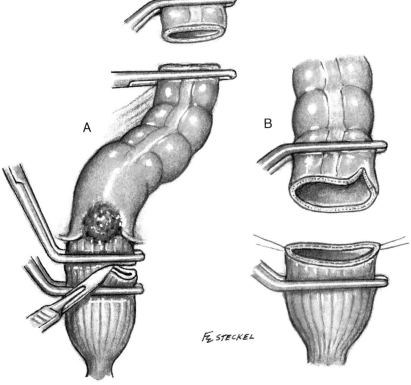

12. RECTOSIGMOID RESECTED

▼

A and *B*, The specimen is now ready to be removed. Noncrushing clamps are placed on the proximal and distal segments of the colon and rectum, and the bowel is divided with a scalpel. A 2- to 3-cm margin distal to the lower border of the tumor is necessary for proper treatment of a malignant lesion. A cuff of bowel controlled by noncrushing angled clamps and measuring 1.5 to 2 cm in length is cleaned of any residual stool with a moistened gauze pad, and the proximal sigmoid colon is approximated to the distal rectum. When a disparity exists between the wide rectal ampulla and the narrow sigmoid colon, the antimesenteric border of the sigmoid colon can be incised for 1 or 2 cm to produce a greater luminal diameter (the Cheatle maneuver).

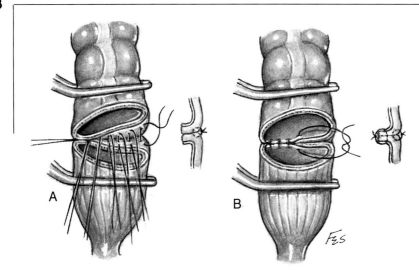

A

B

13. COLORECTOSTOMY

▼

A and *B*, The anastomosis is performed in two layers using an outer
seromuscular layer of interrupted sutures of nylon and an inner inverting
full-thickness layer of interrupted sutures of chromic catgut. The posterior two layers are depicted in this
illustration.

14. ANASTOMOSIS COMPLETED AND DRAINED

▼

A and *B*, The anterior two-layer closure is shown with a full-thickness
layer of sutures of chromic catgut
followed by a seromuscular layer of
interrupted sutures of nylon. The
occluding clamps can be removed
after completion of the inner layer
of sutures of chromic catgut. A flat
Jackson-Pratt suction catheter is
placed behind the anastomosis to remove any potential accumulation of
serum and blood. The pelvic floor
and the rent in the mesocolon are
not closed with sutures.

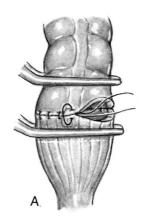

A

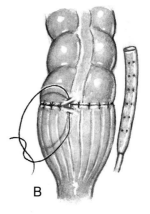

B

15. ABDOMINAL CLOSURE

▼

The abdominal incision is closed
using continuous sutures of long-last-
ing absorbable material to close the
linea alba. The skin is approximated
with either sutures or skin clips, and
a series of small Penrose drains suspended from a silk suture is placed
between the skin sutures to permit
drainage of the subcutaneous space.
The Jackson-Pratt drain, which has
its egress through the lower pole of
the incision, is left in place for six
days.

A complementary colostomy is
used in less than 10 per cent of our
patients, that is, patients in whom the
anastomosis is of questionable security.

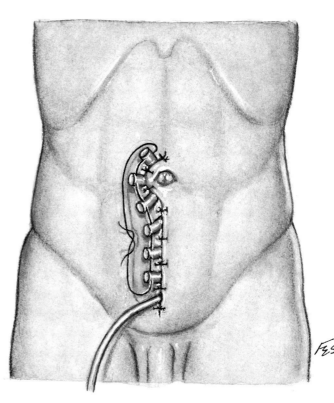

21 | Anterior Resection with Stapled Anastomosis

DAVID J. SCHOETZ, JR., M.D.

▼ IMPORTANT FEATURES
Complete Mobilization of Rectum and Sigmoid Colon
Adequate Proximal and Distal Margins
Anastomosis with Satisfactory Blood Supply without Tension
Circular Staple Line Overlaps Linear Staple Line

▼ STEPS OR PLANS
Complete Mobilization of Rectum
Stapling of Distal Margin of Transection
Placement of Proximal Pursestring Suture
Transanal Insertion of Stapler
Placement of Proximal Colon Over Anvil
Firing of Stapler
Extraction of Stapler
Testing of Anastomosis

Circular Stapled Technique

1. PLACEMENT OF PROXIMAL PURSESTRING

▼

Mobilization of the specimen should proceed in the same way as if the anastomosis were to be hand sewn. The pursestring clamp is placed at the proximal line of transection, and a 2-0 polypropylene (Prolene) suture on a Keith needle is passed through the pursestring clamp. A Kocher clamp is placed distally to prevent fecal soiling during excision of the colon. An alternative method of performing the proximal pursestring technique is to place an atraumatic bowel clamp proximally, transect the specimen, and perform a whipstitch type of pursestring closure on the divided end of the sigmoid colon.

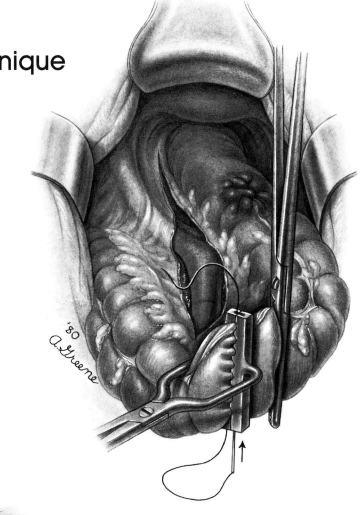

Modified from
W. Baker

2. PLACEMENT OF DISTAL PURSESTRING

▼

After the rectum has been transected at least 2 cm below the most distal extent of the tumor, a whipstitch type of pursestring is placed in the rectum using 2-0 polypropylene (Prolene) suture material. The sutures are started on the anterior wall of the rectum from the outside portion of the rectum to the inside. The pursestring must slide through the rectum so that subsequent complete gathering of the bowel around the shaft of the stapler will occur. The full thickness of the rectal wall is incorporated in each of the bites of the suture. Appropriate spacing is approximately 5 mm from the cut edge and no more than 1 cm apart for each of the sutures of the pursestring.

3. POSITIONING OF STAPLING DEVICE

▼

The size of the cartridge to be used in construction of the anastomosis is critical to avoid subsequent stenosis. The lumen of the colon at the proximal line of transection determines the size of the cartridge to be used; consequently, the sizing devices should be inserted into the colonic lumen. The sizers should be well lubricated, and gentle dilatation of the proximal colon may be accomplished. Care should be exercised in preventing a longitudinal split of the colon proximal to the pursestring. Every attempt should be made to accommodate a 31-mm cartridge. In some instances, the 28-mm cartridge will be necessary, but under no circumstances should a 25-mm cartridge be used in the colon of an adult. When a cartridge of appropriate size has been chosen, the perineal operator passes the stapler with its attached cartridge transanally until the top of the anvil is visible through the rectal pursestring. At this point the stapler

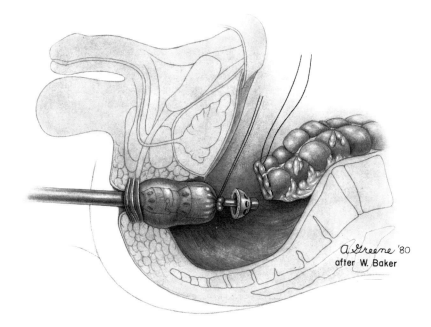

a. Greene '80
after W. Baker

is opened, and the abdominal operator gently guides the anvil through the rectal stump while maintaining upward traction on the rectal pursestring. The pursestring is tied, taking care to ensure that the entire rectum is gathered around the shaft of the instrument with no gaping defects.

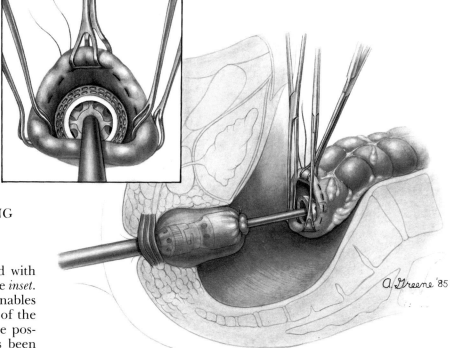

a. Greene '85

4. PROXIMAL PURSESTRING ON ANVIL SECURED

▼

The proximal colon is grasped with Babcock forceps as shown in the *inset*. This triangulation technique enables placement of the posterior lip of the colon over the anvil. When the posterior aspect of the colon has been placed over the anvil, the perineal operator can then direct the stapler posteriorly to facilitate lifting of the anterior lip of the colon over the anvil as well. The Babcock forceps is

removed, and the pursestring is secured, again making certain that the entire colon is drawn tightly around the shaft of the instrument.

5. STAPLER CLOSED

▼

Closure of the stapler is accomplished with some upward traction on the rectum from below and with the abdominal operator being certain that no other tissue is incorporated in the staple line as the instrument is closed.

6. STAPLER FIRED

▼

After the safety latch on the staple gun has been released, the two handles are squeezed together firmly. This maneuver automatically accomplishes firing of a double row of staggered interrupted stainless steel staples with the excision of a doughnut of tissue from both the colon and the rectum.

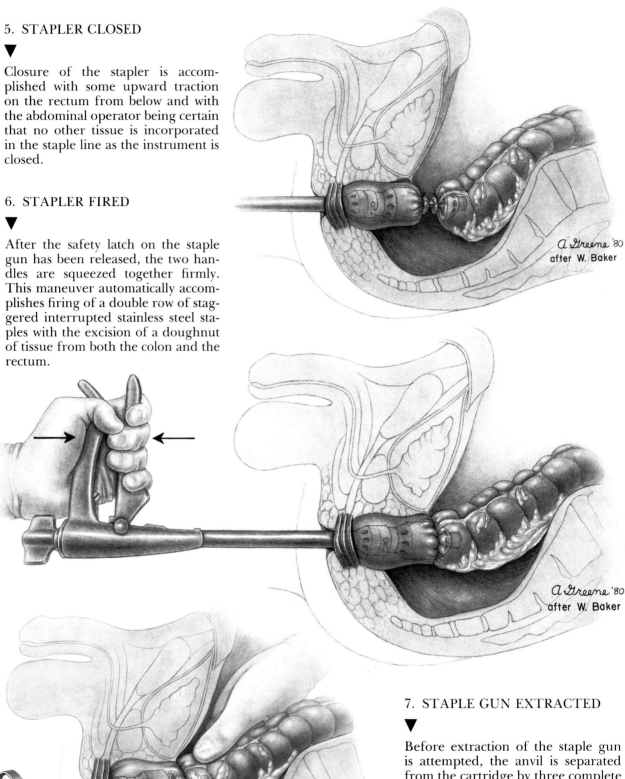

a. Greene '80
after W. Baker

a. Greene '80
after W. Baker

a. Greene '85

7. STAPLE GUN EXTRACTED

▼

Before extraction of the staple gun is attempted, the anvil is separated from the cartridge by three complete turns, thus providing a margin of clearance of approximately 2 cm. A rotational maneuver by the perineal operator frees the cartridge from the anastomosis. When the cartridge rotates freely within the lumen of the bowel, the abdominal operator places

Continued

Figure 7 Continued
downward traction on the colon
while the perineal operator gently
places downward traction on the
staple gun, continuing with both
traction and rotation until the anvil
itself slides through the anastomosis,
and the stapler is removed.

DOUGHNUTS AND ANASTOMOSIS CHECKED

▼

The perineal operator disassembles the staple gun and checks both the proximal
and distal doughnuts, which should be intact. The anastomosis is tested. The
bowel proximal to the anastomosis is occluded and irrigated with full-strength
povidone-iodine (Betadine) solution while the anastomosis is visualized directly.
Interrupted seromuscular sutures can be used to buttress the anastomosis in
the presence of leakage. Individual judgment must be exercised regarding the
addition of a temporary loop colostomy to protect the anastomosis.

Double Stapled Technique

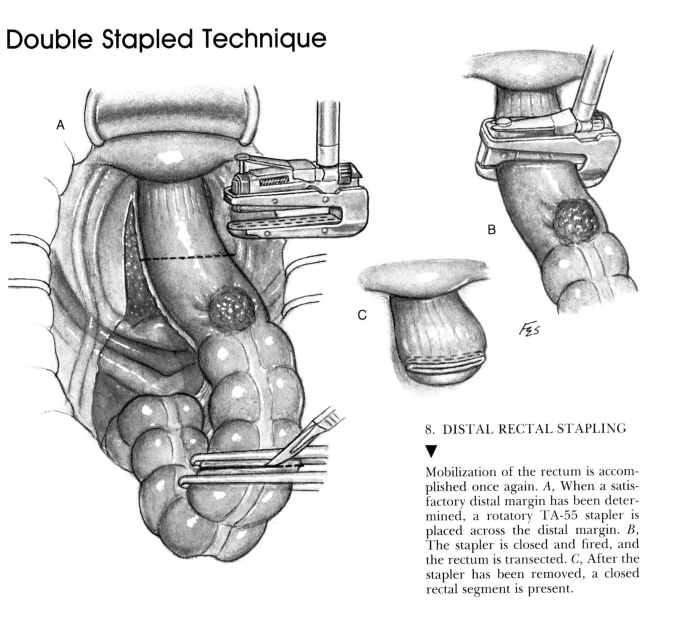

8. DISTAL RECTAL STAPLING

▼

Mobilization of the rectum is accomplished once again. *A,* When a satisfactory distal margin has been determined, a rotary TA-55 stapler is placed across the distal margin. *B,* The stapler is closed and fired, and the rectum is transected. *C,* After the stapler has been removed, a closed rectal segment is present.

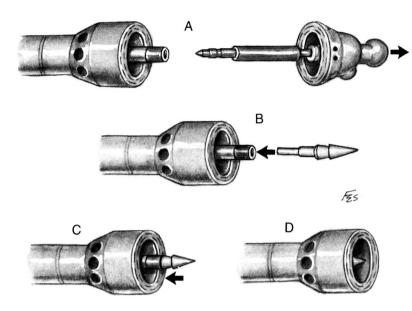

9. PLACEMENT OF TROCAR IN EEA STAPLER

▼

The premium C-EEA stapler is used for the double stapled anastomosis. *A* and *B*, This instrument has a detachable center post and a trocar that is able to fit into the center rod. *C* and *D*, The anvil and center rod are removed, and the trocar is inserted and retracted to below the top of the staple cartridge.

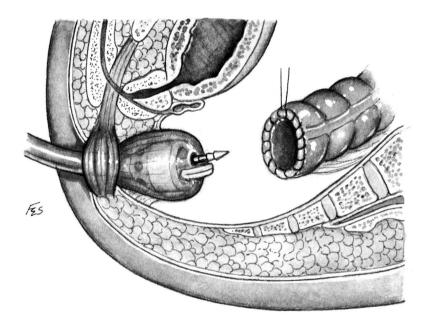

10. ANAL INTRODUCTION OF STAPLER AND PUNCTURING OF RECTUM

▼

The stapler is introduced transanally after gentle dilatation and is guided to the top of the stapled rectal segment. The center rod is extended, and the trocar is used to puncture the top of the rectum, either just anterior or just posterior to the linear staple line.

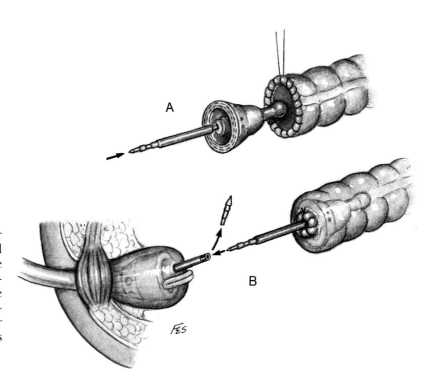

11. ANVIL PURSESTRING SUTURE IN SIGMOID END

▼

A, The anvil with the attached center rod can be placed into the proximal colon under direct vision up on the abdominal wall. *B*, After the pursestring suture has been tied in the groove of the center post and inspected for completeness, the trocar is removed, and the center post is snapped into the center rod.

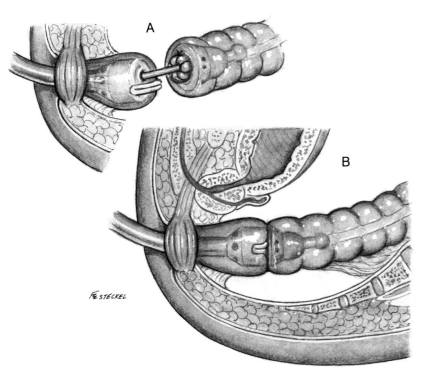

12. INSTRUMENT CLOSED AND FIRED

▼

A and *B*, The instrument is closed, again taking care not to incorporate any extraneous pararectal tissue into the staple line. The circular staple line must overlap the linear staple line to ensure integrity of the anastomosis. After the instrument has been fired, the rest of the steps are carried out as in a conventional circular stapled technique.

22 Colectomy

MALCOLM C. VEIDENHEIMER, M.D.

▼ IMPORTANT FEATURES
Consideration of Blood Supply and Venous Drainage
Wide Excision of Mesocolon with Preservation of Blood Supply to
     Proximal and Distal Bowel
Careful Apposition of Bowel Ends

▼ STEPS OR PLANS
Early Ligation of Artery and Vein, If Possible
Dissection of Mesocolon
Clamping and Dividing Colon
Two-Layer Anastomosis

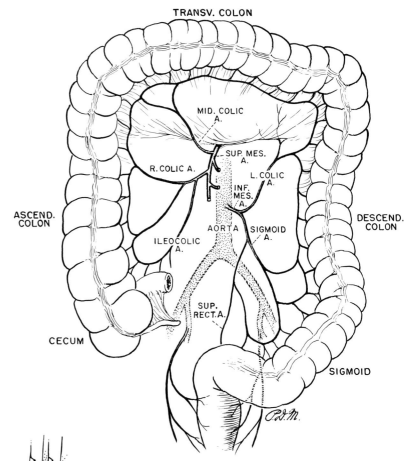

1. VASCULAR ANATOMY OF COLON

▼

The blood supply of the large bowel dictates the extent of mesocolonic resection and determines the extent of bowel to be removed, especially in dealing with neoplastic diseases. Therefore, diseases of the right colon require ligation of the right colic and ileocolic arteries, diseases of the transverse colon require ligation of the middle colic artery, and diseases of the left colon require ligation of either the inferior mesenteric artery at its root or the left colic or sigmoid arteries or both in a more distal site.

2. ARTERIAL LIGATION FOR RIGHT COLECTOMY

▼

For lesions in the right colon, the right colic artery and the ileocolic artery must be ligated, preferably at the origin of the right colic artery from the superior mesenteric artery. Most right colectomies performed for carcinoma should include the right branches of the middle colic artery and vein in the mesocolonic dissection. These ligations may be performed as the initial surgical intervention in thin persons, thus permitting the no-touch approach to a colonic neoplasm. In obese patients, we do not use the no-touch approach but proceed directly to mobilization of the colon.

3. RIGHT COLON MOBILIZATION

The peritoneum lying lateral to the cecum and ascending colon is divided by scissors dissection. Only a few unimportant blood vessels are found in the peritoneum, and ligation of blood vessels is not usually required. As the colon is mobilized and reflected medially, one must be aware of the presence of the ureter as it appears beneath the second and third portions of the duodenum, and care should be taken to avoid injury to the gonadal vessels, which lie in the retroperitoneum close to the ureter. The duodenum must be separated from the hepatic flexure because the incision in the lateral peritoneum is continued superiorly across the cholecystoduodenal colic ligament. In the region of the hepatic flexure, fatty omentum will be encountered, and Kelly clamps are required to control the blood vessels in that structure.

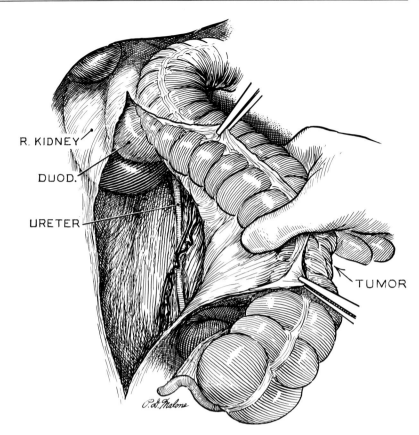

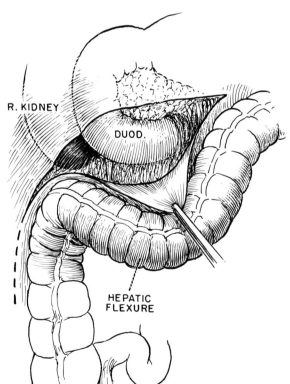

4. DISSECTION OF HEPATIC FLEXURE AND RIGHT TRANSVERSE COLON

The gastrocolic omentum is divided across the inferior aspect of the pancreas and duodenum, extending the dissection medially to the predetermined level of the right branch of the middle colic artery. The greater omentum is divided between Kelly clamps to the border of the colon that has previously been selected for the site of transection.

5. DISSECTION OF MESENTERY AND DIVISION OF BOWEL

▼

After the colon has been mobilized and the blood supply ligated, the mesentery of the terminal ileum and the mesocolon between the major vessels are divided using Kelly clamps, and the colon and ileum are divided. Kocher clamps are placed on the resected specimen side of the intestinal division. Noncrushing Doyen clamps are placed on the remaining segments of ileum and colon to control the contents of the bowel. A cuff of bowel is left that protrudes 1.5 to 2 cm beyond the noncrushing clamps, and the line of division of the intestine is on the Kocher clamps. The bowel may be ligated with umbilical tapes or heavy silk ligatures before manipulation of the intestine or, more commonly, we proceed directly to the use of clamps without any previous ligation of the colon.

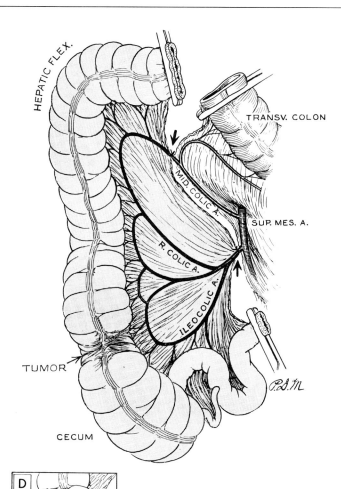

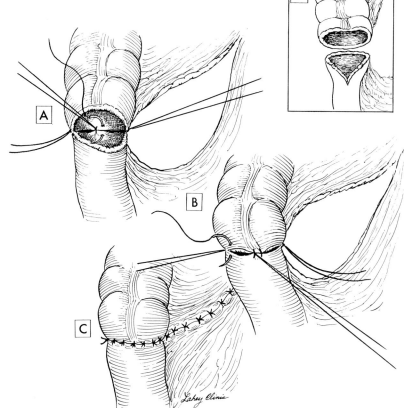

6. ILEOCOLOSTOMY

▼

The colonic anastomosis is performed in two layers using interrupted sutures. *A*, The inner full-thickness layer is of chromic catgut. *B*, The outer seromuscular layer is of fine braided nylon. *C*, The rent in the mesentery is approximated with interrupted or continuous sutures of chromic catgut. *D*, Any disparity between the proximal and distal intestinal circumference is equalized by the use of a Cheatle slit on the antimesenteric border of the intestine that has the smaller circumference.

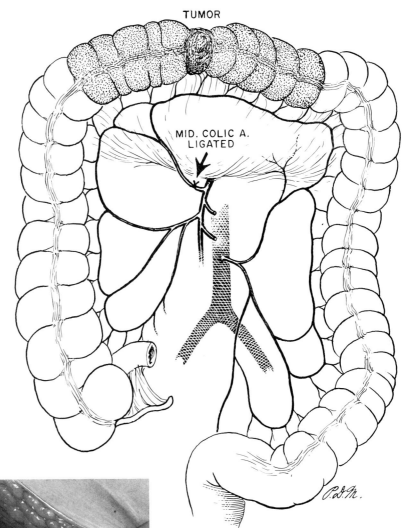

7. TRANSVERSE COLON RESECTION

Resection of the transverse colon is based on ligation of the middle colic artery close to its origin from the superior mesenteric artery. When the lesion in the colon is situated near the hepatic flexure, portions of the right colic artery should also be included in the resected specimen. When the lesion is close to the splenic flexure, branches of the left colic artery as well as the stem of the middle colic artery should be included in the ligated mesentery. Lesions of the transverse colon mandate removal of the entire greater omentum as well as the gastrocolic omentum and the transverse colon mesocolon.

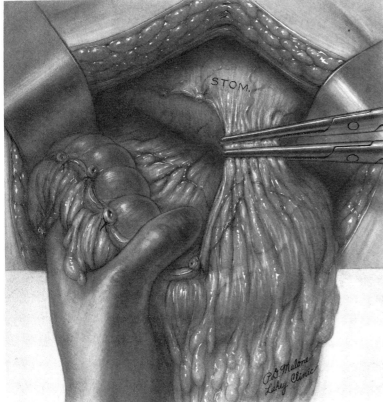

8. DISSECTION OF GASTROCOLIC OMENTUM

The gastrocolic omentum should be divided close to the stomach, including the right gastroepiploic artery in the excised tissue.

9. COLONIC ANASTOMOSIS

▼

The two flexures of the colon are approximated, and the colon anastomosis is performed as previously described.

10 and 11. VASCULAR LIGATION FOR NEOPLASMS NEAR SPLENIC FLEXURE

▼

For neoplasms in the region of the splenic flexure and the upper descending colon, the middle colic *(arrow)* and left colic *(arrow)* and sigmoidal *(arrow)* arteries are divided at sites that are consistent with adequate excision of venous-bearing and lymphatic-bearing mesocolon.

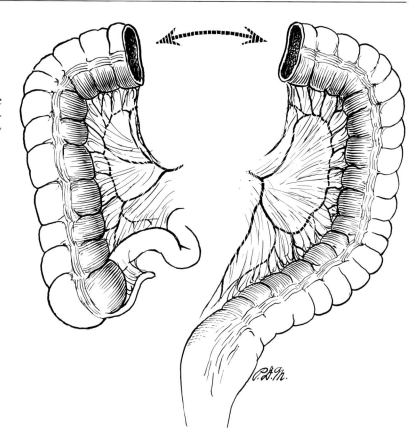

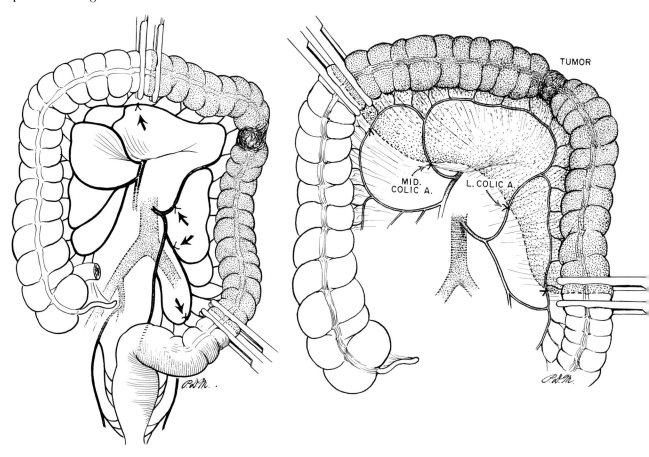

MID. COLIC A.

L. COLIC A.

TUMOR

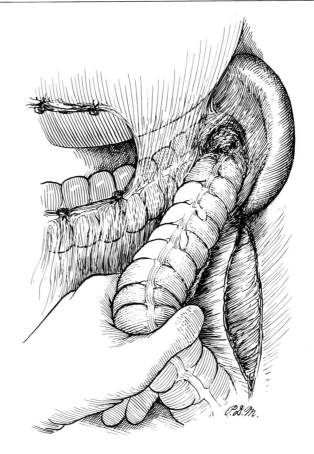

12. SPLENIC FLEXURE MOBILIZATION

▼

Division of the gastrocolic omentum is carried to the left as far as is easily possible, and attention is then turned to the left pericolic gutter where the peritoneum is divided to mobilize the upper descending colon. Care is taken to avoid heavy traction on the splenic flexure lest the splenic capsule be torn by traction on its peritoneal adhesions.

13. FURTHER DISSECTION OF SPLENIC FLEXURE

▼

The splenic flexure may be adherent to the spleen. However, mobilization of the transverse colon close to the splenic flexure, and mobilization of the peritoneum lateral to the descending colon, permit gentle traction on the colon and careful dissection of the splenic flexure and its mesentery. Thus, the colon and its mesentery can be mobilized away from the spleen and out onto the abdominal wall. There, the blood vessels within the mesocolon may be dealt with easily without risk of injury to the spleen and its circulation.

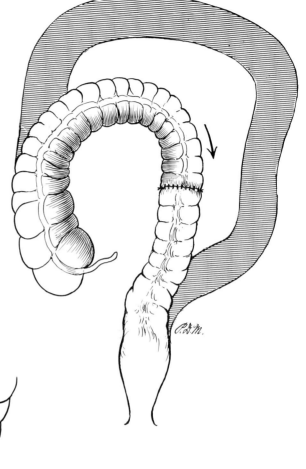

14. COLOCOLOSTOMY

Anastomosis is performed in the usual fashion after resection of the splenic flexure. It is sometimes awkward to close the rent in the mesocolon after this dissection, and care must be taken when approximating the mesocolon in the region of the ligament of Treitz.

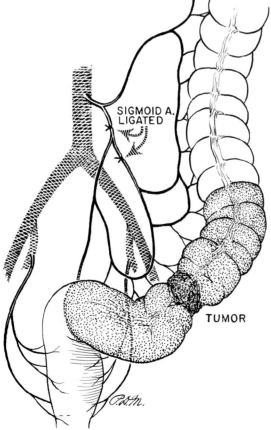

SIGMOID A. LIGATED

TUMOR

15. SIGMOID NEOPLASMS

Carcinoma of the sigmoid colon is managed by ligating the sigmoidal artery either after it has arisen from the inferior mesenteric artery or immediately after the superior rectal branch has been given off by the sigmoidal artery. High ligation of the inferior mesenteric artery does not enhance survival in dealing with carcinoma of the left colon.

16. SIGMOID COLON MOBILIZATION

▼

The sigmoid colon is mobilized, with care taken not to injure the ureters. The peritoneal surfaces of the mesocolon on either side of the sigmoid are incised, and the blood vessels lying within the mesocolon are doubly clamped, divided, and ligated. The anastomosis is performed as has been described.

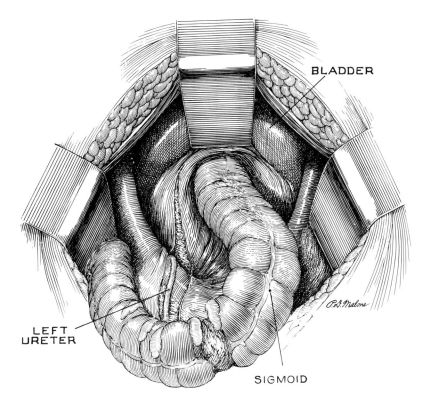

BLADDER

LEFT
URETER

SIGMOID

23 Mucosal Proctectomy, Ileal J-Reservoir, and Ileoanal Anastomosis

MALCOLM C. VEIDENHEIMER, M.D.

▼ IMPORTANT FEATURES
Total Abdominal Colectomy
Formation of Ileal Reservoir
Mucosal Proctectomy
Anastomosis of Reservoir to Anus

▼ STEPS OR PLANS
Total Abdominal Colectomy with Preservation of Ileal Branches and
    Ileocolic Artery
Scoring Retroperitoneum and Mobilization of Root of Mesentery
Elongation of Ileal Mesentery with Ligation of Vascular Arcades
Construction of Ileal J-Reservoir
Exposure of Perineum
Dissection of Rectal Mucous Membrane Free from Submucosa and
    Muscularis
Excision of Rectum and Mucosal Tube
Anastomosis of J-Reservoir to Dentate Line
Loop Ileostomy

1. DIVISION OF ILEUM AND MOBILIZATION OF RECTUM

▼

The patient is placed in stirrups in a position similar to that used for abdominoperineal resection. The operation starts by performing total abdominal colectomy. Care is taken to preserve the ileal branches of the ileocolic artery. The ileum is divided with a GIA stapler. The dissection is carried distally through the pelvic floor to mobilize the rectum down to the level of the levator muscles. This dissection is carried out close to the rectal wall to preserve the nerves that have a role in sexual function.

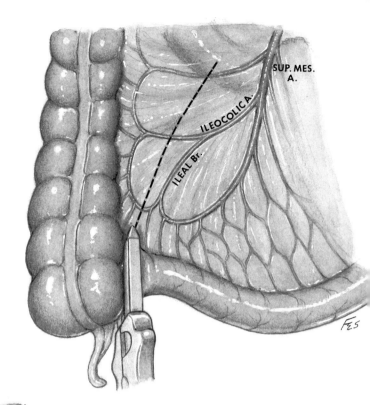

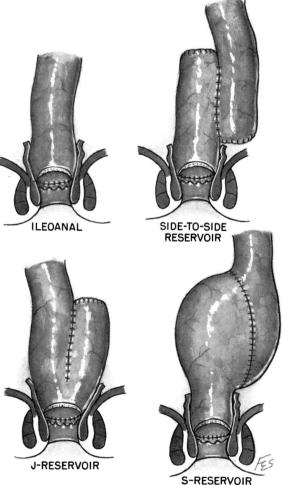

ILEOANAL

SIDE-TO-SIDE RESERVOIR

J-RESERVOIR

S-RESERVOIR

2. RESERVOIRS

▼

Several types of anal reconstruction have been used. The use of an ileoanal anastomosis without any reservoir has not proved to be satisfactory in adults. Keeping some reservoir capacity appears to be important to the success of the operation. The types of reservoirs shown have been used. The reservoir most commonly used by us is the J-shaped one.

3. LENGTHEN SMALL BOWEL MESENTERY

▼

At the conclusion of rectal mobilization, the mesentery of the small bowel is lengthened to permit approximation of the terminal ileum to the anal canal. Division of the anterior leaf of the mesenteric peritoneum has taken place.

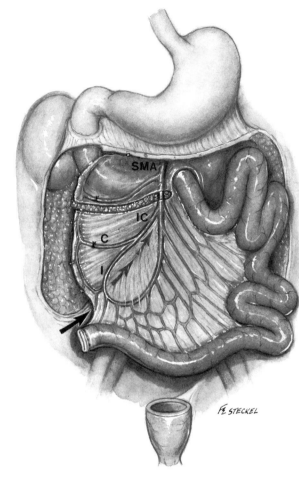

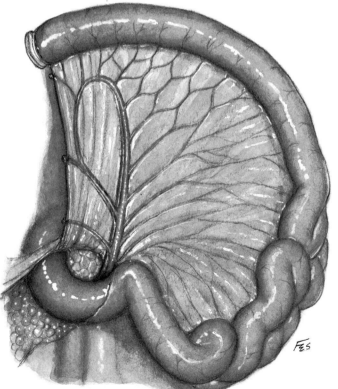

4. LENGTHEN SMALL BOWEL MESENTERY *(Continued)*

▼

The small bowel mesentery is mobilized posteriorly along the root of the mesentery up to the duodenum.

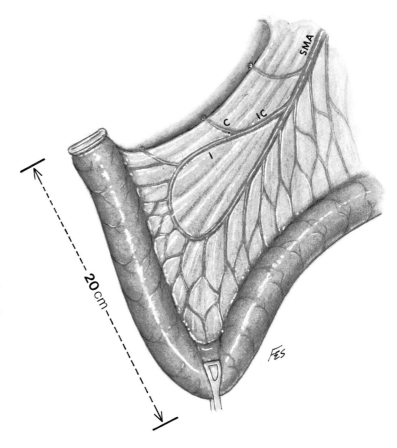

5. FORMATION OF J-LOOP

The distal ileum is grasped with Babcock clamps to form a J-shaped loop. Each limb of the loop measures 20 cm.

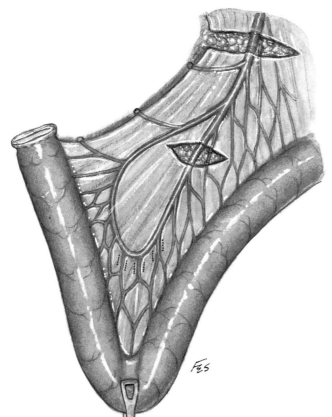

6. FORMATION OF J-LOOP
(Continued)

The peritoneum of the anterior and posterior leaves of the mesentery is scored in several places to lengthen the mesentery. The arcades of the mesenteric vessels leading to the apex of the J-shaped limb are delineated and divided. This usually results in sufficient lengthening of the mesentery to permit the apex of the J-loop to reach the dentate line of the anal canal.

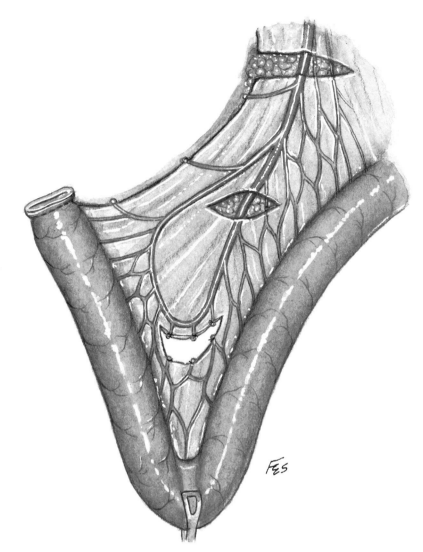

7. FORMATION OF J-LOOP
(Continued)

▼

When division of the arcades along the ileal artery does not permit sufficient lengthening of the mesentery, the ileal branch of the ileocolic or the major branch of the superior mesenteric artery may be divided to produce sufficient lengthening. When the apex of the J-loop can be stretched to reach four fingerbreadths below the symphysis pubis, the length is sufficient to achieve anastomosis to the dentate line.

A   B   C

8. CREATION OF J-RESERVOIR

▼

A to C, The ileum is now turned on itself. The walls of the bowel are approximated with stay sutures. The common wall between the two limbs of the J-reservoir is divided by means of GIA staplers. The common wall is divided by two separate applications of the 90-mm GIA stapler placed through the apex of the J-loop. The apical enterotomy is later sutured to the dentate line as the ileoanal anastomotic site. The J-reservoir is shown as it is placed within the muscular sleeve and sutured to the dentate line.

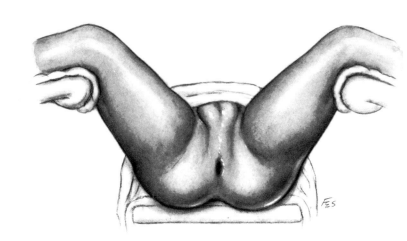

9. PERINEAL DISSECTION

After the rectum has been mobilized and as the abdominal surgeon begins to construct the J-reservoir, a second team of operators begins the perineal dissection.

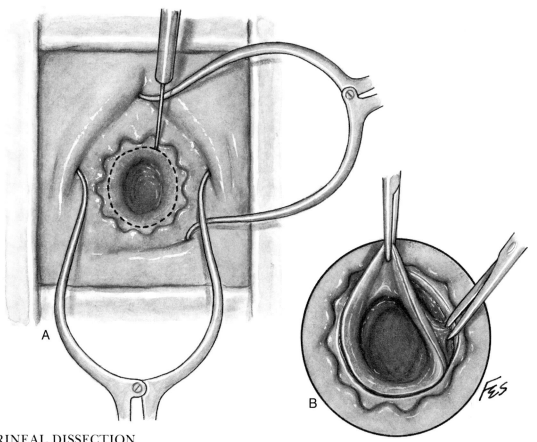

10. PERINEAL DISSECTION
(Continued)

A and *B*, The rectum is cleaned with a solution of povidone-iodine (Betadine), and Gelpi retractors are placed in an anteroposterior and lateral plane to display the dentate line. A long spinal needle is used to inject saline solution with epinephrine (1:200,000) into the submucosa from the dentate line to the level of the levator muscles. The mucosa is dissected free from the internal sphincter muscle by sharp dissection with scissors aided by blunt dissection with peanut pledgets.

11. MUCOSAL DISSECTION

▼

A and B, The dissection is carried proximally to the level of the levator muscles. This area of submucosa is often characterized by a small collection of fatty tissue. A silk ligature is placed around the mucosal tube at that level.

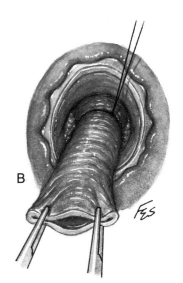

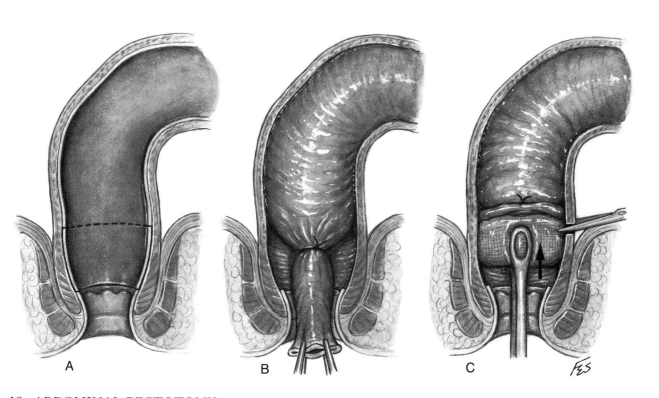

12. ABDOMINAL RECTOTOMY

▼

A to C, The mucosa is dissected out of the rectal muscular sleeve, and the perineal operator passes a sponge on a stick through the anus to elevate the mucosal sleeve and to form a firm palpable object on which the abdominal operator may then cut. Thus, the rectum is entered distal to the mucosal dissection.

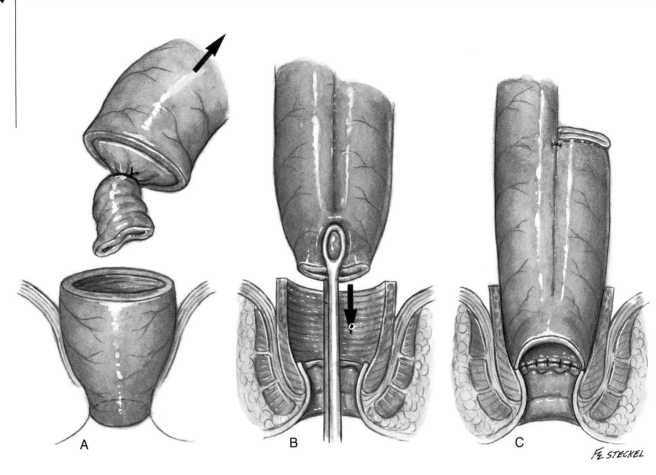

A   B   C   *F*. STECKEL

13. PLACEMENT OF RESERVOIR IN RECTAL SLEEVE

A to *C*, The abdominal operator has now mobilized the rectum by dividing it distal to the upper limits of the mucosal dissection, and the specimen is removed. A sponge-holding forceps is passed by the perineal operator through the anus and up the muscular anorectal sleeve. The J-reservoir is grasped by the sponge-holding forceps, drawn into the anal canal, and fixed in place by interrupted sutures of chromic catgut.

DRAINAGE AND ILEOSTOMY

The lumen of the reservoir is drained with a soft Penrose drain left in place for four or five days. The pelvis is drained by bilateral suprapubic suction drains that are passed out through separate stab wounds on the left lower anterior abdominal wall. These drains are left in place until the drainage has ceased, usually in four to six days. A loop ileostomy is performed proximal to the reservoir. The patient does not use the J-reservoir and ileoanal anastomosis for eight weeks, at which time digital, endoscopic, and barium examinations of the reservoir are carried out. When all the suture lines are intact, the patient is readmitted to the hospital for closure of the loop ileostomy.

S-Reservoir Segment

JOHN A. COLLER, M.D.

The colectomy and mucosal proctectomy dissections are similar whether a J-reservoir or S-reservoir is anticipated. An S-reservoir may be employed in an effort to gain an additional 1 or 2 cm of length in the case of a foreshortened mesentery. To maximize the potential benefit of the S-reservoir, the ileum is divided close to the ileocecal junction. However, to minimize obstructive complications, as little terminal ileum as possible (2 to 4 cm) is used as the efferent limb from the reservoir.

14. PREPARATION OF ILEUM

▼

The apex of the reservoir is selected by placing traction on the distal ileum and locating the point that reaches farthest in the direction of the symphysis pubis. This point will usually be along the line of direct extension of the superior mesenteric artery, approximately 25 cm from the cut margin of the terminal ileum. It is likely that several centimeters of ileum will appear to reach an equally maximal distance. In such cases, the most proximal point should be selected as the apex. The apex will therefore be approximately 25 to 30 cm proximal to the cut margin of the ileum and will provide 12- to 15-cm lengths in each of the three limbs of the S-reservoir. Additional apical length is obtained by scoring the mesenteric peritoneal investment and dividing one or more arcades as described for the J-reservoir. Whereas division of the ileocolic vessels may be optional with the J-reservoir, it is required for the construction of an S-reservoir. This permits the terminal ileum to be reflected caudad to form the first

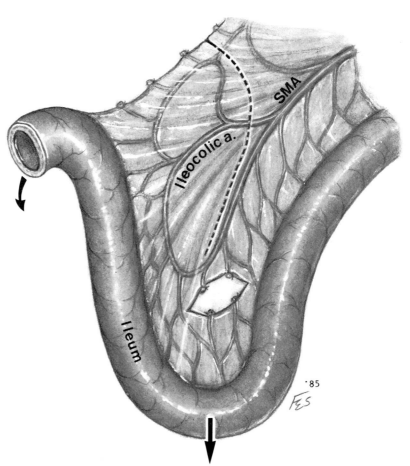

limb of the reservoir and the efferent limb. The division should be made proximal to any arcades that communicate with the cut margin unless the cut margin is tethered by the arcade.

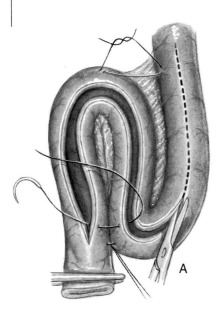

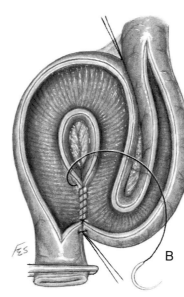

15. CONSTRUCTION OF RESERVOIR

▼

A, The three reservoir limbs are aligned with stay sutures. The stay suture between the apex and first limb should be placed no more than 3.5 to 4 cm proximal to the ileal cut margin, which will be used for the ileoanal anastomosis. A longer efferent segment would contribute to the development of reservoir outlet obstruction. A continuous enterotomy along the antimesenteric border of each of the three limbs is made from the stay suture at the efferent limb to the stay suture at the afferent limb. *B*, The adjacent cut edges of the first and second limbs are approximated with a continuous submucosal suture of 2-0 Vicryl.

16. CONSTRUCTION OF RESERVOIR *(Continued)*

▼

A, Similarly, the adjacent edges of the second and third limbs are approximated. *B*, The resulting large confluent mucosal surface is closed by a continuous submucosal suture, which starts at the level of the apical stay suture.

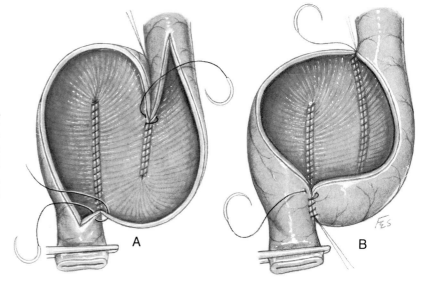

17. COMPLETION OF RESERVOIR

▼

A, As this continuous submucosal suture is placed, the remaining cut edges of the first and third limbs are brought into approximation, and the reservoir closure is completed. The completed reservoir is positioned with the efferent limb situated ventrally as it is directed into the pelvis. *B*, In this fashion, the mesentery will bridge the pelvis from the sacral promontory with the reservoir situated primarily to the left and posterior of the mesentery. Orientation is maintained by the perineal operator during placement by guiding the efferent limb with a sponge forceps. An end-to-end anastomosis is performed between the cut margin of the efferent limb and the pectinate line, incorporating a small depth of internal sphincter. Approximately 12 to 16 interrupted sutures of 3-0 Vicryl are usually required. When an excess length of efferent limb is present, it should be amputated so as to minimize the development of efferent limb obstruction. Suction drainage is provided in the same manner as for the J-reservoir.

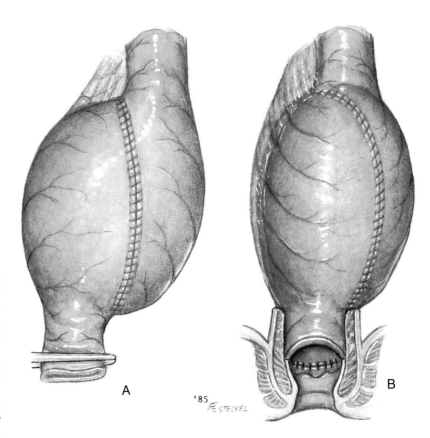

24 Rectal Prolapse

DAVID J. SCHOETZ, Jr., M.D.

▼ IMPORTANT FEATURES
Document Full-Thickness Prolapse by Direct Examination
Exclude Proximal Neoplasm by Endoscopy and Radiography
Assess Overall Operative Risk to Decide Whether Transabdominal
  Procedure or Circumanal Procedure Is More Appropriate
Complete Mechanical and Antibiotic Preparation Required for All
  Teflon Sling Repairs

▼ STEPS OR PLANS
Transabdominal Teflon Sling Repair
  Normal and Pathologic Anatomy
  Mobilization of Rectum
  Placement of Teflon Mesh Sling
Circumanal Silastic Sling Repair
  Exposure In Prone Jackknife Position
  Incisions Over Both Ischiorectal Fossae
  Dissect Anterior and Posterior Tunnels
  Insert Silastic Sheet to Form Sling
  Staple Ends of Sling and Close Incision

Transabdominal Teflon Sling Repair

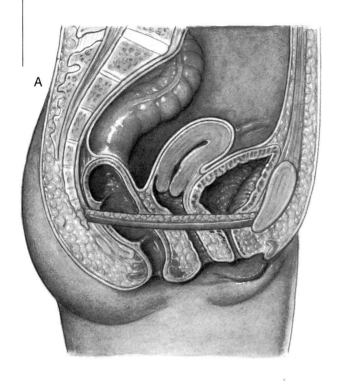

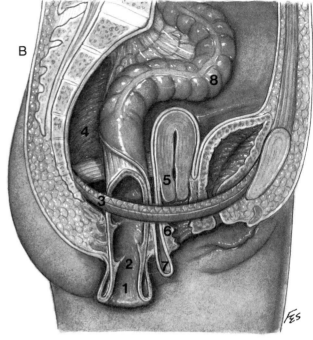

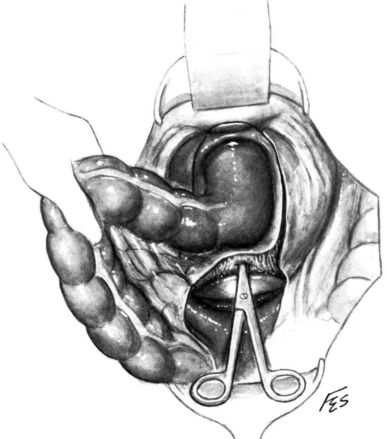

1. ANATOMY

▼

A, Normal anatomy of the pelvis. *B,* Pathologic anatomy of rectal prolapse. 1, Prolapsed rectum. 2, Lax external sphincter. 3, Attenuation of the levator muscle. 4, Increased retrorectal space with a long mesorectum. 5, Associated uterine prolapse. 6, Weakness of the endopelvic fascia and associated rectocele. 7, Abnormally deep cul-de-sac of Douglas. 8, Redundant sigmoid colon.

2. INITIAL DISSECTION

▼

After standard mechanical and antibiotic bowel preparation, the abdomen is entered through a lower abdominal midline incision. Exploratory laparotomy is completed. The patient is placed in the deep Trendelenburg position, the small bowel
Continued

Figure 2 *Continued*

is packed superiorly, and upward traction is placed on the redundant rectosigmoid. An incision is made in the peritoneum on both sides of the rectum beginning at the level of the sacral promontory. Care is taken to keep the incision close to the rectum to avoid injury to the ureters and the autonomic nerve supply within the pelvis.

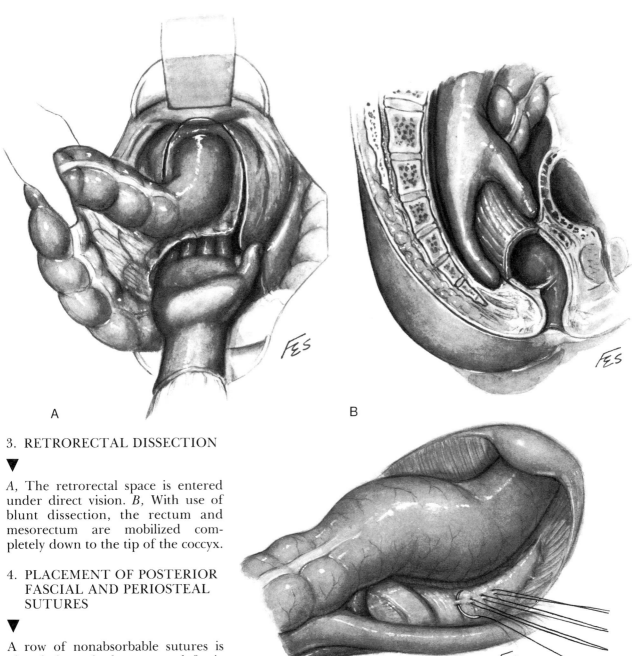

A

B

3. RETRORECTAL DISSECTION

▼

A, The retrorectal space is entered under direct vision. *B,* With use of blunt dissection, the rectum and mesorectum are mobilized completely down to the tip of the coccyx.

4. PLACEMENT OF POSTERIOR FASCIAL AND PERIOSTEAL SUTURES

▼

A row of nonabsorbable sutures is placed through the presacral fascia and the periosteum of the sacrum to the right of the midline. Care must be taken at this point not to enter any visible presacral veins. The uppermost suture is placed approximately 2 cm below the sacral promontory, and the sutures are spaced 1 cm apart. If a presacral vein is entered, the suture should be removed and pressure applied. When this is not sufficient to control the bleeding, suture ligatures of absorbable material should be placed.

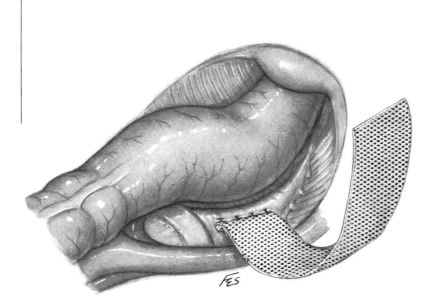

5. ATTACHMENT OF TEFLON SLING

▼

A sling of presterilized Teflon mesh 4–cm wide is fashioned. It is much easier to place the sutures in the mesh before tying them. This maneuver permits accurate placement of the sutures in the mesh.

6. ATTACHMENT OF SLING TO RECTUM

▼

Upward traction is placed on the rectum to maintain it as taut as possible, and nonabsorbable sutures are placed from the mesh to the seromuscular layer of the rectum at the level of the peritoneal reflection. Care should be taken not to gather the sling because this reduces the surface area of contact between the rectum and the sling itself.

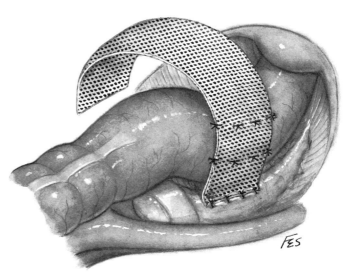

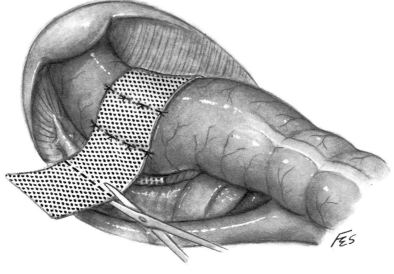

7. SLING TAILORED

▼

The sling is wrapped around the rectum and secured. The mesh is cut to the appropriate length. To prevent subsequent stenosis, the surgeon must be able to insert two fingers alongside the rectum inside the sling.

8. ATTACHMENT OF SLING TO LEFT PERIOSTEUM

▼

Heavy nonabsorbable sutures are placed through the sling and secured to the sacral periosteum to the left of the midline. All sutures should be placed before tying to ensure adequate visualization of any bleeding point secondary to the placement of the sutures.

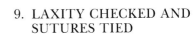

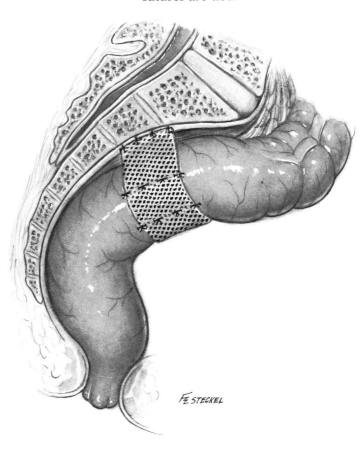

9. LAXITY CHECKED AND SUTURES TIED

▼

Before the sutures are tied, the sling should be brought into position. Two fingers are placed posterior to the rectum inside the sling. When adequate laxity has been ensured, the sutures are tied.

10. LATERAL VIEW

▼

In this lateral view, the rectum is shown secured to the sacrum, thus restoring posterior fixation.

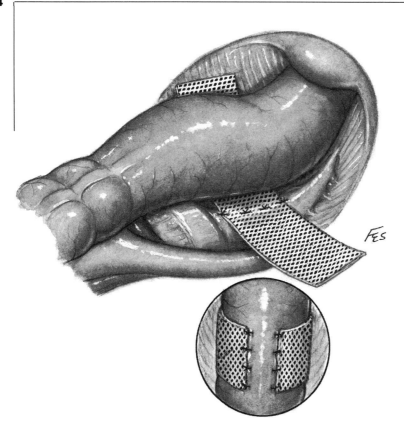

11. ALTERNATIVE PROCEDURE

▼

This alternative operative technique shows the sling fixed in the midline posteriorly by heavy nonabsorbable sutures, partially wrapped on either side, and secured in position on the anterior seromuscular layer of the rectum. The potential advantages of this alternative technique include fewer sutures placed in the presacral fascia and sacral promontory with a resultant decreased chance of bleeding and the absence of a circumferential wrap, thereby lessening the incidence of impaction above the sling.

Circumanal Silastic Sling Repair

12. PREPARATION

▼

Although it is possible to perform this operation under local anesthesia, general or spinal or epidural anesthesia is preferred. As with the abdominal procedure, the patient is prepared with a standard mechanical bowel preparation as well as oral and parenteral antibiotic agents. The patient is placed in the prone jackknife position to afford exposure of and access to the coccyx, the external sphincter musculature, the vagina, and both ischiorectal fossae.

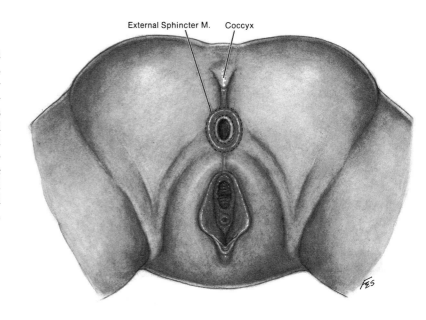

External Sphincter M.   Coccyx

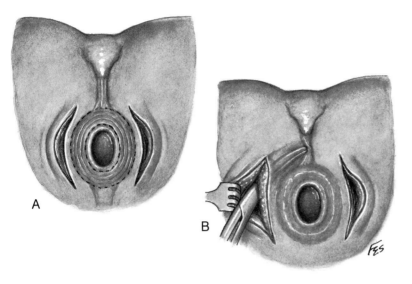

13. INITIAL PERINEAL DISSECTION

▼

A, Incisions of approximately 4 cm are made over each ischiorectal fossa, and the incisions are deepened by blunt and sharp dissection under direct vision. The entire sphincter mechanism is encompassed. *B,* The posterior aspect of the tunnel is made using blunt dissection.

14. ANTERIOR AND POSTERIOR TUNNELS

A and *B,* The anococcygeal raphe must be disrupted to complete the tunnel posteriorly. The anterior tunnels are completed in similar fashion. Insertion of the index finger in the vagina aids in ensuring that the tunnel is made in the appropriate plane within the rectovaginal septum. It is important not to penetrate either the anal mucosa or the vaginal mucosa during this dissection.

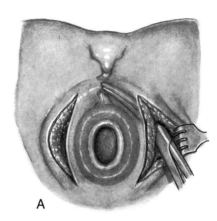

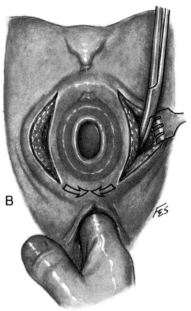

15. PREPARATION OF SILASTIC SLING

▼

A, The tunnels are marked with ¼–inch Penrose drains. The material used for the sling is a Dacron-impregnated Silastic sheet with elasticity along its longitudinal axis. After the tunnels have been completed, a 2-cm strip of the sheet is cut for use as the sling. The elasticity must be in the longitudinal axis of the sling to permit expansion during defecation. *B,* After the sling has been cut, a Kelly clamp is passed through the posterior tunnel using the Penrose drain as a guide.

16. PLACEMENT OF SILASTIC SLING

▼

A, The Silastic sheet is grasped and pulled through the tunnel, taking care to avoid twists. *B*, The Kelly clamp is passed through the anterior tunnel in a similar fashion, and once again the Silastic sheet is grasped and pulled through the tunnel. As a result, the sling will encompass the entire sphincter mechanism.

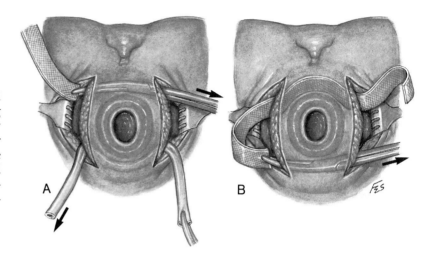

17. SLING SECURED AND CLOSURE

▼

The sling is checked once again to be sure that it is flat within the tunnels. *A*, The two ends of the Silastic sheet are overlapped and held so that the sphincter is snug around the index finger of the operator. *B*, A TA-30 stapling device is placed across the overlapped sling and fired. *C*, The wounds are irrigated, and a layered closure is performed with absorbable interrupted sutures of a synthetic material. Closure of the subcutaneous tissue as well as the subcutaneous portion of the external sphincter provides adequate protection against erosion of the sling through the skin.

25 Operations for Fecal Incontinence

DAVID J. SCHOETZ, JR., M.D.

▼ IMPORTANT FEATURES

Detailed History and Physical Examination to Discover Cause of
Incontinence

Utilization of Anal Manometry, Electromyography, and
Defecography to Refine Diagnosis

Direct Sphincter Repair for Patients with Functional Muscle Around
50 Per Cent or More of Circumference

Posterior Proctopexy for Patients with Pelvic Floor Abnormalities

Consider Circumanal Silastic Sling for Major Neurologic Cause of
Incontinence

Complete Mechanical Preparation and Antibiotics Preoperatively

Postoperative Confinement of Bowels Will Avoid Need for Colostomy

▼ STEPS OR PLANS

Direct Sphincter Repair
Excise Skin and Scar Over Sphincters
Reconstitute Sphincter
Mobilize Dermis Laterally for Closure
Posterior Proctopexy
Incision Posterior to Anal Canal
Intersphincteric Plane Dissection of Puborectalis
Plicate Puborectalis Sling and External Sphincter
Subcutaneous and Skin Closure

Direct Sphincter Repair

Disruption of the sphincter muscle is most often the result of operative trauma. Surgical procedures designed to treat fistula in ano are the most common causes, although many other anal operative procedures may result in division of substantial portions of the sphincter muscle and subsequent incontinence. Direct trauma to the sphincters by blunt or penetrating injuries is less frequently seen. Direct sphincter repair is considered the operative procedure of choice regardless of the delay in performance of the operation as long as a palpable contractile external sphincter is present around at least 50 per cent of the circumference of the anus.

When a colostomy has not been performed before the operative procedure, a full mechanical and antibiotic bowel preparation should be administered. We do not divert the fecal stream routinely; rather, confinement of the bowels in the immediate postoperative period, with pharmacologic agents and liquids and a low-residue diet, is sufficient to result in early postoperative healing without appreciable fecal contamination.

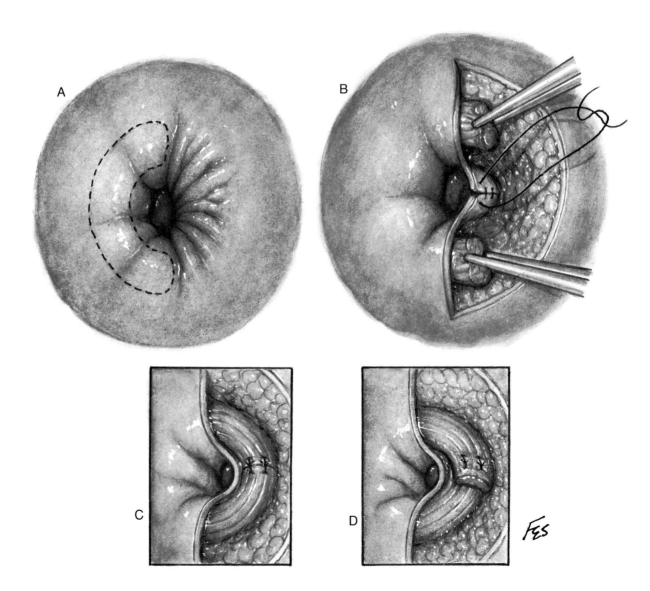

1. TECHNIQUE (*Opposite page*)

A, With the patient in the prone jackknife position and after adequate preparation and draping, inspection of the perianal region reveals the palpable muscle mass *(broken line)* and on the opposite side an accentuation of the laxity of the perianal skin owing to the lack of underlying muscular support. In addition, relative gaping of the anus is present. *B,* The skin and subcutaneous tissue with attached scar are removed over the entire sphincter defect. The anoderm is mobilized for adequate exposure of the musculature. Careful dissection of the divided sphincter musculature is undertaken, care being exercised to identify the muscle ends and to leave some scar tissue attached to the muscle to hold the sutures. After the transected ends of the muscle have been identified and freed from the surrounding tissues, the anoderm is reapproximated with continuous sutures of chromic catgut. *C,* At this point, the muscle is approximated. Although some surgeons directly appose the muscle ends, we believe the ends should be overlapped *(D)* and transfixion sutures of a nonabsorbable monofilament material placed to achieve an overlap of approximately 2 cm. At the termination of the muscle repair, wounds are irrigated with a dilute povidone-iodine (Betadine) solution, and the dermis is mobilized laterally over the buttock and advanced medially to achieve primary closure of the skin. When the defect is too large to permit closure of the skin without tension, the wound should be packed open and permitted to granulate.

Posterior Proctopexy for Idiopathic Fecal Incontinence

2. INCISION

With the patient in the lithotomy position, after standard preparation and draping, a semicircular incision is made posterior to the anal canal.

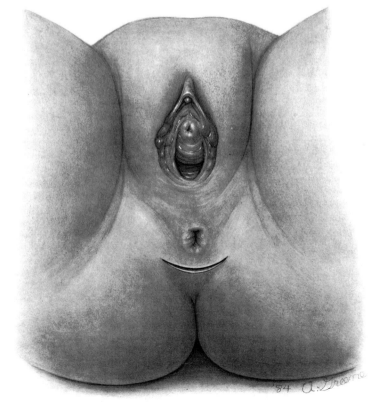

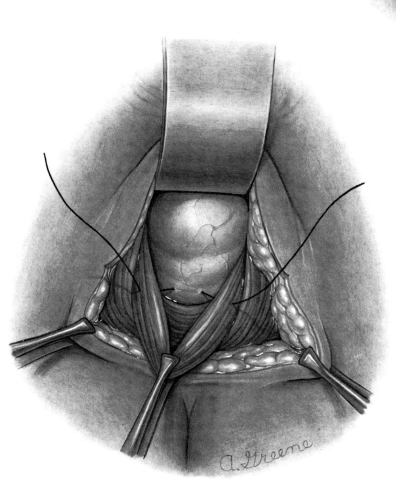

3. PUBORECTALIS MUSCLE EXPOSED

▼

After dissection through the subcutaneous tissue, the lower borders of the internal and external sphincters are exposed, and the intersphincteric plane is identified. Even though this embryonic plane is entered sharply, dissection of the internal sphincter off the external sphincter is a bloodless procedure that proceeds superiorly, lifting the rectum off the external sphincter. The puborectalis muscle is thus exposed.

4. PUBORECTALIS MUSCLE SUTURED

▼

With anterior traction on the rectum, the puborectalis sling is demonstrably lax. The absorbable apical suture of heavy synthetic material is placed incorporating the puborectalis muscle on either side and Waldeyer's fascia in the midline.

5. EXTERNAL SPHINCTER PLICATED

▼

The entire puborectalis sling is reefed with interrupted sutures of a similar material. The remainder of the external sphincter is plicated in a similar fashion to buttress the rest of the external sphincter below the puborectalis closure.

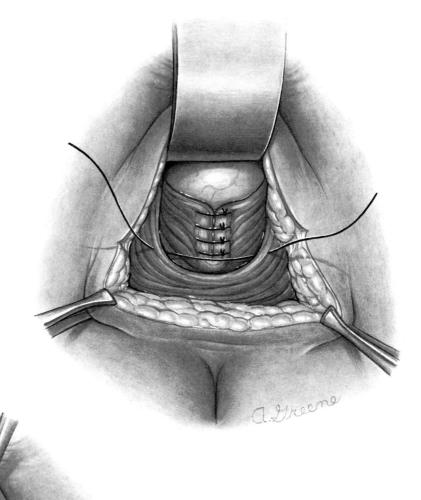

6. CONFIRMATION OF ANTERIOR DISPLACEMENT OF ANORECTAL ANGLE

▼

After both layers of the postanal repair have been completed, a digital rectal examination confirms anterior displacement of the anorectal angle. The wound is irrigated with a dilute povidone-iodine (Betadine) solution, and the subcutaneous tissue is approximated with absorbable interrupted sutures of synthetic material.

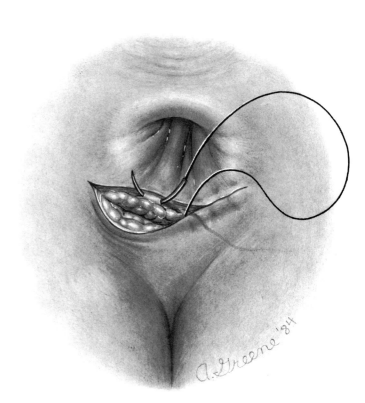

7. CLOSURE

The skin is closed with an absorbable running subcuticular suture of synthetic material. A digital rectal examination confirms anterior displacement of the anal canal and restoration of the rectoanal angle.

Operations for Abscess and Fistula

DAVID J. SCHOETZ, JR., M.D.

▼ IMPORTANT FEATURES
Thorough Knowledge of Anatomy, Particularly Puborectalis Muscle
and Perirectal Spaces
Accurate Identification of Site and Extent of Abscess
Examination Under Anesthesia for Suspected, Deep-Seated, or
Extensive Abscess
Precise Anatomic Definition of Fistulous Tract
Simple Fistulotomy for Low-Lying Fistulas
Avoid Operative Extensions of Tracts That May Complicate
Management
Reserve Fistulotomy at Initial Drainage Procedure for Low-Lying,
Easily Identifiable Fistulas
Adequate Drainage
Use of Seton as Marker for Possible Supralevator Fistulas

▼ STEPS OR PLANS
Anorectal Abscess
    Sites of Abscesses
    Simple Drainage
    Intermuscular Abscess Drained into Anal Canal
    Supralevator Abscess Drained Transrectally
Anorectal Fistula
    Pertinent Anatomy
    Goodsall's Rule
    Intersphincteric—Divide Intervening Tissue
    Transsphincteric—Simple Division
    Demonstrate Fistula with Probe or Methylene Blue Injection
    Unroof Fistula
    Combined Internal Closure with External Drainage
    Use Seton with Supralevator Extension
    Horseshoe Abscess and Fistula

Anorectal Abscess

1. VARIETIES OF ABSCESS

▼

A, Perianal abscess, the most common site of perianal suppuration. *B,* Ischiorectal abscess. *C,* Intermuscular abscess presenting with anal pain and no external sign of infection. *D,* Supralevator abscess presenting with complaints of pelvic pain and fever and no external sign of infection.

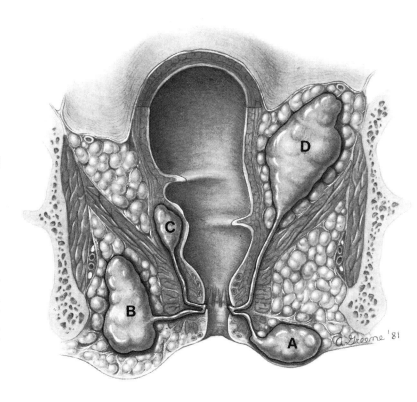

2. POSITION AND INCISION

▼

The appropriate position of the patient for drainage of the abscess is dictated by the surgeon's and the patient's comfort. The lithotomy position is best when draining the abscess under general or spinal anesthesia. When the abscess is drained under local anesthesia in the office, the prone jackknife position is more comfortable for the patient. Incision and drainage are performed over the area of fluctuance. However, the incision should be made as close to the the anal verge as possible because in approximately 50 per cent of patients a subsequent fistula in ano will develop. Making the incision close to the anal verge results in a shorter fistulous tract for subsequent definitive fistulotomy. The incision must be made parallel to the sphincter mechanism to minimize damage to the sphincteric muscle. Aerobic and anaerobic bacterial cultures should be obtained routinely.

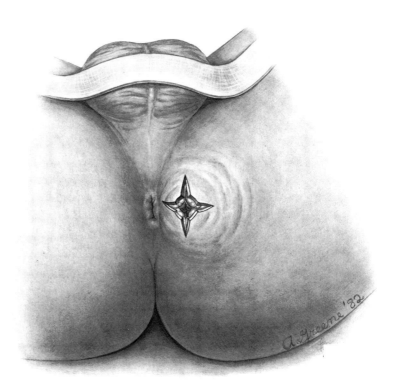

3. ENLARGED INCISION

A cruciate incision is made after digital exploration of the abscess cavity. The skin edges are trimmed to provide a satisfactory opening without the necessity for packs or drains. The only reason for packing the wound is to provide hemostasis.

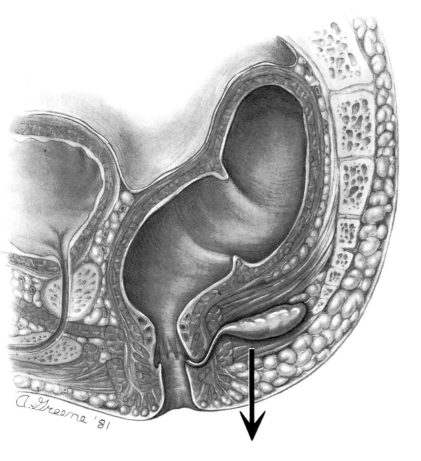

4. POSTANAL ABSCESS

The postanal space is in the midline posteriorly and is separated into superficial and deep compartments. The superficial postanal space is the location of the midline posterior perianal abscess and is entirely below the superficial external sphincter. The deep postanal space is between the superficial external sphincter and the levator muscle. An unrecognized and undrained abscess deep in the postanal space is the most common cause of persistent or recurrent horseshoe abscess and fistula. The appropriate avenue of drainage of the abscess deep in the postanal space is by way of an extrarectal incision between the anus and coccyx (arrow).

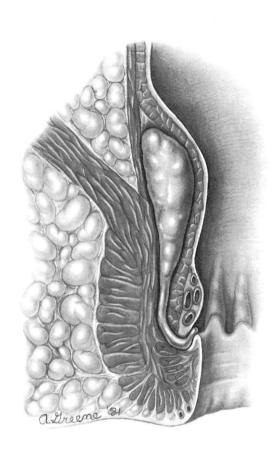

5. INTERMUSCULAR ABSCESS

The abscess lies between the internal and external sphincters and represents superior extension of the suppurative process in the intermuscular plane. Patients complain of pain and may have a fever, but on examination they have no external sign of infection. Diagnosis requires a high index of suspicion.

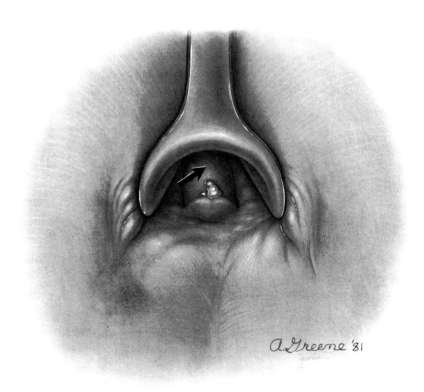

6. INTERMUSCULAR ABSCESS
(Continued)

An examination with the patient under anesthesia or with use of a complete circumferential perianal block and pudendal nerve blocks is necessary to establish the diagnosis. After a Hill-Ferguson retractor has been inserted, inspection reveals an indurated swelling extending superiorly from the dentate line with purulence exuding from the crypt of origin.

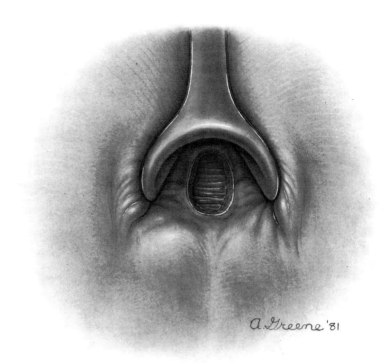

7. DRAINAGE OF INTERMUSCULAR ABSCESS

▼

Appropriate drainage of the intermuscular abscess requires excision of the mucosa, submucosa, and internal sphincter to afford complete drainage into the anal canal and rectum.

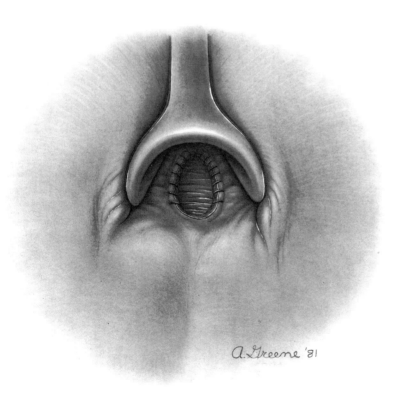

8. SUTURE FOR HEMOSTASIS

▼

Marsupialization by means of a continuous suture of chromic catgut may be added to achieve hemostasis. In most instances however hemostasis will be adequate without the addition of a foreign body that may result in prolonged local inflammatory changes.

9. TRANSRECTAL ASPIRATION OF SUPRALEVATOR ABSCESS

A high index of suspicion is required to establish a diagnosis of supralevator abscess. Patients complain of pelvic pain and fever, but inspection of the perianal region and digital examination of the rectum will not reveal anal abnormality. Tenderness may be present as the abscess cavity is palpated above the level of the anorectal ring. Examination under anesthesia is required and reveals a fluctuant mass above the levator muscle, depicted here in the anterior position. Appropriate therapy requires documentation of the abscess by transrectal aspiration to confirm the presence of a purulent collection.

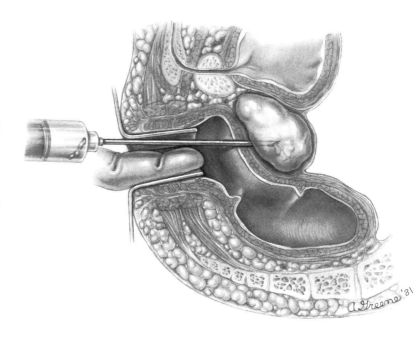

10. CATHETER PLACEMENT IN ABSCESS CAVITY

Appropriate therapy is incision over the area of fluctuance and insertion of a drainage catheter directly into the abscess cavity. A large Foley catheter or a Silastic de Pezzer catheter is left in place for drainage and subsequent irrigation. The supralevator abscess may represent an intra-abdominal suppurative process, such as diverticulitis, perforated appendicitis, tubo-ovarian abscess, or Crohn's disease. The drainage catheter can be used for subsequent contrast studies to delineate intra-abdominal abnormality.

Anorectal Fistula

11. ANAL ANATOMY

▼

Accurate identification of the pubo-rectalis muscle is the single most important step in the operative therapy of fistula in ano. Although division of the internal sphincter and the subcutaneous and superficial portions of the external sphincter will not result in total incontinence, minor degrees of soiling are common after simple fistulotomy.

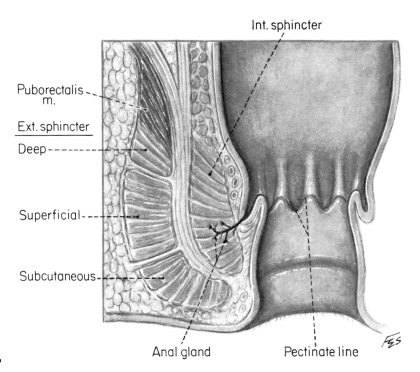

Int. sphincter

Puborectalis m.

Ext. sphincter

Deep

Superficial

Subcutaneous

Anal gland

Pectinate line

Post.

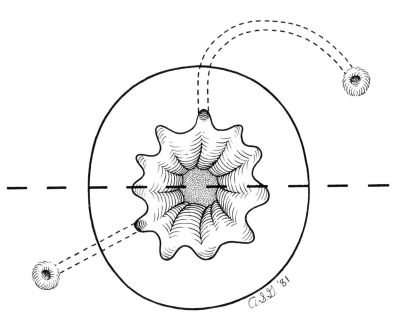

Ant.

12. GOODSALL'S RULE

▼

Goodsall pointed out that the site of the internal opening can be predicted by the position of the external opening of the fistula in ano. When the external orifice is posterior to a line bisecting the anus, the internal opening is most often at the midline posteriorly. On the other hand, external openings anterior to this line have a fistulous tract that pursues a direct radial course to its internal opening. Exceptions to this rule are known, particularly with external openings farther than 3 cm from the anal verge. Nevertheless, knowledge of Goodsall's rule is essential for defining the anatomy of fistulas.

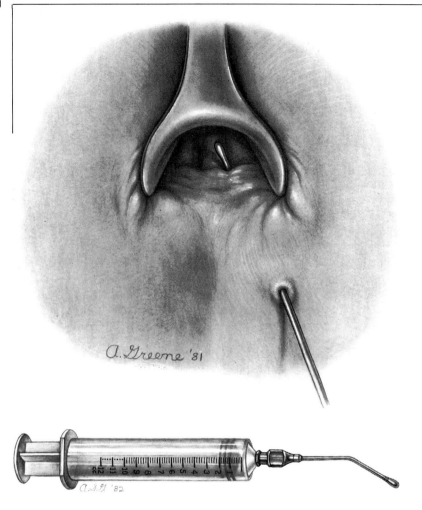

13. BASIC MANEUVERS

▼

All fistula surgery is performed under general or spinal anesthesia. The use of either the lithotomy position or the prone jackknife position is acceptable and is dictated by the preference of the operating surgeon. The external opening is gently explored with a flexible probe. Care must be taken not to create a false passage. In most instances of chronic fistula, the probe slides easily along the epithelialized tract and appears at the crypt of origin at the dentate line.

14. CONTRAST RECOGNITION OF FISTULA

▼

In some cases, the course of the fistula will be difficult to delineate by use of a probe. Insertion of a blunt-tipped needle into the external opening followed by gentle instillation of milk will often reveal the internal opening. When the internal opening is identified, the probe can be passed easily.

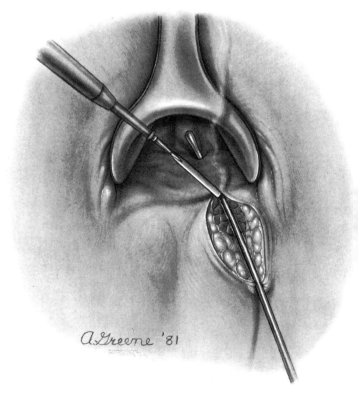

15. UNROOFING FISTULA

▼

The tract is opened after identifying the puborectalis muscle in relationship to the top of the probe. The electrocautery is used to provide hemostasis during the procedure.

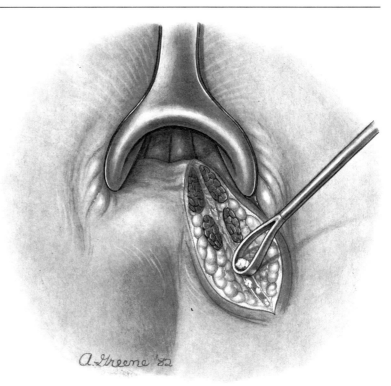

16. CURETTAGE AND CONTROL OF HEMORRHAGE

After the fistula has been unroofed completely, a curet is used to remove excess granulation tissue from the tract. Any accessory tracts are probed and opened. Control of bleeding is provided by the electrocautery. Iodoform gauze is gently laid into the wound and left in place for 24 hours. Packing the wound tightly merely adds to the patient's discomfort.

17. INTERSPHINCTERIC FISTULA

The acute presentation of simple intersphincteric fistula, which is the most common anal fistula seen, is that of a perianal or perirectal abscess. Surgical treatment of this fistula involves identification of the tract followed by division of the intervening tissue, including internal and subcutaneous external sphincters.

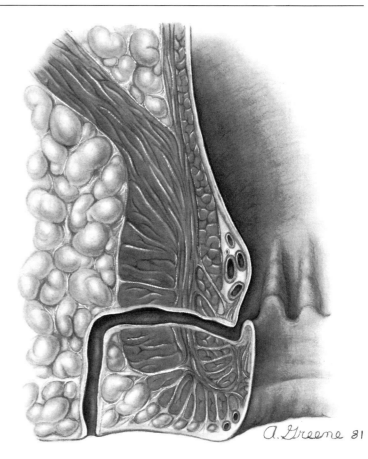

18. END RESULT OF DRAINAGE OF ISCHIORECTAL ABSCESS

This fistula is treated by simple division of the tissue between the internal and external openings.

19. INFRALEVATOR FISTULA

This anatomic arrangement is a frequent result of drainage of a large ischiorectal abscess. More important, the infralevator nature of the blind extension must be recognized and maintained. Vigorous probing and curettage may result in a supralevator abscess or even perforation of the rectum. Proper treatment includes simple fistulotomy of the transsphincteric component of the fistula and debridement with packing of the superior extension.

20. SUPRALEVATOR TRANSSPHINCTERIC FISTULA

▼

Rarely seen, this fistula presents a challenge to recognition. Often it is the result of excessive probing of the previously described fistula. After the supralevator component has been identified, great care must be exercised not to extend the fistula into the rectum, thereby creating an extrasphincteric fistula. Appropriate operative treatment of the supralevator extension includes fistulotomy of the transsphincteric fistula, debridement of the ischiorectal fossa, and enlargement of the levator opening to permit placement of a mushroom type of catheter for long-term drainage and daily irrigation.

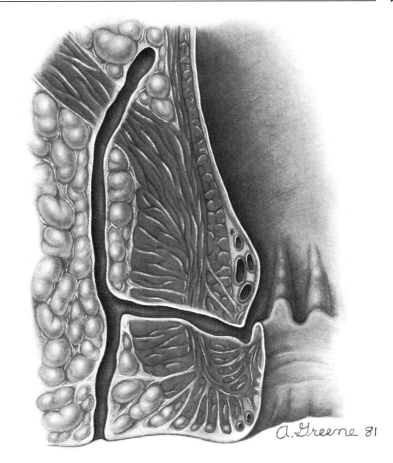

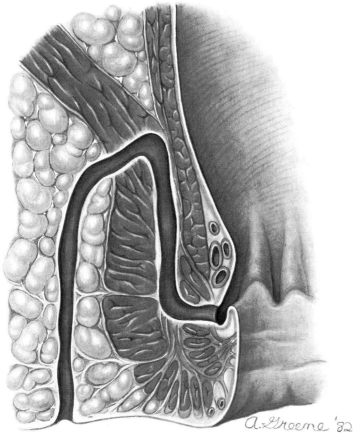

21. SUPRASPHINCTERIC FISTULA

▼

Failure to recognize a suprasphincteric fistula may result in division of the puborectalis muscle during the course of simple fistulotomy. When probing of internal and external openings reveals any suggestion of a supralevator fistula, a seton should be passed through the fistulous tract without division of muscle.

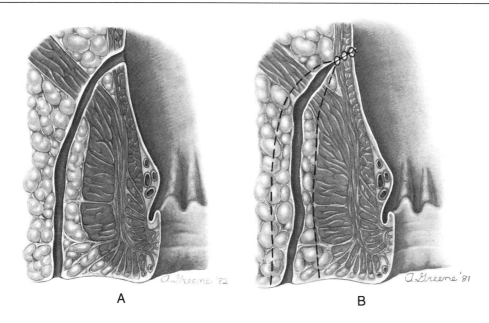

A

B

22. SUPRALEVATOR FISTULA

▼

A, When probing of the fistulous tract demonstrates an extrasphincteric course, the first consideration should be that the origin of the fistula is either an intrapelvic or an intraabdominal abscess. When no rectal opening is demonstrable, a mushroom type of catheter should be left in situ to provide adequate drainage, and appropriate contrast study is obtained after the patient recovers from anesthesia. B, When a rectal opening is identified, resection of the internal opening with careful layered closure permits drainage through the mushroom catheter similar to the blind supralevator extension.

23. USE OF SETON

▼

A, When probing of the fistulous tract indicates a possible supralevator extension, the most prudent course of action is to pass a No. 5 silk tie through the tract. Initially, the seton is tied loosely, and the patient is reexamined after recovery from anesthesia. With active contraction of the sphincter apparatus, the seton can be palpated to identify the relationship between the superior aspect of the tract and the puborectalis muscle. When the fistula is infralevator in position, the fistulotomy can be performed safely on an elective basis. B, On the other hand, when a supralevator fistula is present, the seton can be tied tightly under local anesthesia. Over time, the seton will cut through the puborectalis muscle by the process of extrusion. The remaining fistula can be divided when the superior aspect of the tract is below the puborectalis muscle. In this way, continence can be preserved.

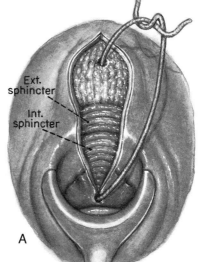

Ext. sphincter

Int. sphincter

A

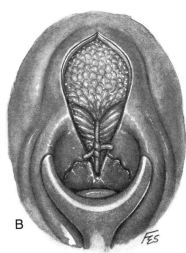

B

24. POSTANAL SPACE SUPPURATION

▼

Anterior extension of a suppurative process with its origin deep in the postanal space may occur unilaterally or bilaterally. The ischiorectal space is traversed with a horseshoe extension. In the acute stage, the presentation is that of an ischiorectal abscess. Unless the deep postanal space is drained, the subsequent clinical course will be that of recurrent abscesses and extension of the fistulous tracts. After repetitive drainage procedures, multiple external openings will result in a horseshoe configuration.

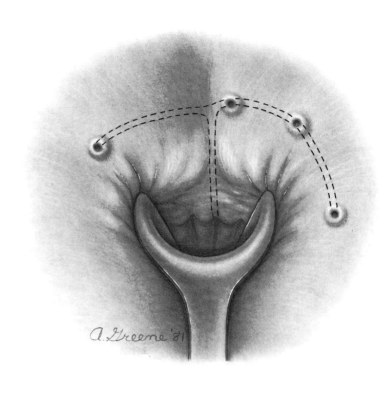

25. COMPLEX MULTIPLE POSTERIOR TRACTS

▼

Drainage of the postanal space is an essential part of therapy. After the internal opening has been identified, a generous posterior internal sphincterotomy is made into the deep postanal space, and the abscess cavity is curetted. Trimming the edges of the wound provides adequate drainage without packing. Bleeding from the anoderm is controlled with a continuous suture of catgut. External openings are then probed and curetted. Rather than performing complete fistulotomy with the resultant large perianal wound and considerable patient morbidity, soft latex rubber drains are inserted into each fistulous tract and secured to the skin. For horseshoe abscess, counterincisions are made over the concomitant ischiorectal abscess, and similar drains are placed. By disconnecting the extensions from the source, the tracts will close without creating extensive soft tissue wounds.

27 Operations for Anal Fissure

DAVID J. SCHOETZ, JR., M.D.

▼ IMPORTANT FEATURES
   Complete Anorectal Examination to Exclude Coincident Conditions
   Trial of Medical Therapy with Stool Softeners
   Local Wound Care Before Operative Approach

▼ STEPS OR PLANS
   Lateral Subcutaneous Internal Sphincterotomy
        Positioning
        Local Anesthesia
        Palpation of Intersphincteric Groove
        Knife Sphincterotomy
   Fissurectomy and Posterior Sphincterotomy
        Indication
        Excision

Lateral Subcutaneous Internal Sphincterotomy

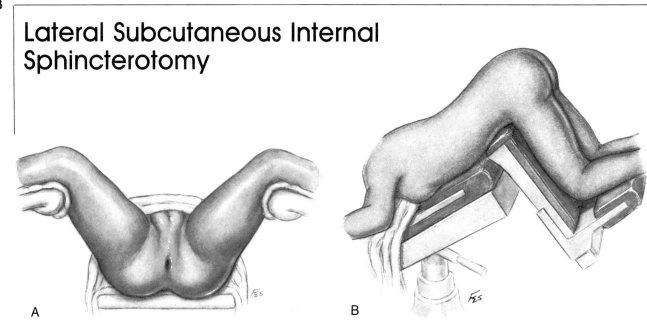

A

B

1. POSITION

Although this operative procedure can be performed with the patient in many positions, the lithotomy position (A) is preferred with either general or regional anesthesia. Relaxation of the external sphincter combined with the lithotomy position results in effacement of the musculature so that the intermuscular groove is easily palpable on the perianal skin, simplifying the procedure. B, The prone jackknife position is more convenient for performance of the procedure under local anesthesia as an office procedure. The standard examining table provides excellent support for the patient and maximizes comfort.

2. SUPERFICIAL INFILTRATION ANESTHESIA

A, After the perianal skin has been prepared with a suitable antiseptic agent, skin wheals are raised in four quadrants with a solution of 1 per cent lidocaine (Xylocaine) and 100,000:1 to 200,000:1 epinephrine through a 25-gauge needle. B, With a 21-gauge needle, the wheals are joined by circumferential injection of the same anesthetic agent.

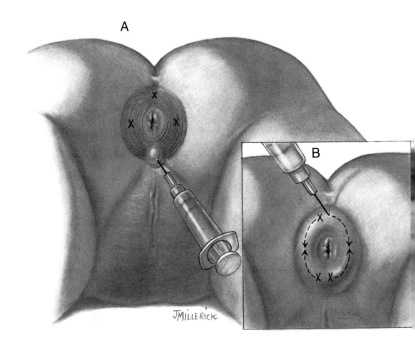

A

B

3. INTERNAL PUDENDAL NERVE BLOCK

▼

A bilateral internal pudendal nerve block is achieved by insertion of the needle into the ischiorectal fossa on either side with the operator's finger in the rectum as a guide. The internal pudendal nerve, which terminates at the anus as the inferior hemorrhoidal nerve, will be blocked by the injection of 7 to 10 ml of local anesthesia at the apex of the ischiorectal fossa. Satisfactory anesthesia is ensured by observing complete relaxation of the sphincter musculature.

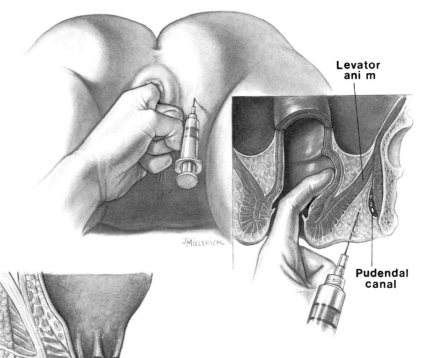

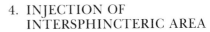

A   B

4. INJECTION OF INTERSPHINCTERIC AREA

▼

A, After the perianal skin and the anal canal have been prepared, the intersphincteric groove between the internal and external sphincters is palpated on the patient's right side. The right side is preferred because this avoids the potential for injury to the left lateral hemorrhoidal plexus. B, Routine injection of 5 to 10 ml of 25 per cent bupivacaine (Marcaine) with 100,000:1 to 200,000:1 epinephrine into the space decreases pain in the immediate postoperative period even when general anesthesia is used.

B

C

A

5. INTERNAL SPHINCTEROTOMY

▼

A and B, After the intersphincteric groove has been palpated, a No. 11 knife blade is passed into the intermuscular plane with the blade parallel to the sphincter. The index finger of the operator's left hand is placed into the anal canal as a guide. C, The blade is then turned toward the index finger.

6. INTERNAL SPHINCTEROTOMY

Satisfactory results are achieved only when the superior edge of the divided internal sphincter is above the apex of the fissure. *A,* Most often, this point is at the dentate line. *B,* Division of the internal sphincter is accomplished by a to-and-fro motion of the knife blade against the operator's index finger. Care should be taken not to buttonhole the anoderm because of the potential for subsequent development of abscess and fistula. Pressure is applied for one or two minutes, and the dressing is placed. No packs are used.

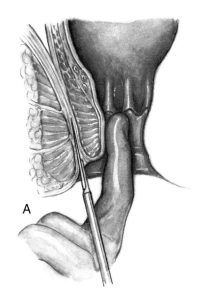
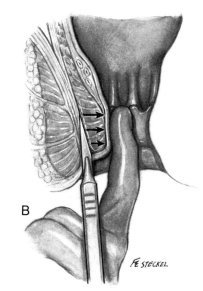

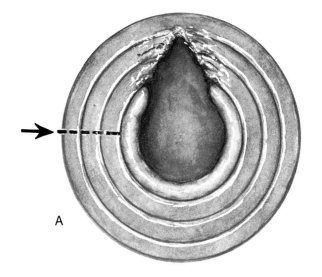
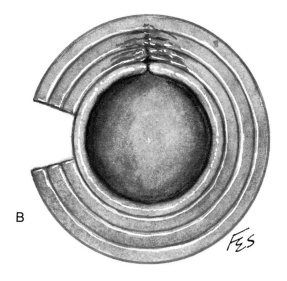

7. EFFECT OF SPHINCTEROTOMY

A, Before the sphincterotomy is performed, a chronic anal ulcer is palpable, most often in the posterior midline. *B,* After the sphincterotomy has been carried out *(arrow),* a wedge-shaped defect in the internal sphincter is palpable, and spasm of the internal sphincter is relieved.

Fissurectomy and Posterior Sphincterotomy

8. EXCISION

▼

Although this operative procedure is rarely indicated, an occasional fissure does not heal despite repeated lateral internal sphincterotomies. This situation probably results from fixation of the ulcer to the internal sphincter, along with induration of the edges, that prevents reepithelialization. Total excision of the indurated edges back to soft pliable mucosa and submucosa is essential. An elliptical wound is preferable.

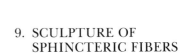

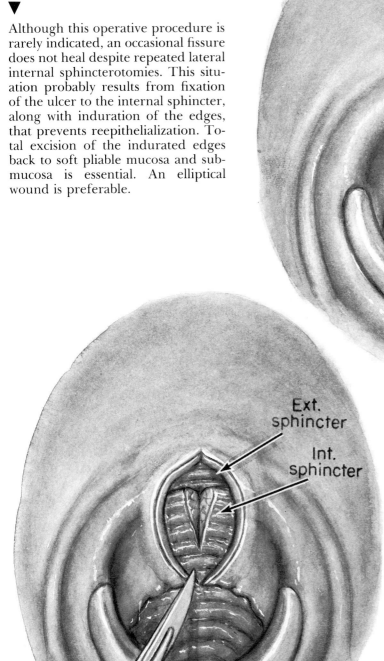

Ext. sphincter

Int. sphincter

9. SCULPTURE OF SPHINCTERIC FIBERS

▼

Indurated internal sphincter fibers that had formed the base of the fissure are carefully sculptured. The full thickness of the internal sphincter is not divided because of the potential for development of a keyhole deformity and subsequent permanent fecal soilage. Postoperative care of this wound is similar to that of any open anal wound, that is, sitz baths and stool softeners. Digital examination at weekly postoperative visits prevents premature bridging of the healing wound, with a resultant chronic fistula.

28 | Operations for Hemorrhoids

DAVID J. SCHOETZ, JR., M.D.

▼ IMPORTANT FEATURES
Understanding of Pathologic Anatomy
Clinical Grading of Hemorrhoids
    Grade 1: Bleed, No Prolapse
    Grade 2: Prolapse, Spontaneously Reduced
    Grade 3: Prolapse, Manually Reduced
    Grade 4: Always Prolapsed
Rubber Ring Ligation for Grades 1 and 2 and Some Grade 3
    Hemorrhoids
Hemorrhoidectomy for Some Grade 3 and All Grade 4 Hemorrhoids
Complete Anorectal Examination to Exclude Coincident Conditions
Radiographic Examination of Colon When Appropriate

▼ STEPS OR PLANS
Anatomy
Excisional Hemorrhoidectomy
    Positioning
    Submucosal Injection
    Excision
    Hemostasis
    Closure
Rubber Ring Ligation
    Positioning
    Equipment
    Application of Band

Anatomy

1. ANATOMY

Hemorrhoids are classified as internal or external. Internal hemorrhoids represent abnormalities of the superior hemorrhoidal plexus, which is a part of the portal venous system. These hemorrhoids lie predominantly within the anal canal and distal rectum. As they enlarge, they may prolapse out of the anal verge during straining and defecation. The symptoms of internal hemorrhoids are bleeding and prolapse. External hemorrhoids are enlargements of the inferior hemorrhoidal plexus, which is the terminal branch of the hypogastric veins and thus the systemic venous circulation. Symptoms of external hemorrhoids include pain and swelling resulting from episodes of thrombosis.

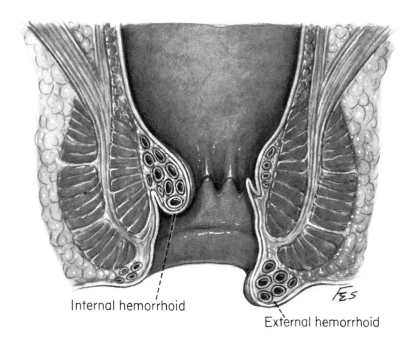

Internal hemorrhoid

External hemorrhoid

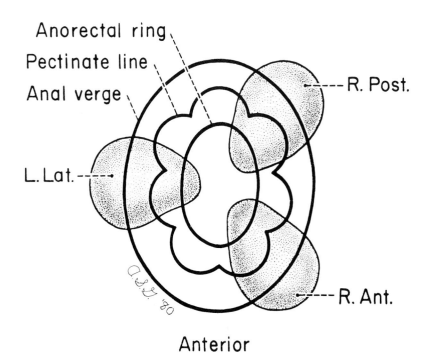

Anorectal ring

Pectinate line

Anal verge

R. Post.

L. Lat.

R. Ant.

Anterior

2. ANATOMY *(Continued)*

The three major anatomic positions of internal hemorrhoids are right posterior, right anterior, and left lateral. The base of the hemorrhoid is within the distal rectum. A hemorrhoid seen in a simple inspection in the primary internal hemorrhoidal position represents considerable enlargement of the internal hemorrhoid with an external component and is referred to as a combined hemorrhoid.

Excisional Hemorrhoidectomy

3. POSITIONING

Under general or spinal anesthesia, the patient is placed in the prone jackknife position, and the buttocks are taped apart to enhance operative exposure. The perianal region and rectum are prepared with a solution of povidone-iodine (Betadine), and the patient is draped in the standard fashion.

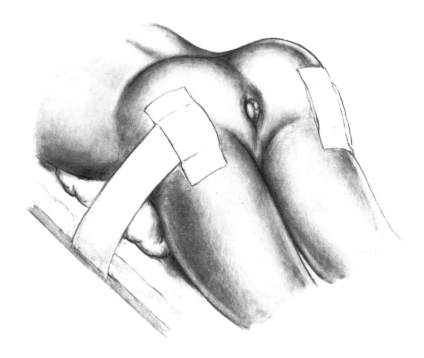

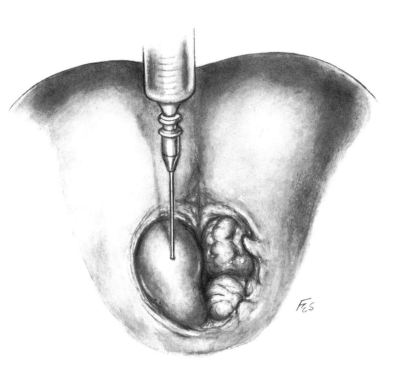

4. SUBMUCOSAL INJECTION

Submucosal injections of approximately 5 ml of 25 per cent bupivacaine (Marcaine) with 100,000:1 to 200,000:1 epinephrine facilitate subsequent dissection and help alleviate immediate postoperative pain.

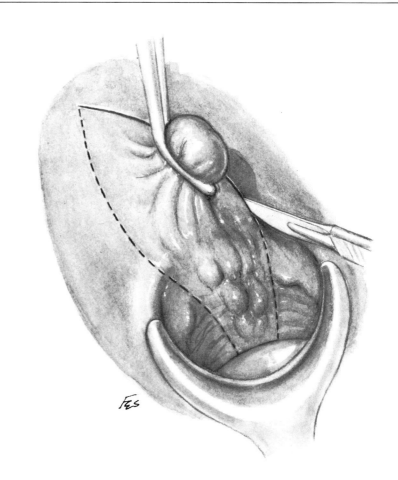

5. INCISION

▼

With the Hill-Ferguson retractor in place acting as an exclusion retractor and exposing only the hemorrhoid to be excised, the hemorrhoid is grasped, and an elliptical incision is made from the perianal skin into the distal rectum.

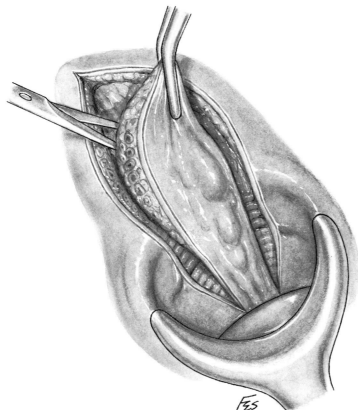

6. INITIAL DISSECTION

▼

The apex of the skin incision is grasped, and submucosal resection of hemorrhoidal tissue is performed. The subcutaneous fibers of the external and internal sphincters are preserved during excision, and the dissection is limited to the submucosal plane.

7. FURTHER DISSECTION AND SUTURE OF PEDICLE

The dissection is continued into the rectal ampulla. Care is taken to preserve as much anoderm as possible to prevent subsequent stenosis. A transfixion suture of the pedicle is placed with 2-0 chromic catgut.

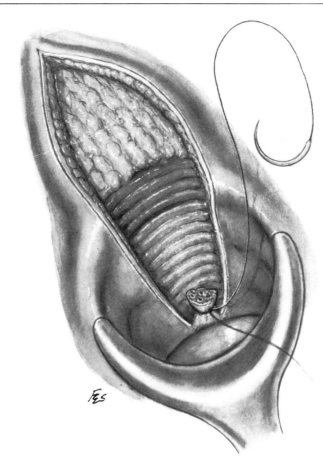

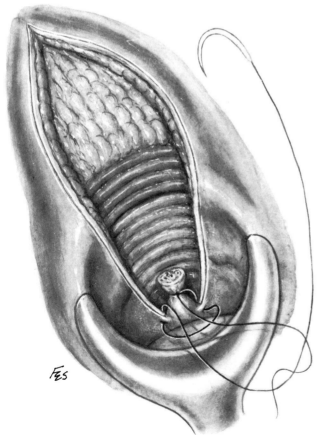

8. RESUTURING OF PEDICLE

Because immediate postoperative hemorrhage is almost always from the pedicles, care is taken to buttress the pedicles with the same suture.

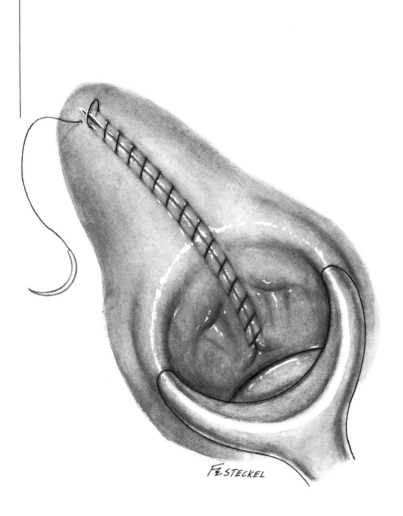

FESTECKEL

9. CLOSURE

The same suture is then used for continuous closure of the entire wound.

Each hemorrhoid is excised in a similar fashion, with care taken to preserve adequate mucosal bridges between each of the excision sites. At the termination of the procedure, a ¼-inch Penrose drain is placed into the rectal ampulla to prevent the accumulation of blood within the rectum. This drain is left in position for 12 to 24 hours. A pack is not used because it will not substantially improve hemostasis and will add to the patient's discomfort. The Penrose drain permits early detection of postoperative bleeding that otherwise may accumulate in the rectum and not be visible externally.

Rubber Ring Ligation

10. PREPARATION AND POSITIONING

This simple office procedure can be performed without the use of an anesthetic and has largely supplanted operative hemorrhoidectomy for symptomatic internal hemorrhoids. The patient is given an enema before being placed in the prone jackknife position on an examining table.

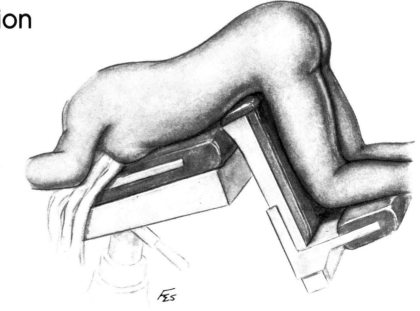

FES

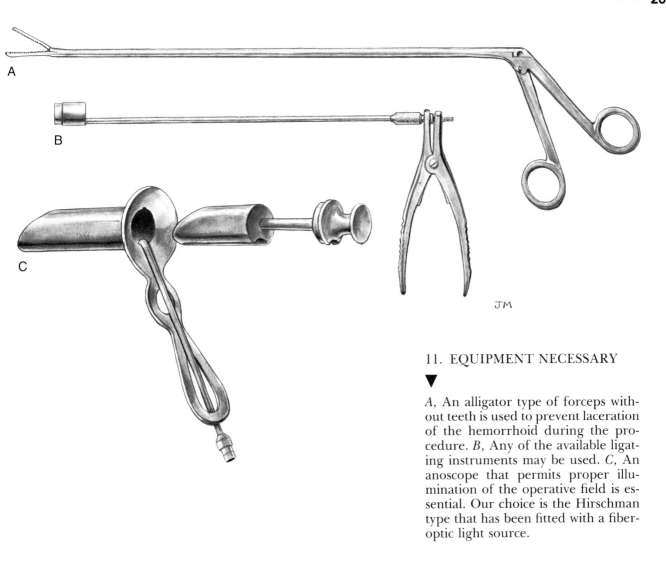

11. EQUIPMENT NECESSARY

▼

A, An alligator type of forceps without teeth is used to prevent laceration of the hemorrhoid during the procedure. *B*, Any of the available ligating instruments may be used. *C*, An anoscope that permits proper illumination of the operative field is essential. Our choice is the Hirschman type that has been fitted with a fiberoptic light source.

12. GRASPING THE HEMORRHOID

A, The base of the hemorrhoid is grasped above the dentate line and is tested for sensation. Pain may be felt 2 to 3 cm above the dentate line; if this is the case, either the hemorrhoid must be grasped higher within the distal rectum or operative hemorrhoidectomy is recommended. The patient is asked to perform the Valsalva maneuver to facilitate prolapse of the redundant mucosa into the anoscope before it is grasped. *B*, When the mucosa has been grasped at a pain-free level, the mucosa is tented up and pulled toward the drum of the ligator.

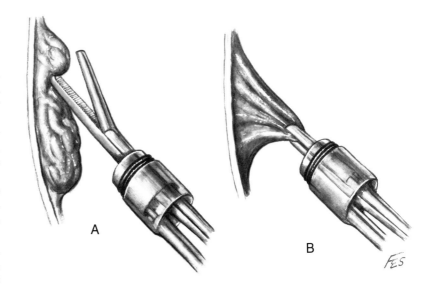

13. CORONAL VIEW

The coronal view demonstrates the grasping of mucosa above the dentate line with the anoscope in position.

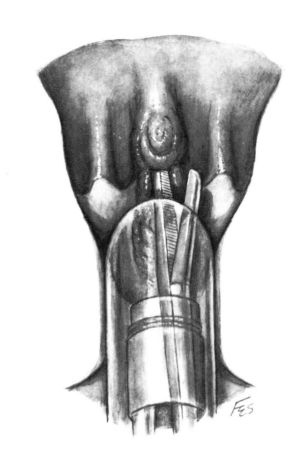

14. BANDING

A, As much of the redundant mucosa as possible is pulled into the drum, and the ligator is activated, releasing two bands around the base of the hemorrhoid. Two bands are used in case one breaks. *B,* The instrument is removed, and the ligated hemorrhoid is examined to ensure a good tourniquet effect around the redundant mucosa.

A

B

29 | Anoplasty Techniques

DAVID J. SCHOETZ, JR., M.D.

▼ IMPORTANT FEATURES
Exact Assessment of Anatomic and Functional Defect Preoperatively
Choose Simplest Operative Procedure to Achieve Complete
      Correction of Defect
Preoperative Colon Preparation Is Proportional to Extent of
      Operative Procedure
Prone Jackknife Position Affords Greatest Access to Buttock Area for
      Local Flap Reconstruction
Broad-Based Full-Thickness Flaps Minimize Ischemic Necrosis
Diversion of Colostomy Is Rarely Necessary Because Postoperative
      Confinement of Bowels Prevents Fecal Contamination

▼ STEPS OR PLANS
Local Excision
> *Simple Excision*
> *Subcutaneous Closure*

Posterior Advancement Flap
> *Excision of Ulcer*
> *Sphincterotomy*
> *Advance Flap*

Keyhole Deformity
> *Excise Posterior Defect*
> *Raise Flap*
> *Single-Layer Closure*

Bilateral Advancement Anoplasty
> *Remove All Scar Tissue*
> *Undermine Edges for Tension-Free Closure*

Z-Plasty
> *Bilateral Flaps Not Extending onto Buttocks*

Anoplasty with Sphincter Repair
> *Excise Rectovaginal Fistula*
> *Excise Redundant Vaginal Mucosa and Anoderm*
> *Plicate Pillars of Levator Muscles*
> *Reconstitute Perineal Body*
> *Interdigitate Flaps of Perineal Skin*

Circumferential Perianal Skin Graft
> *Biopsies to Plan Extent of Excision*
> *Excise Lesion*
> *Skin Graft with Stent*

Local Excision

1. LOCAL EXCISION

▼

A, Simple excision of indolent benign anal wounds and of lesions of the perianal skin represents the simplest of anoplastic procedures. This technique is also appropriate for some neoplasms involving the perianal region. An elliptical excision is planned to encompass the entire lesion. *B,* When the lesion has been excised back to supple normal tissue, undermining of the skin permits closure with a continuous absorbable suture in a subcuticular fashion.

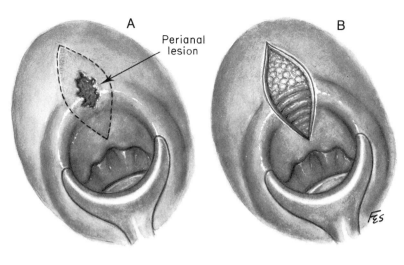

Posterior Advancement Flap

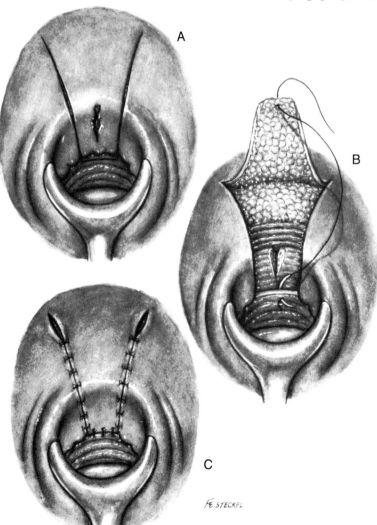

2. POSTERIOR ADVANCEMENT FLAP

▼

In some cases, chronic anal fissure may result in mild stenosis at the anal verge. This is true particularly when surgical excision of the fissure has been attempted previously. Under these circumstances, excision of the fissure should be combined with sphincterotomy, as well as advancement of additional normal skin into the anal canal, to overcome stenosis at the anal verge. *A,* A single posterior advancement flap can be designed that includes excision of the fissure itself up to the dentate line. The portion of the flap that contains the fissure is then excised. *B,* A posterior internal sphincterotomy performed under direct vision at the base of the wound extends up to the dentate line. The full-thickness flap is advanced into the anal canal using absorbable sutures of synthetic material. *C,* With the wide-based flap advanced into the anal canal, the corners of the skin are left open for drainage of serosanguineous fluid that would otherwise accumulate under the flap, thus preventing adherence to underlying structures. No drains are required, and confinement of the bowels is not necessary.

Keyhole Deformity

3. DEFORMITY

Fissurectomy with full-thickness posterior sphincterotomy is accompanied by an appreciable incidence of the keyhole deformity. This anatomic defect results from a posterior opening in the internal sphincter that permits leakage of fecal material in the resting state because of incomplete closure of the anal canal.

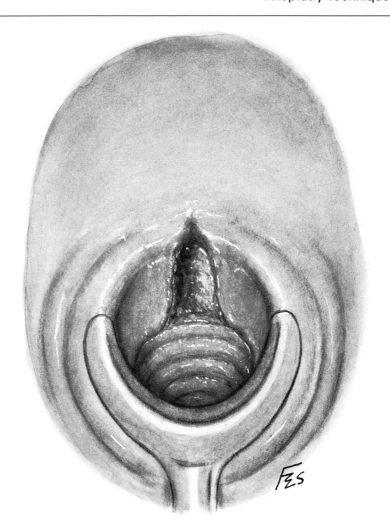

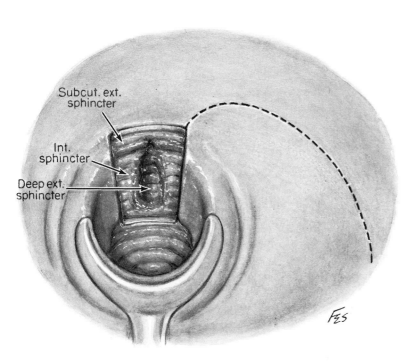

Subcut. ext. sphincter

Int. sphincter

Deep ext. sphincter

4. CHARACTERISTICS OF FLAP

The posterior defect is excised with indurated muscle. To achieve closure of the flap without tension, the edge of the rotation flap must measure between 8 and 12 cm and provide both skin and subcutaneous tissue.

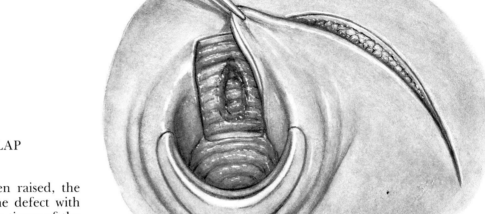

5. ROTATION OF FLAP

▼

After the flap has been raised, the apex is rotated into the defect with as little handling of the tissue of the flap as possible.

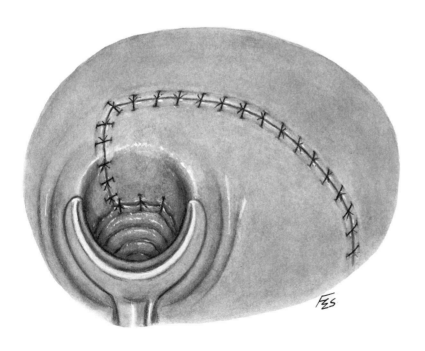

6. CLOSURE

▼

Single-layer closure of the full thickness of the flap is completed with absorbable interrupted sutures of synthetic material. Hemostasis must be absolutely perfect to prevent accumulation of a hematoma that will disrupt the flap. Drains are unnecessary, and confinement of the bowels for a period of three days ensures minimal fecal contamination.

Bilateral Advancement Anoplasty

7. BILATERAL ADVANCEMENT ANOPLASTY

▼

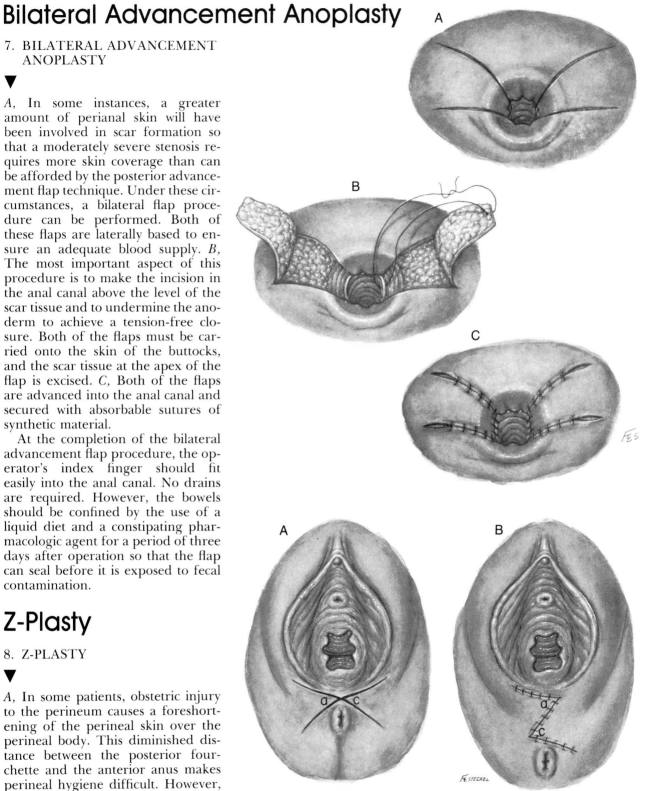

A, In some instances, a greater amount of perianal skin will have been involved in scar formation so that a moderately severe stenosis requires more skin coverage than can be afforded by the posterior advancement flap technique. Under these circumstances, a bilateral flap procedure can be performed. Both of these flaps are laterally based to ensure an adequate blood supply. *B*, The most important aspect of this procedure is to make the incision in the anal canal above the level of the scar tissue and to undermine the anoderm to achieve a tension-free closure. Both of the flaps must be carried onto the skin of the buttocks, and the scar tissue at the apex of the flap is excised. *C*, Both of the flaps are advanced into the anal canal and secured with absorbable sutures of synthetic material.

At the completion of the bilateral advancement flap procedure, the operator's index finger should fit easily into the anal canal. No drains are required. However, the bowels should be confined by the use of a liquid diet and a constipating pharmacologic agent for a period of three days after operation so that the flap can seal before it is exposed to fecal contamination.

Z-Plasty

8. Z-PLASTY

▼

A, In some patients, obstetric injury to the perineum causes a foreshortening of the perineal skin over the perineal body. This diminished distance between the posterior fourchette and the anterior anus makes perineal hygiene difficult. However, the transverse perineal musculature is still intact. A simple Z-plasty is performed to restore the perineal skin. Simple bilateral flaps are planned using the full thickness of the perineal skin but not requiring extension of the flaps onto the buttocks. *B*, Interdigitation of the flaps and closure with absorbable interrupted sutures of synthetic material restore the distance between the posterior fourchette and the anterior anal verge. Postoperative care requires no confinement of the bowels.

Anoplasty with Sphincter Repair

9. THE PROBLEM

▼

In its severe form, obstetric injury to the perineum results in disruption of the transverse perineal musculature with resultant fecal incontinence, a low rectovaginal fistula, and deficient perineal skin. This injury is often caused by disruption of an episiotomy repair or of repair of a third-degree perineal laceration. The operative procedure is deferred until local sepsis has cleared, and it may take several months for satisfactory formation of a scar to occur before primary repair. *A,* Examination of the patient in the prone jackknife position reveals an absence of perineal body, deficiency of perineal skin, and a low rectovaginal fistula. *B,* Operative intervention requires development of the rectovaginal septum

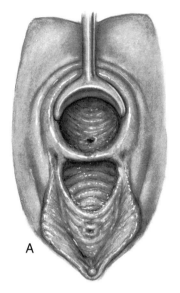 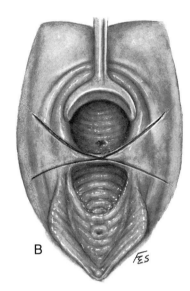

along with excision of the rectovaginal fistula and construction of bilateral flaps for subsequent reconstitution of the perineal skin.

10. THE REPAIR

▼

After the incision has been made over the attenuated rectovaginal septum, the dissection proceeds superiorly to the level of the levators. Care is taken to keep a margin of scar tissue on the divided transverse perineal musculature. The pillars of the levator muscles are plicated with absorbable interrupted sutures of heavy synthetic material. Reconstitution of the perineal body is performed with the same suture material, using the scar on the transected edges of the transverse perineal muscles to achieve a strong closure. Meticulous attention paid to hemostasis will prevent formation of hematomas with resultant breakdown. *A,* The redundant vaginal mucosa and anoderm, including the rectovaginal fistula if present, are excised. *B,* The perineal skin is closed by interdigitating the flaps and closing with absorbable interrupted sutures of fine synthetic

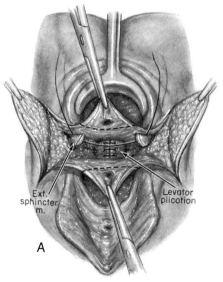 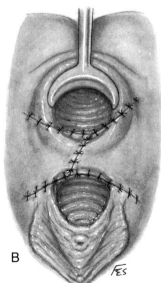

material. Postoperatively, the bowels are confined by pharmacologic measures for a period of three to five days.

Circumferential Perianal Skin Graft

11. THE PROBLEM

▼

Some conditions, specifically Bowen's disease and Paget's disease, may diffusely affect the perianal skin from the dentate line for variable distances onto the perianal skin. Greatest success in the treatment of these diffuse diseases is achieved by full-thickness excision of the entire lesion. Both of these diseases have a high incidence of recurrence and may cause death. Other neoplastic diseases involving the perianal region may also leave a defect after a large enough excision of the tumor to require split-thickness skin grafting as well. The techniques described are as applicable to partial circumference wounds as they are to complete circumferential excisions.

Excisional biopsies are made from both the inner and outer margins of the proposed excisional area to ensure that the entire lesion is encompassed by the planned excision. Fro-

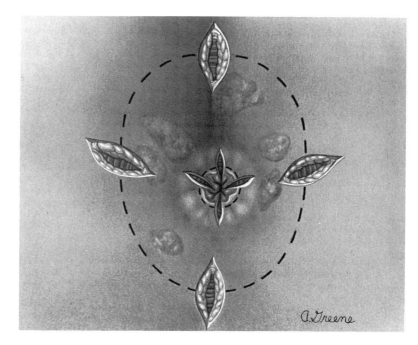

zen section analysis of all margins is obtained, and when appropriate the planned excision is extended as dictated by histologic examination.

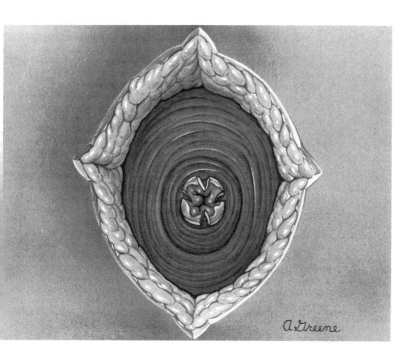

12. EXCISION

▼

Full-thickness skin and subcutaneous tissue have been excised from the perianal region, thus exposing the subcutaneous external sphincter. The excision may extend proximally up to the level of the dentate line. After the excision has been completed, a standard split-thickness skin graft is obtained. Because the patient is in the prone jackknife position, the skin of the posterior thigh and buttocks is a convenient site from which to harvest the graft. Every attempt should be made to obtain a graft large enough to cover the entire defect.

13. PLACEMENT OF GRAFT

▼

The mucocutaneous junction is fashioned with absorbable interrupted sutures of synthetic material, suturing the full thickness of the dentate line to the internal sphincter and to the skin graft. Sutures are left long for subsequent stenting. The outer margin of the graft is secured to the dermal margin with interrupted sutures of nylon, again with the ends left long.

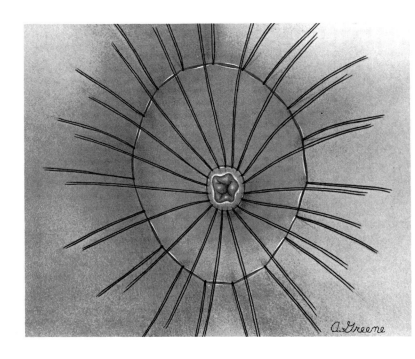

14. IMMOBILIZATION

▼

A stent of cotton soaked in mineral oil is placed over the graft, and the sutures are tied over the dressing. The buttocks are approximated by the use of Montgomery straps to prevent shearing through the motion of the buttocks on the stent itself.

Postoperatively, the patient is given a constipating regimen and is kept at bed rest. Under ideal conditions, the stent is removed on the seventh postoperative day, and the constipating regimen is discontinued. When fever or drainage is noted, the stent is removed, and local wet-to-dry dressings are applied to salvage as much of the graft as possible.

Liver, Biliary Tract, Pancreas, Spleen, Adrenal Glands, and Abdominal Wall Hernias

Drainage of Liver Abscess

30

J. LAWRENCE MUNSON, M.D.

▼ IMPORTANT FEATURES

Search for an Intra-Abdominal Cause of Liver Abscess and Treat It Before Draining the Abscess

Wall Off Surrounding Viscera to Minimize Contamination from the Abscess

Aspiration of the Abscess to Verify the Absence of Echinococcosis

Drainage with Closed-Suction Catheters and Debridement

▼ STEPS OR PLANS

Incision and Exposure

Exploration and Treatment of the Underlying Source of Sepsis

Packing Viscera Away from the Right Upper Quadrant

Mobilization of the Liver Sufficient to Guarantee Free Drainage of the Abscess

Aspiration for Gram Stain and Culture, Scoleces, and Infusion of Hypertonic Saline Solution for Echinococcosis

Unroofing, Drainage of the Abscess, and Debridement

Closed-Suction Catheter Perihepatic Drainage

Closure of the Wound

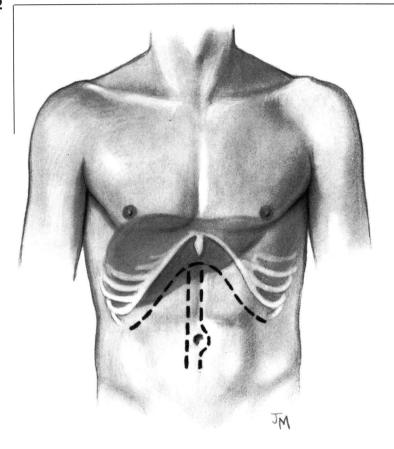

1. INCISION

▼

The abdomen is entered through a long subcostal incision. Alternatively, an upper midline or right paramedian incision can be used. An impermeable wound protector is placed, and the abdomen is explored for an intra-abdominal source of the liver abscess. Usually, preoperative investigations have isolated a probable source of the liver sepsis; however, in the absence of a preoperative diagnosis, the usual sources are diverticular disease, intestinal neoplasia, inflammatory bowel disease, periappendiceal abscess, or biliary tract disease. After appropriate treatment of the intestinal or biliary tract disease, attention is turned to the liver abscess.

2. ASPIRATION

▼

Laparotomy pads moistened with saline solution are placed about the viscera in the right upper quadrant to isolate the liver and thus minimize contamination by drainage from the abscess. The subcutaneous tissue is protected by laparotomy pads or a plastic ring protective sheet. A self-retaining retractor is placed to elevate the rib cage anteriorly and superiorly and to permit full exposure of the liver and its appropriate mobilization. The liver is mobilized from its posterior and superior ligamentous attachments only enough to permit free drainage of the abscess without unnecessarily opening up the subphrenic areas for loculation of further infection.

Because echinococcosis cannot definitely be ruled out preoperatively, an aspirating syringe on a stopcock is used to puncture the abscess. Immediate microscopic examination is carried out for bacteria and scoleces. When echinococcosis is suspected, the abscess is aspirated and refilled with an infusion of 20 per cent saline solution, which is left intracystic for 10 minutes. The abscess is incised, suction is applied quickly, the daughter cysts are evacuated, and the major cyst wall is excised.

Abscess cavity

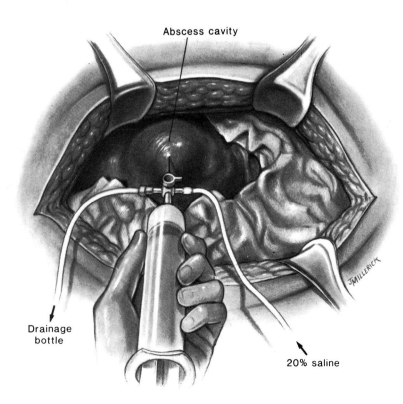

Drainage
bottle

20% saline

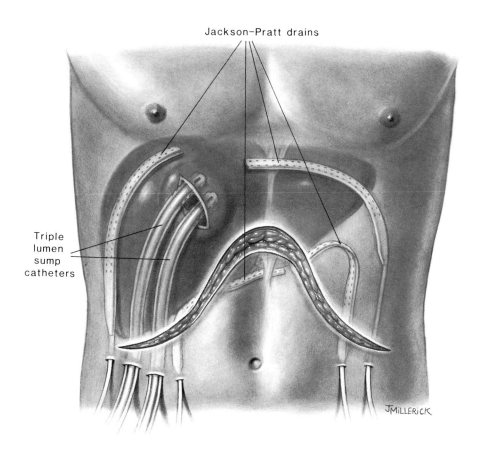

Jackson-Pratt drains

Triple
lumen
sump
catheters

JMiLLERiCK

3. DRAINAGE

▼

When the aspirated sample confirms bacterial abscess, the abscess is unroofed, debrided, and drained. Sump catheters are placed within the abscess cavity, and closed suction drains are placed about the liver and brought out through separate lateral counterincisions. The wound is closed with an absorbable monofilament suture material. The fascia and the skin are closed with a delayed primary technique or with surgical staples, depending on potential contamination.

31

Operation for Simple Liver Cyst

J. LAWRENCE MUNSON, M.D.

▼ IMPORTANT FEATURES
Verification That the Lesion Is a Simple Cyst and Not a Cystic
    Neoplasm, Abscess, or Echinococcal Cyst
Drainage of Cyst and Biopsy of Cyst Wall
Marsupialization
Drainage

▼ STEPS OR PLANS
Incision and Exposure
Walling Off Surrounding Viscera
Aspiration of the Cyst for Gram Stain, Culture, and the Presence of
    Bile
Unroofing of the Cyst, Biopsy of the Cyst Wall, and Search for Bile
    Leakage
Intraoperative Cholangiography
Internal Marsupialization

1. INCISION

The incision for drainage of a simple cyst of the liver is dictated by the preoperative assessment of its location. However, for most purposes, a long right subcostal incision is useful. After careful exploration of the abdomen, the viscera bordering the upper quadrants are packed off with laparotomy pads moistened with saline solution.

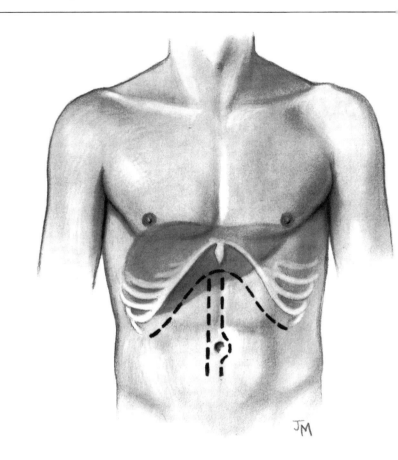

Cyst

Drainage bottle

20% saline

2. ASPIRATION

Despite the preoperative diagnosis of simple cyst of the liver, it is imperative to verify the absolute nature of the cystic lesion; this is best accomplished by aspirating the cyst using a closed aspirating system with drainage tubing and an inflow port. The aspirate is examined for the presence of bile and sent to the laboratory for Gram stain and culture, cytology, and the presence or absence of scoleces. The fluid from the cyst may be clear, cloudy, or bile stained or show evidence of past or recent hemorrhage.

3. UNROOFING AND DRAINAGE

▼

When a determination has been made that the lesion is a simple cyst, Glisson's capsule is cauterized over the cyst, and the liver substance is entered to unroof the cyst. After evacuation of all cyst contents, a careful inspection is made of the cyst wall, and any excrescences are submitted for biopsy to rule out a cystic neoplasm. A portion of the cyst wall itself is also sent for pathologic examination to verify the benign, flattened, or atrophic epithelium of the benign simple cyst. Careful inspection is also made for evidence of bile leakage, and intraoperative cholangiography is performed to verify the integrity of the biliary tree, especially if the cyst fluid is bilious. Mattress sutures of chromic catgut are placed about the saucerized cyst to appose Glisson's capsule to the cyst wall. When a connection to the biliary tree is present, this must be closed or a Roux-en-Y loop of jejunum brought up for anastomosis to the cyst wall. When the unroofing and saucerization of the cyst have been adequate or when the cyst lies superficially within the liver substance, an omental pack is not necessary before closure. However, when the edges of the cyst appear to fall together, a large ped-

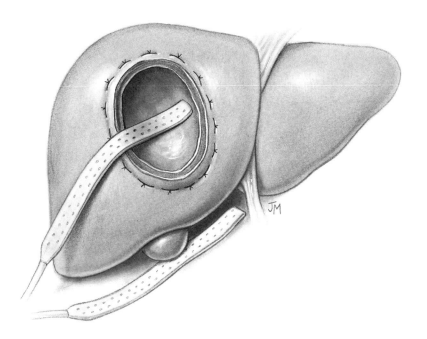

icle of omentum can be developed off the transverse colon, inserted into the depths of the cyst, and held there with a chromic catgut suture. When the unroofed cyst gapes open, a closed suction drain can be placed within the cyst and another in the subhepatic space. These drains are brought out through lateral counterincisions. After hemostasis has been verified, the incision is closed in the usual fashion.

Local Resection of Solitary Liver Lesion

32

J. LAWRENCE MUNSON, M.D.

▼ IMPORTANT FEATURES
Search for Evidence of Disseminated Disease
Search for Other Hepatic Lesions
Overlapping Hemostatic Suture Technique

▼ STEPS OR PLANS
Incision and Exposure
Exploration for Disseminated Disease
Search for Other Hepatic Lesions
Placement of Hemostatic Sutures
Excision of the Lesion
Drainage and Closure

1. INCISION AND EXPLORATION

Either the solitary lesion of the liver has been found on routine exploration during another intra-abdominal procedure or the location of the hepatic lesion is known from preoperative investigations. Because exploration of the liver can evolve into formal hepatic lobectomy, placement of the hepatic artery catheter, or local wedge excision, the incision of preference is a long right subcostal incision, which can be extended into a bilateral subcostal incision to provide full exposure of the liver.

After careful exploration of the abdomen has ruled out disseminated disease and confirmed a solitary lesion of the liver, a self-retaining retractor is placed, and the costal margin is elevated upward and cephalad. A careful search is made for other hepatic lesions, detaching the falciform, triangular, and coronary ligaments as necessary to perform bimanual palpation of the entire liver. Intraoperative ultrasonography can be used for finer definition of intrahepatic pathologic conditions.

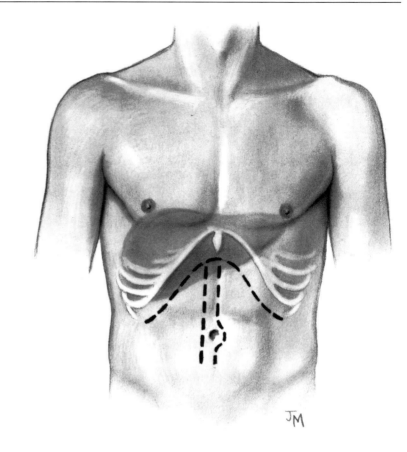

2. WEDGE OR LOCAL EXCISION

With confirmation of a solitary lesion at the edge of the liver, a wedge excision can be planned. Full-thickness mattress sutures of 0 chromic catgut are placed in an overlapping fashion 2 cm from the visible edge of the lesion. The sutures are tied firmly without crushing into hepatic parenchyma, rendering the circumscribed area ischemic. The lesion is excised with the Bovie electrocautery, and suture ligatures are used to occlude any ductules or blood vessels not secured by the overlapping mattress sutures.

For other lesions not on the edge of the liver, biopsy is appropriate when the lesion is large. For indeterminate lesions, local excision is often possible with local control of bleeding or bile leakage.

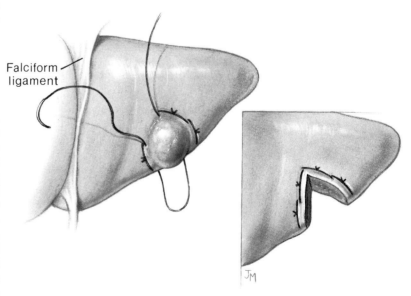

Falciform ligament

Microfibrillar collagen or other topical hemostatic agents can be used to complete hemostasis. A closed-suction type of drainage catheter is placed in the subhepatic space, subjacent to the excision, and brought out through a separate counterincision. The wound is closed in layers.

Resection of Biliary Cystadenoma

33

J. LAWRENCE MUNSON, M. D.

▼ IMPORTANT FEATURES

Preoperative Hepatic Arteriography

Full Mobilization of the Liver in Preparation for Possible Resection

Dissection and Identification of the Portal Structures

Establishment of the Correct Plane of Dissection External to the Cystadenoma

Search for and Correction of Bile Leakage After Enucleation of the Cystadenoma

Formal Resection When Malignant Disease Is Proved on Pathologic Examination of the Resected Specimen

▼ STEPS OR PLANS

Incision and Exposure

Mobilization of the Liver

Cholecystectomy, Cholangiography, and Isolation of the Common Bile Duct, Hepatic Artery, and Portal Vein

Establishment of the Proper Dissection Plane External to the Cystadenoma and Careful Enucleation of the Tumor

Search for Bile Leakage and Oversewing of Severed or Communicating Bile Ducts

Careful Intraoperative Pathologic Examination of the Excised Cystadenoma with Attention to Areas of Firm Capsular Attachment to the Hepatic Parenchyma

Formal Hepatic Resection When Cancer Is Determined

1. INCISION

The incision of choice for resection of biliary cystadenoma is the bilateral subcostal incision with vertical extension to the sternum to permit adequate retraction and elevation of the costal margins. The self-retaining retractor is invaluable in providing adequate exposure when this incision is used.

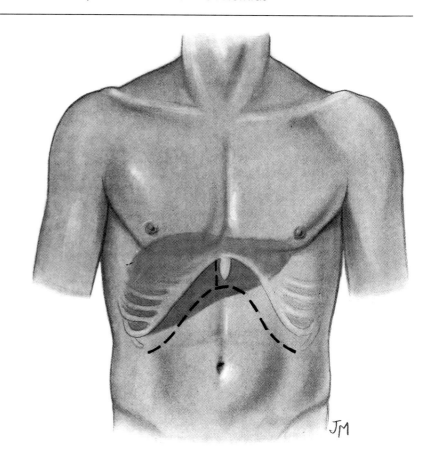

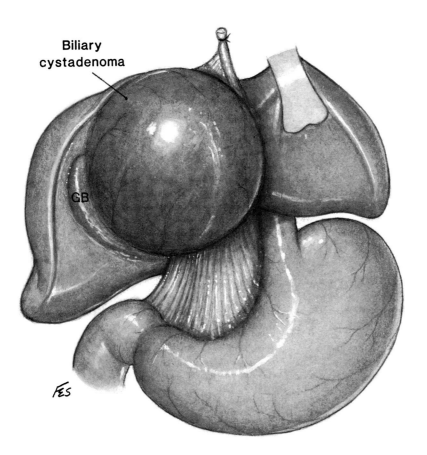

Biliary cystadenoma

GB

2. APPEARANCE OF CYSTADENOMA

The cystadenoma often presents as a rounded bulging mass at the antero-inferior aspect of the liver, often tenting the gallbladder over the lesion and displaying the cystic duct and artery along the surface of the cyst.

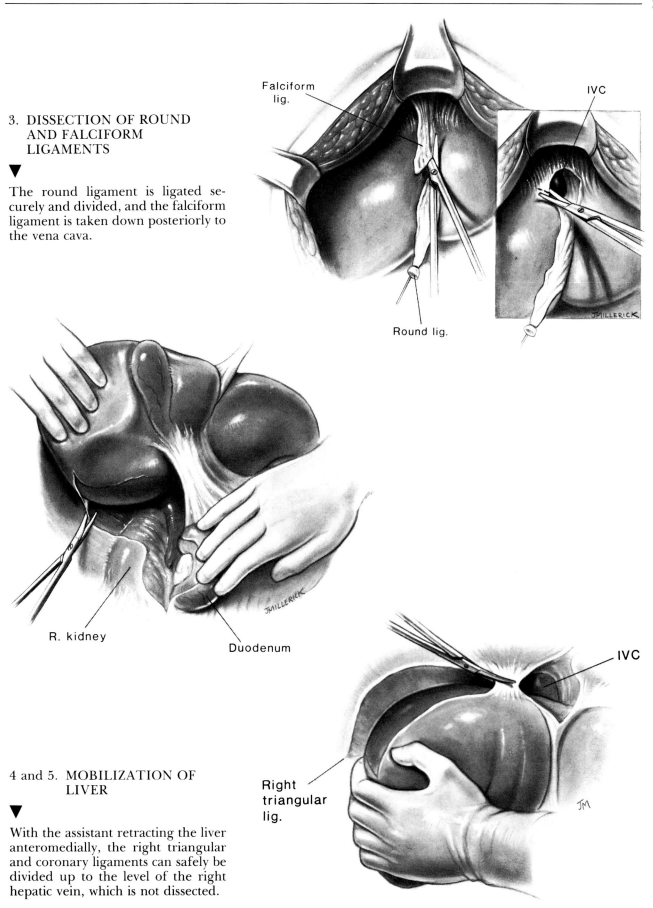

3. DISSECTION OF ROUND AND FALCIFORM LIGAMENTS

▼

The round ligament is ligated securely and divided, and the falciform ligament is taken down posteriorly to the vena cava.

4 and 5. MOBILIZATION OF LIVER

▼

With the assistant retracting the liver anteromedially, the right triangular and coronary ligaments can safely be divided up to the level of the right hepatic vein, which is not dissected.

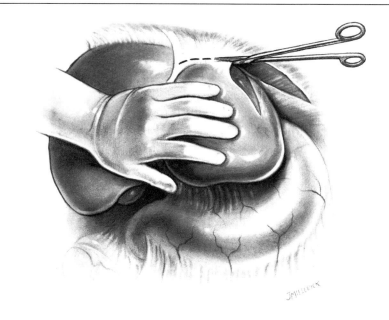

6. MOBILIZATION OF LIVER
(*Continued*)

In similar fashion, the liver can be retracted anterolaterally, and the triangular ligaments to the left lobe are divided up to the level of the left hepatic vein. Often, subphrenic vessels will have to be controlled with ligatures at this point.

CHOLECYSTECTOMY

Cholecystectomy is performed with careful dissection of the cystic duct back to its junction with the common bile duct, which facilitates further exposure of the porta hepatis. After placement of a vascular clamp across the distal bile duct, cholangiography of the cystic duct is performed to define the biliary ductal anatomy and to demonstrate any communication (albeit rare) with the cystadenoma. Large volumes of contrast material may be necessary because any communication will rapidly dilute the contrast material, and failure to demonstrate a communicating duct will result. The portal structures are identified, although their full mobilization and control with a vascular tape are not necessary.

7. EXCISION OF ADENOMA

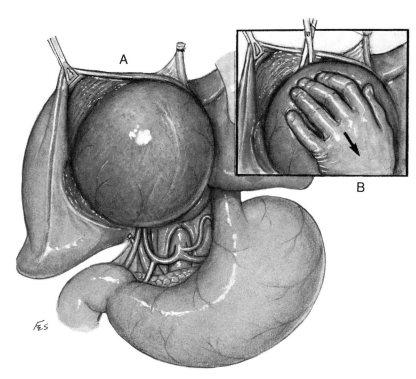

A and *B,* Careful dissection along the junction of the compressed liver parenchyma with the cyst capsule using a combination of blunt and sharp dissection will permit the proper plane of separation to be entered. When this plane has been developed, the edges of the liver are grasped with Pennington or Duval clamps, and steady traction is applied to them away from the capsule of the cystadenoma. This dissection should be relatively avascular, although fine vessels can course from the cyst wall to the liver parenchyma. The dissection is continued circumferentially so that the operator can maintain full view of the proper plane of dissection.

At the completion of the enucleation, the entire cyst is sent for immediate pathologic examination. A careful search is made of areas firmly adherent to the liver for the presence of invasive tumor. The cyst wall is also carefully inspected for papillary excrescences that have signs of carcinoma.

8. POSTRESECTION HEMOSTASIS

At the completion of enucleation, the hepatic and portal veins and ducts and branches of the hepatic artery are all displayed in relief on the compressed liver substance. The cut surface of the liver is inspected for hemostasis or leakage of bile. Small ductules are ligated, but any major peripheral ductal structures subtending viable liver parenchyma may be considered for biliary enteric reconstruction using a Roux-en-Y limb.

9. MAJOR RESECTION FOR CARCINOMA

▼

When carcinoma has been determined on biopsy of the capsule of the cystadenoma, formal resection is performed. This can be carried out without further dissection of the liver because the portal structures have been mobilized and the hepatic veins can be seen in relief in the posterior wall of the cavity of enucleation. The portal structures are doubly suture ligated, and the level of devitalized hepatic parenchyma can be determined. With careful finger fracture technique proceeding posteriorly, the hepatic veins are isolated and doubly suture ligated. The preoperative arteriogram should be reviewed before this resection because the cystadenoma often will cause severe displacement of the normal vascular structures. T-tube drainage is not necessary unless the remaining ductal structures have been entered in the course of the resection. All vascular and biliary structures encountered during resection are ligated, and final hemostasis is obtained with microfibrillar collagen or a similar topical hemostatic agent. Closed-suction drainage in the right upper quadrant is essential. After the drains are brought out through counterincisions, the abdominal wound is closed in the usual fashion.

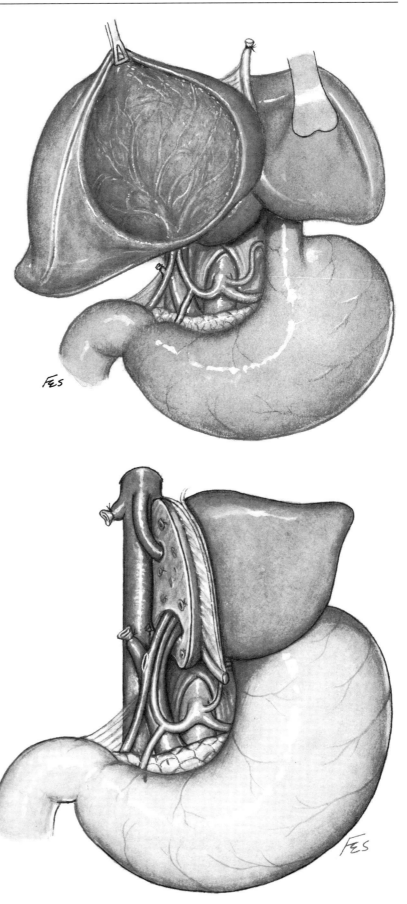

34 Hepatic Resection

RICARDO L. ROSSI, M.D.
STEPHEN G. ReMINE, M.D.

▼ IMPORTANT FEATURES
Conserve as Much Functioning Liver Tissue as Is Consistent with Treatment
Hepatic Lobar and Segmental Anatomy
Hepatic Arterial and Venous Blood Supply
Preliminary Control of Blood Supply and Biliary Tract
Sectioning of Liver
Control of Bleeding and Bile Leakage from Cut Surface

▼ SURGICAL ANATOMY
Lobar Division
Inferior View
Distribution of Portal Vein
Hepatic Venous Drainage
Variations in Origins of Hepatic Arteries
Posterosuperior Attachments
Lines of Resection

▼ SPECIAL SITUATIONS
Right Hepatic Lobectomy
Extended Right Hepatic Lobectomy
Left Hepatic Lobectomy
Left Lateral Segmentectomy

Surgical Anatomy

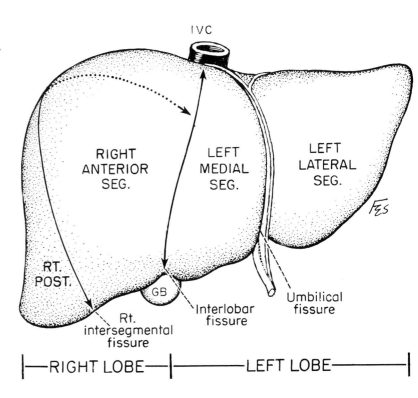

1. MAJOR FISSURES, LOBES, AND SEGMENTS

The main portal fissure divides the liver into left and right lobes. The right portal fissure divides the right lobe into anterior and posterior segments. The right hepatic vein courses in this fissure. The left portal fissure divides the left lobe into medial and lateral segments and contains the left hepatic vein. The middle hepatic vein is located in the main portal fissure between the right and left lobes.

After Soupault and Couinaud

2. SEGMENTAL DISTRIBUTION

Inferior view of the liver showing its segments.

3. PORTAL VEIN BRANCHES
(opposite page)

Bile ducts and arteries have the same distribution as do the portal vein branches.

4. DISTRIBUTION OF HEPATIC VEINS
(opposite page)

Hepatic veins are found in interlobar and segmental fissures. A variant of the middle hepatic vein joins the left hepatic vein at a distance from the inferior vena cava.

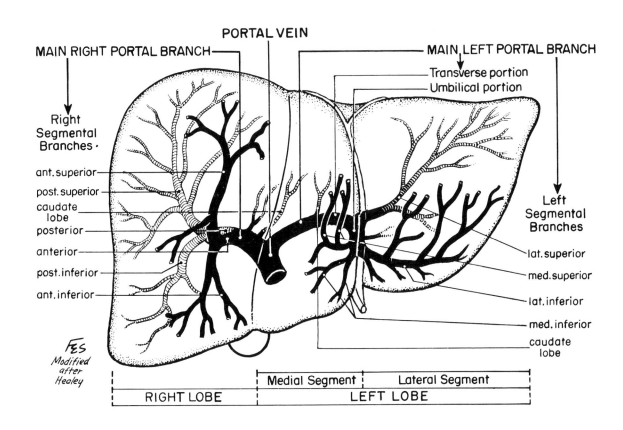

PORTAL VEIN

MAIN RIGHT PORTAL BRANCH

MAIN LEFT PORTAL BRANCH

Transverse portion
Umbilical portion

Right
Segmental
Branches·

ant. superior
post. superior
caudate
lobe
posterior
anterior
post. inferior
ant. inferior

Left
Segmental
Branches

lat. superior
med. superior
lat. inferior
med. inferior
caudate
lobe

FES
Modified
after
Healey

Medial Segment	Lateral Segment
RIGHT LOBE	LEFT LOBE

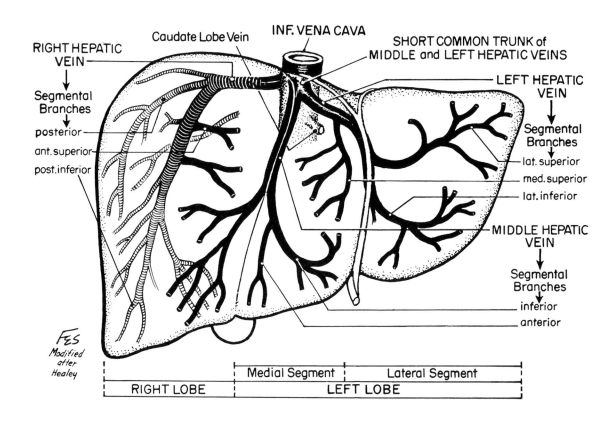

Caudate Lobe Vein

INF. VENA CAVA

SHORT COMMON TRUNK of
MIDDLE and LEFT HEPATIC VEINS

RIGHT HEPATIC
VEIN

LEFT HEPATIC
VEIN

Segmental
Branches

posterior
ant. superior
post. inferior

Segmental
Branches

lat. superior
med. superior
lat. inferior

MIDDLE HEPATIC
VEIN

Segmental
Branches

inferior
anterior

FES
Modified
after
Healey

Medial Segment	Lateral Segment
RIGHT LOBE	LEFT LOBE

VARIATIONS IN HEPATIC ARTERIAL BLOOD SUPPLY

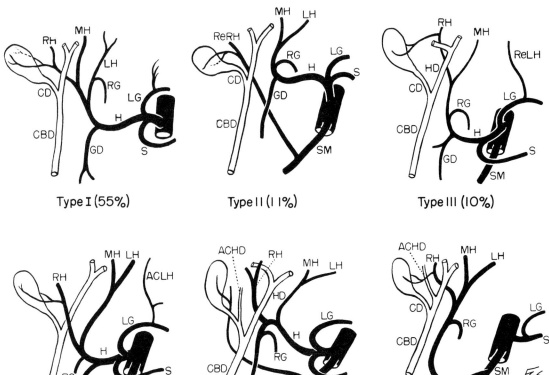

Type I (55%)   Type II (11%)   Type III (10%)

Type IV (8%)   Type V (7%)   Type VI (4.5%)

5. ORIGIN AND COURSE OF HEPATIC ARTERIES

In only 55 per cent of patients are the origin and distribution traditional, and in 22 per cent of patients, all or some part of the hepatic artery originates from the superior mesenteric artery. The left hepatic artery originates from the left gastric artery in about 20 per cent of subjects. AC = accessory, CBD = common bile duct, CD = cystic duct, GD = gastroduodenal artery, H = common hepatic artery, HD = hepatic duct, LG = left gastric artery, LH = left hepatic artery, MH = middle hepatic artery, Re = replaced, RG = right gastric artery, RH = right hepatic artery, S = splenic artery, SM = superior mesenteric artery.

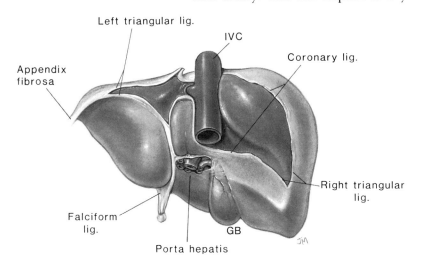

Left triangular lig.

IVC

Coronary lig.

Appendix fibrosa

Right triangular lig.

Falciform lig.

GB

Porta hepatis

6. LIGAMENTS OF LIVER

The posterosuperior surface and attachments of the liver are shown.

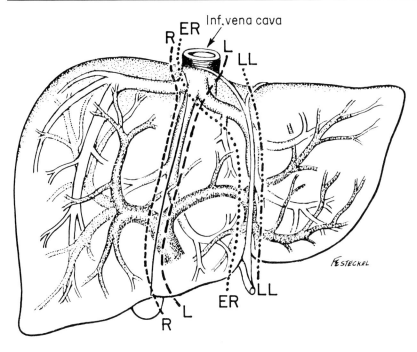

7. LINES OF RESECTION

▼

Lines of resection for right and left hepatectomy and extended right and left lateral lobectomy are based on vascular branching in the liver, especially the distribution of the hepatic veins. ER = extended right, L = left, LL = left lateral, R = right.

Right Hepatic Lobectomy

8. INCISION

▼

Bilateral subcostal incision with midline extension to the xiphoid process is shown.

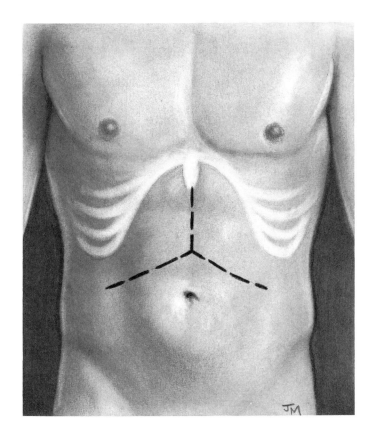

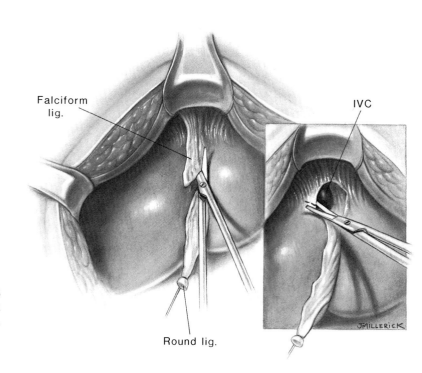

9. DIVISION OF FALCIFORM LIGAMENT

Lysis of the liver attachments is shown with division of the falciform ligament up to the inferior vena cava.

10. FURTHER MOBILIZATION OF RIGHT LOBE

Division of the attachments to the right lobe of the liver is shown with lysis of the attachment of the posterior border of the liver to the inferior vena cava.

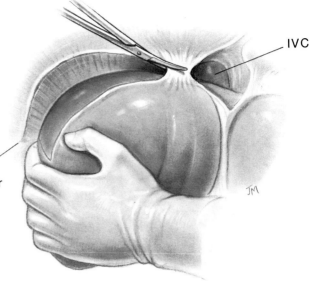

11. FURTHER SUPERIOR MOBILIZATION

▼

Division of the right triangular ligament and the coronary ligament is shown.

Right triangular lig.

IVC

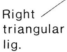

IVC

Adrenal gland

R. kidney

12. DISSECTION OF VENA CAVA POSTERIORLY

▼

Division of the attachment of the liver to the lateral inferior vena cava and retroperitoneum is shown. Some hepatic veins may require ligation and transection.

13. CHOLECYSTECTOMY

▼

Cholecystectomy is performed in the usual fashion.

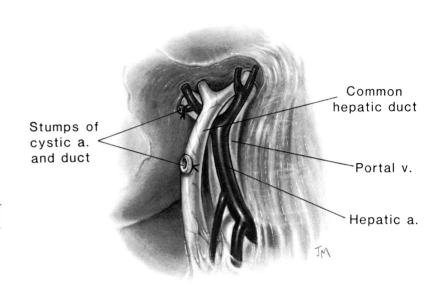

Common
hepatic duct

Stumps of
cystic a.
and duct

Portal v.

Hepatic a.

14. HILAR STRUCTURES

▼

Dissection of the hilar structures of
the liver is shown. This is an optional
step.

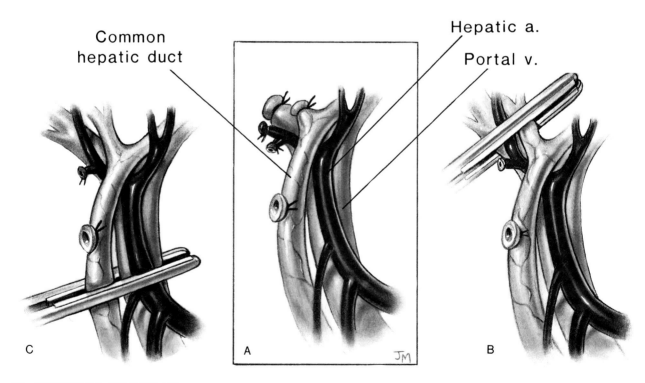

Common
hepatic duct

Hepatic a.

Portal v.

C   A   B

15. CONTROL OF LOBAR
ARTERY, VEIN, AND DUCT

▼

Hepatic hilar dissection is necessary
to perform individual ligation of the
right branches of the hepatic artery,
portal vein, and common hepatic
duct before resection. Three options
for control of hilar vessels are shown.
A, Ligation. *B,* Clamp. *C,* Clamp on
duodenohepatic ligament.

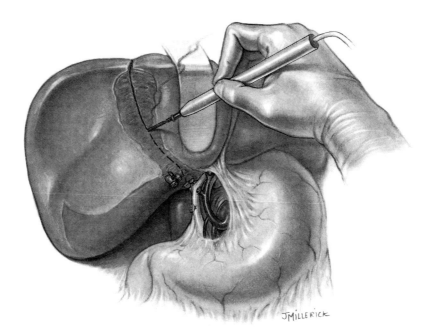

16. PLANE OF TRANSECTION

The line of transection of the liver is marked on its inferior surface with the electrocautery. This plane is from the gallbladder fossa to the vena cava.

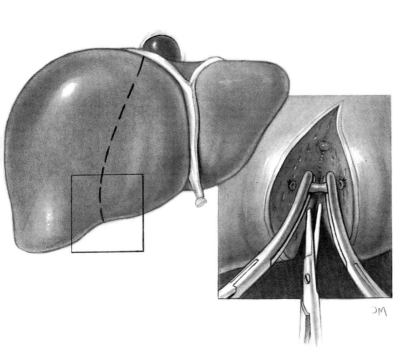

17. PLANE OF TRANSECTION
(Continued)

The anterior and superior surfaces are shown.

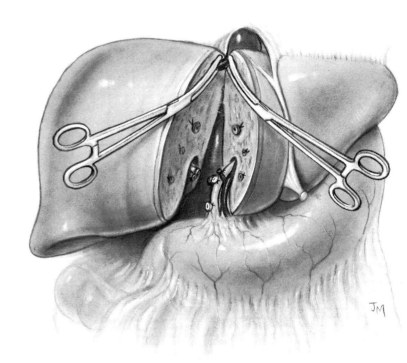

18. TECHNIQUE OF SECTIONING LIVER

Right lobectomy is performed with the finger fracture technique, with the tip of an instrument, or with the Cavitron instrument. Vascular and ductal structures are identified, clamped or clipped, and divided from the anterior surface of the liver toward the inferior vena cava. Posteriorly, the right hepatic vein is identified, clamped, and divided.

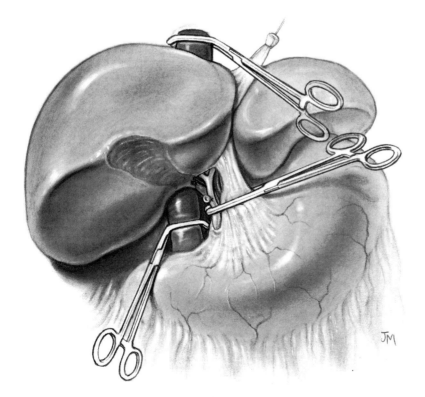

19. TECHNIQUE OF VASCULAR ISOLATION

Vascular isolation is used selectively in some patients when major bleeding is anticipated (that is, involvement by tumor of one hepatic vein at the level of the inferior vena cava). A vascular clamp is placed in the inferior vena cava between the liver and the renal veins. An atraumatic vascular clamp is placed in the hepatoduodenal ligament. A vascular clamp is placed in the inferior vena cava at the level of the diaphragm.

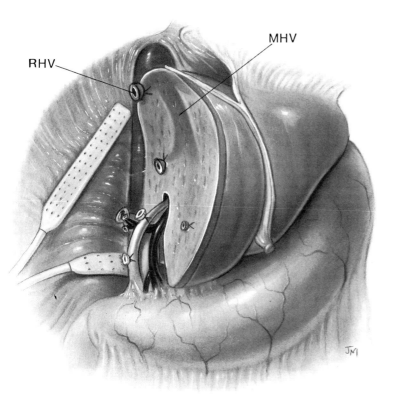

RHV

MHV

20. HEMOSTASIS AND DRAINAGE

▼

After the transection has been completed, the ductal and vascular structures are religated when necessary. Suture ligatures are preferred for larger structures. Mattress sutures to approximate the anterior and posterior borders of the transection are placed rarely and only when needed for hemostasis because, with this technique, the middle hepatic vein and hilar structures are at risk of compression or injury. Microfibrillar collagen (Avitene) is placed on the transected surface.

Extended Right Hepatic Lobectomy

21. EXTENT OF RESECTION

▼

The technique of liver dissection is similar to that of right hepatectomy. The left hepatic vein must be preserved as shown.

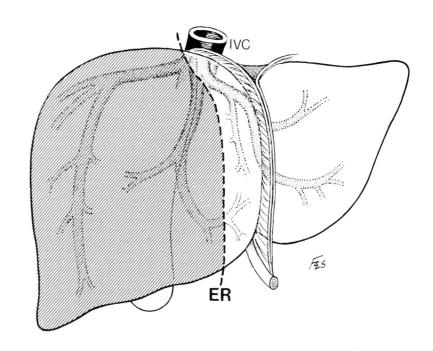

IVC

ER

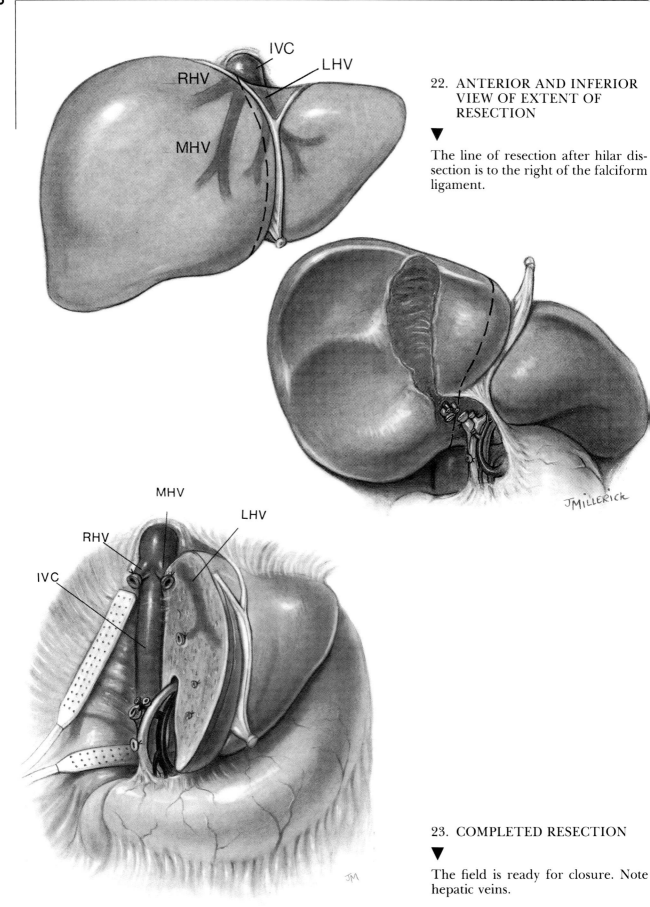

22. ANTERIOR AND INFERIOR VIEW OF EXTENT OF RESECTION

▼

The line of resection after hilar dissection is to the right of the falciform ligament.

23. COMPLETED RESECTION

▼

The field is ready for closure. Note hepatic veins.

Left Hepatic Lobectomy

24. INCISION

▼

The incision can be either bilateral subcostal or midline extended.

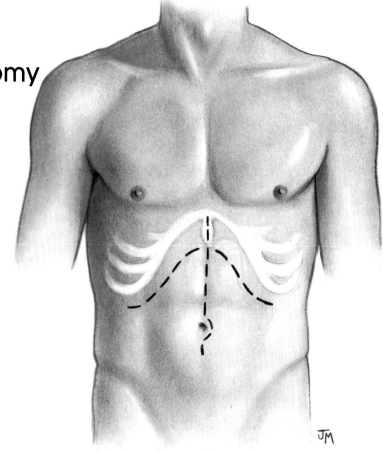

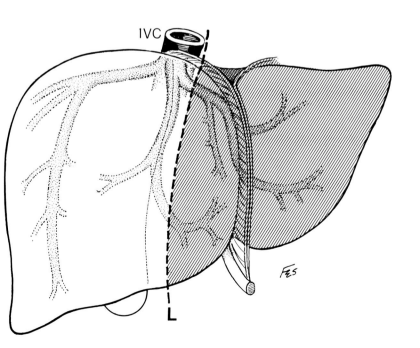

25. EXTENT OF LEFT HEPATECTOMY

▼

The area removed by left hepatectomy is shown in the shaded area. Note preservation of the middle hepatic vein.

26. EXTENT OF MOBILIZATION

▼

This illustration depicts the dissection necessary for mobilization of the liver. The round ligament, ligamentum teres, and falciform ligament are disconnected *(a)*. The attachments of the lateral segment of the left lobe of the liver are dissected *(b)*. For formal left hepatectomy, it is advisable to mobilize the right lobe of the liver as for right hepatectomy *(c)*.

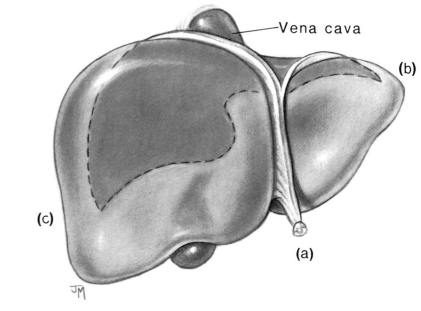

Vena cava

(b)

(c)

(a)

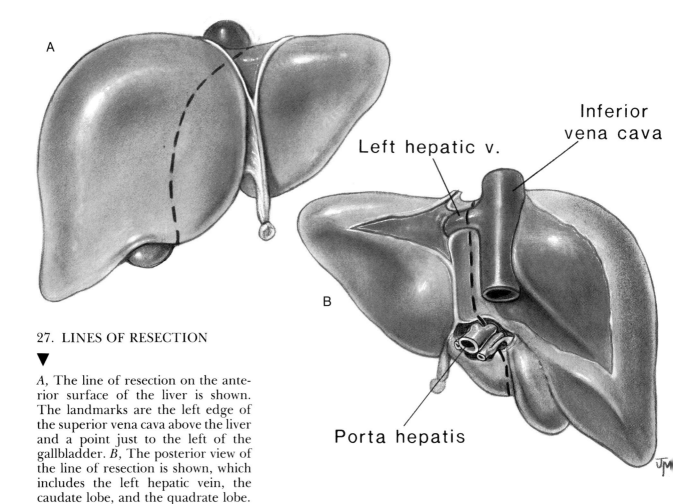

A

Inferior vena cava

Left hepatic v.

B

Porta hepatis

27. LINES OF RESECTION

▼

A, The line of resection on the anterior surface of the liver is shown. The landmarks are the left edge of the superior vena cava above the liver and a point just to the left of the gallbladder. *B,* The posterior view of the line of resection is shown, which includes the left hepatic vein, the caudate lobe, and the quadrate lobe.

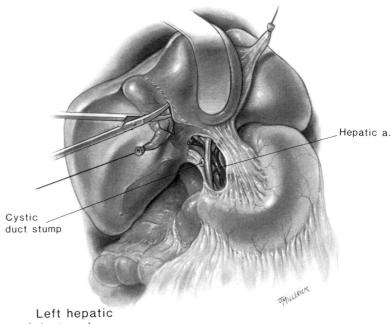

Hepatic a.

Cystic
duct stump

28. CHOLECYSTECTOMY

Cholecystectomy is followed by dissection of the hilus of the liver as for right hepatectomy.

Left hepatic
duct and a.

Left portal v.

Stumps of
cystic a.
and duct

Portal v.

29. HILAR DISSECTION

The hilar dissection is as shown. The left portal vein, hepatic artery, and hepatic duct are severed. These structures, especially the portal vein and artery, should be suture ligated.

Hepatic a.

Common
bile duct

Ischemic region

30. TECHNIQUE OF LIVER DISSECTION

The line of resection is defined with the electrocautery just to the left of the bed of the gallbladder and to the left of the border of ischemia after hilar ligation. Resection is begun anteriorly using the finger fracture technique or the tip of a scissors or a dissector.

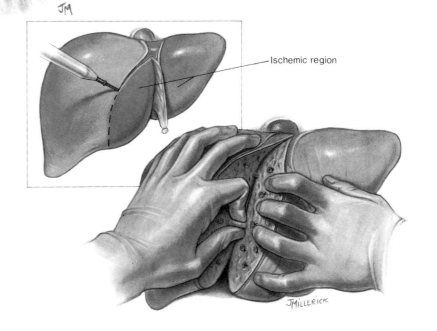

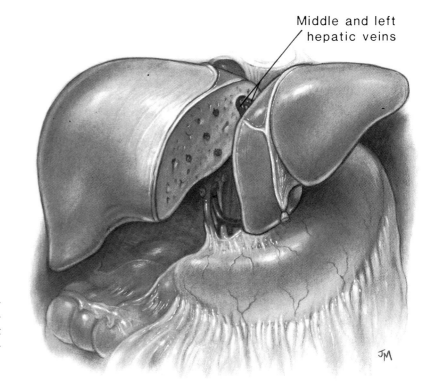

Middle and left hepatic veins

31. MANAGEMENT OF HEPATIC VEINS

The dissection is continued posteriorly. Branches of the middle hepatic vein and the entire left hepatic vein are occluded, divided, and suture ligated.

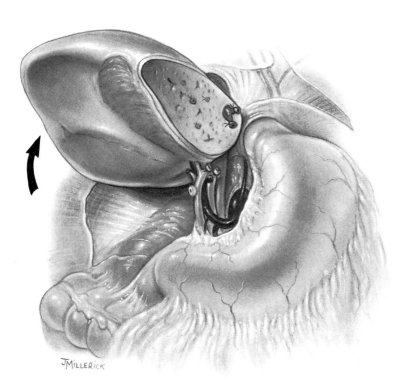

32. HEMOSTASIS AND DRAINS

This illustration depicts the field after completion of total left hepatectomy. Great effort must be extended to dry the cut edge of the liver. Ligation, electrocautery, Gelfoam soaked in thrombin, or microfibrillar collagen (Avitene) powder is useful in obtaining a dry field. Drains are placed, and the incision is closed.

Left Lateral Segmentectomy (Removal of Segments II and III)

33. INCISION

▼

A bilateral subcostal incision is made with or without vertical extension to the xiphoid process or midline.

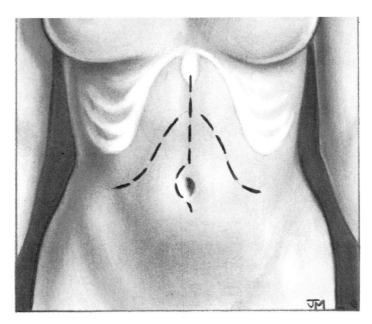

Coronary ligament

Left triangular ligament

(a)

34. MOBILIZATION

▼

The liver is mobilized as shown. Division of the ligamentum teres and falciform ligament to the inferior vena cava is shown *(a)*. Division of the left triangular ligament and the left coronary ligament up to the inferior vena cava is shown *(b)*.

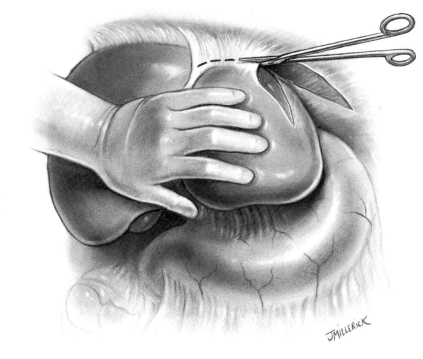

35. MOBILIZATION *(Continued)*

The lateral segment is rotated to the right, and dissection is continued to the inferior vena cava.

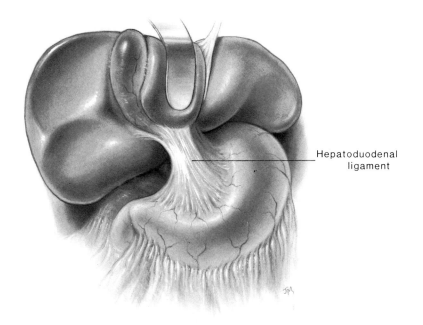

Hepatoduodenal ligament

36. PREPARATION OF LIVER HILUM

The hepatoduodenal ligament is identified, and the foramen of Winslow is opened. Usually its structures do not need to be dissected for left lateral segmentectomy. Occasionally, an atraumatic vascular clamp should be placed across the hepatoduodenal ligament.

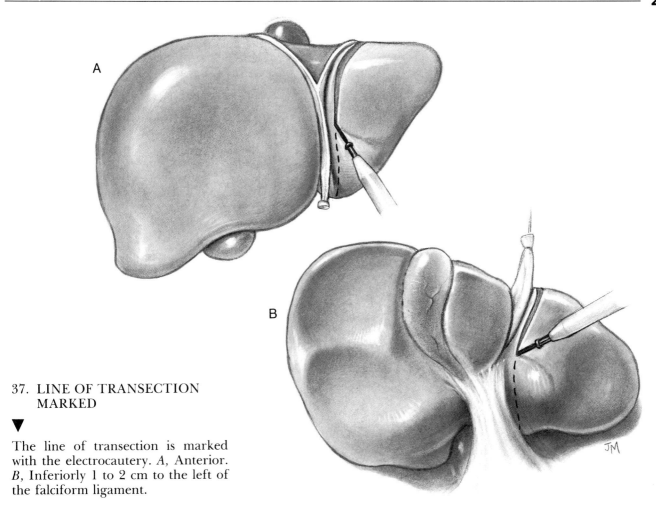

37. LINE OF TRANSECTION MARKED

▼

The line of transection is marked with the electrocautery. *A,* Anterior. *B,* Inferiorly 1 to 2 cm to the left of the falciform ligament.

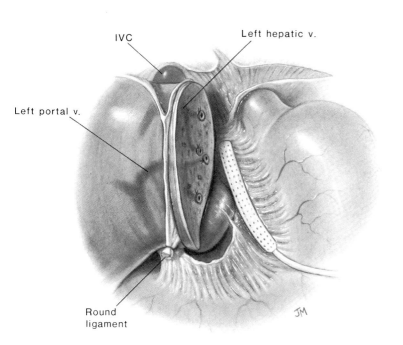

38. DISSECTION OF LIVER AND HEMOSTASIS

▼

The finger fracture technique or the tip of a scissors is used to transect the liver, starting in the anterior and superior locations and carrying the transection posteriorly and inferiorly. Vascular and ductal structures are clamped and divided. Posteriorly, the left hepatic vein is identified, clamped, and divided. At times, an assistant may pinch off the liver near the transection for hemostasis. The specimen is removed, and vascular and ductal structures are suture ligated. The illustration depicts the completed procedure.

Hepatic Transplantation

35

C. WRIGHT PINSON, M.D.
W. DAVID LEWIS, M.D.
ROGER L. JENKINS, M.D.

▼ IMPORTANT FEATURES
Donor Operation
Evaluation of the Liver and Arterial Supply
Mobilization of the Graft
Cannulation and Irrigation
Excision of the Graft
Recipient Hepatectomy
Mobilization of the Liver
Institution of Venovenous Bypass
Resection of the Liver
Control of Retroperitoneal Hemorrhage
Implantation of the Graft
Inferior Vena Caval Anastomosis Above the Liver
*Inferior Vena Caval Anastomosis Below the Liver and Irrigation of
the Graft to Remove Preservation Solution*
Portal Vein Anastomosis
Reconstruction of Hepatic Arterial Inflow
Cholecystectomy and Reconstruction of Biliary Drainage

▼ STEPS OR PLANS
Donor Operation
*Donor Incision and Evaluation of the Graft and Arterial Blood
Supply*
*Mobilization of the Left Lobe of Liver by Division of the Falciform
Ligament, the Left Triangular Ligament, and the Hepatogastric
Ligament*
*Dissection of the Celiac Axis and Hepatic Artery with Ligation and
Division of Branches*
Division of the Common Duct and Irrigation of the Biliary Tree
*Cannulation of the Splenic Vein, Control of the Superior Mesenteric
Vein, and Ligation of the Inferior Mesenteric Vein*
Cattell Maneuver and Control of the Superior Mesenteric Artery
Mobilization of the Infrahepatic Inferior Vena Cava
*Cannulation of the Aorta and Inferior Vena Cava at Their
Bifurcation*

Donor Operation

1. INCISION

▼

The vertical midline incision extends from the suprasternal notch to the symphysis pubis. The sternum is divided with a saw. The round and falciform ligaments are divided. The diaphragm is divided bilaterally on an angle beginning near the midline and extending posterolaterally to permit wide displacement of both sternal and abdominal retractors. The pericardium can be opened to expose the heart. The liver and other abdominal viscera are exposed for evaluation.

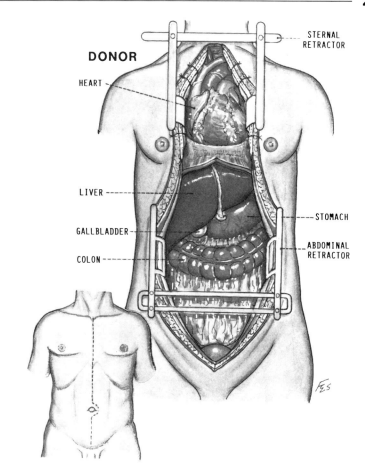

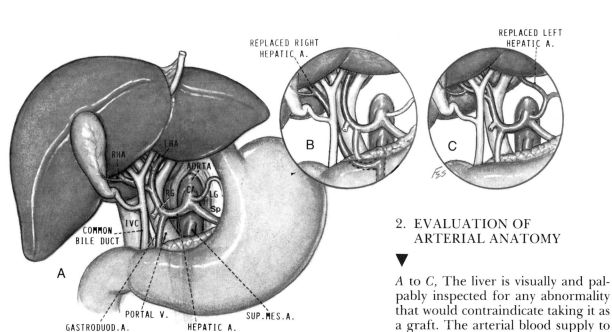

2. EVALUATION OF ARTERIAL ANATOMY

▼

A to C, The liver is visually and palpably inspected for any abnormality that would contraindicate taking it as a graft. The arterial blood supply to the liver is assessed. Careful notation of either a replaced right hepatic artery (as shown in *B*) or a replaced left hepatic artery (as shown in *C*) is made.

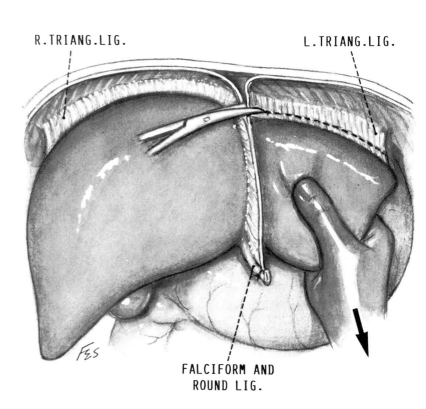

R.TRIANG.LIG.   L.TRIANG.LIG.

FALCIFORM AND
ROUND LIG.

3. DIVISION OF LEFT TRIANGULAR LIGAMENT

With the left lateral segment of the liver in the surgeon's right hand, the left triangular ligament is put on the stretch and divided. This division is extended to the right over the supra-hepatic inferior vena cava.

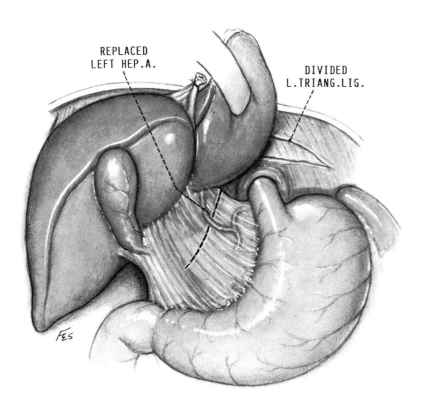

REPLACED
LEFT HEP.A.

DIVIDED
L.TRIANG.LIG.

4. DIVISION OF HEPATOGASTRIC LIGAMENT

With the left lateral segment mobilized, it is possible to visualize the hepatogastric ligament. A thin portion adjacent to the hepatoduodenal ligament is opened, and division of the ligament is carried superiorly to the diaphragm, just to the left of the inferior vena cava. Within the hepatogastric ligament is where a replaced left hepatic artery would be located, and caution not to divide this artery is in order.

5. DISSECTION OF CELIAC AORTA

▼

An assistant elevates the left lateral segment of the liver, exposing the crura of the diaphragm overlying the aorta and celiac axis. The peritoneum is divided as shown. Muscular fibers of the crura of the diaphragm are picked up by the surgeon and assistant and divided with the electrocautery to the level of the aorta. Approximately 3 cm of aorta is dissected around the takeoff of the celiac axis.

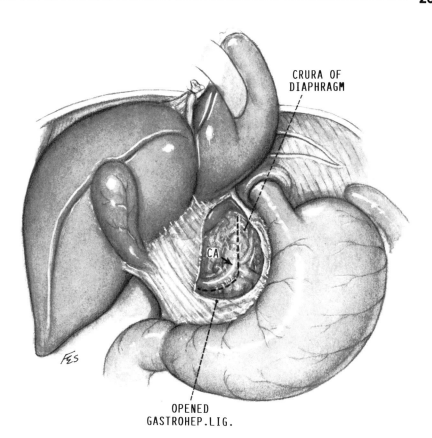

CRURA OF DIAPHRAGM

CA

OPENED GASTROHEP.LIG.

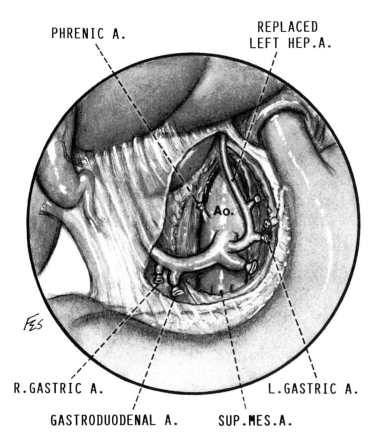

PHRENIC A.

REPLACED LEFT HEP.A.

Ao.

R.GASTRIC A.

L.GASTRIC A.

GASTRODUODENAL A.

SUP.MES.A.

6. DISSECTION OF HEPATIC ARTERY

▼

The hepatic artery is identified by palpation and dissected in retrograde fashion along its anteroinferior border. Four branches—the right gastric, the gastroduodenal, the splenic, and the left gastric arteries—are encountered and ligated. The illustration depicts the completed dissection of the hepatic artery and celiac aorta in a patient who has a replaced left hepatic artery.

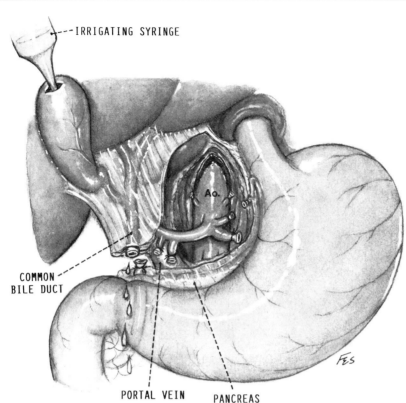

COMMON
BILE DUCT

PORTAL VEIN   PANCREAS

7. DISSECTION OF COMMON DUCT AND IRRIGATION OF BILIARY TREE

▼

The right lateral aspect of the hepatoduodenal ligament is divided just above the level of the duodenum and pancreas. Care is taken to note in this area a replaced right hepatic artery, when present. The common duct is encircled with minimal dissection and divided at this level. The fundus of the gallbladder is opened with an electrocautery. Saline solution is irrigated through the gallbladder, exiting the common duct. The common duct is irrigated in retrograde fashion using a blunt needle on a syringe. Soft tissues over the portal vein are divided between ligatures.

8. CANNULATION OF SPLENIC VEIN, CONTROL OF SUPERIOR MESENTERIC VEIN, AND LIGATION OF INFERIOR MESENTERIC VEIN

▼

A and B, Dissection in the hepatoduodenal ligament is carried inferiorly on the anterior surface of the portal vein. Sometimes retraction of the pancreas inferiorly permits adequate exposure of the splenic vein. If not, it is possible for the surgeon to pass a finger gently under the neck of the pancreas. At this level, two heavy silk sutures are placed around the pancreas, and the pancreas is ligated and divided between these sutures. Gentle traction laterally on each suture exposes the portal vein and superior mesenteric vein–splenic vein confluence. The coronary vein and inferior mesenteric vein are ligated and divided. Two ligatures are passed around the proximal portion of the splenic vein. The splenic side is ligated, and gentle traction is placed on the portal side. A small vascular clamp can be placed on the portal side. A venotomy is made in

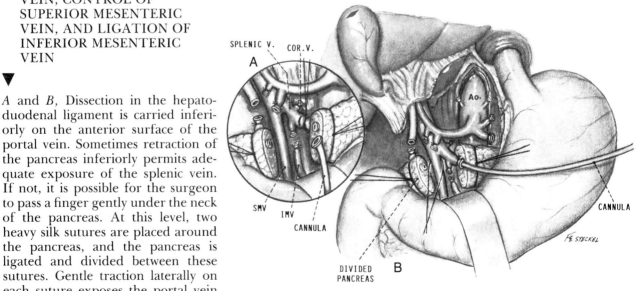

SPLENIC V.   COR.V.

A

SMV   IMV
      CANNULA

CANNULA

DIVIDED
PANCREAS   B

the splenic vein through which a flanged cannula is inserted and held snugly by tying the second suture. The splenic vein is divided beyond the cannula. Finally, the superior mesenteric vein just below the confluence is dissected and encircled for control with a silk suture, which is not yet tied.

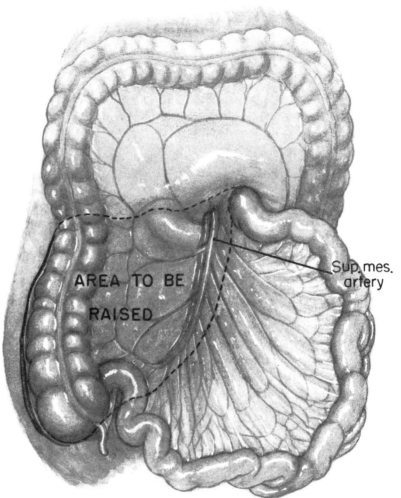

9. THE CATTELL MANEUVER

▼

An incision made along the hepatic flexure of the colon is extended down the white line of Toldt around the cecum and up the base of the mesentery and is stopped at the lower border of the pancreas. With blunt dissection, the right colon, small bowel, and mesentery are mobilized and elevated anterosuperiorly. The duodenum is also mobilized extensively in this process.

10. CONTROL OF SUPERIOR MESENTERIC ARTERY

▼

The superior mesenteric artery, which is identified at the base of the mesentery by palpation, is dissected out from either above or below the mesentery and circled with a heavy silk suture but not tied. This view from below shows a replaced right hepatic artery, which is dissected; the suture on the superior mesenteric artery must be distal to this branch as shown. Also shown in *broken lines* is the Carrel patch, incorporating the origin of both the celiac axis and the superior mesenteric artery that will be required in this circumstance.

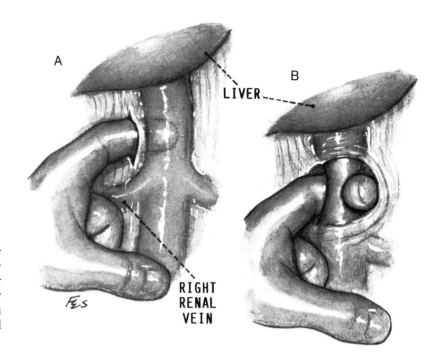

11. CONTROL OF INFRAHEPATIC INFERIOR VENA CAVA

▼

The inferior vena cava just posterior to the portal vein is dissected out by first (A) dividing the peritoneum for 3 or 4 cm and (B) with blunt finger dissection encircling the inferior vena cava above the level of the right renal vein.

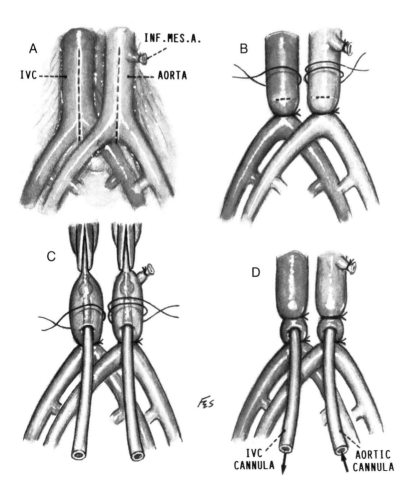

12. CANNULATION OF AORTA AND INFERIOR VENA CAVA

▼

A, The distal aorta and inferior vena cava are dissected. B, Two heavy silk sutures are passed two times around the distal aorta, and two more heavy silk sutures are placed around the distal inferior vena cava. The distal aorta is ligated after heparin is administered. C, A vascular clamp is placed across the aorta just above the inferior mesenteric artery. An aortotomy, 1 cm in length, is made through which a flanged catheter is inserted cephalad. D, The superior suture is tied quickly while the vascular clamp is removed. In a completely analogous fashion, the inferior vena caval catheter can be inserted.

13. IRRIGATION OF LIVER (KIDNEY AND PANCREAS) GRAFTS

▼

The aorta at the level of the diaphragm is clamped, and the previously placed sutures around the superior mesenteric artery and superior mesenteric vein are tied. The aortic cannula is flushed with preservation solution, totaling 1 or 2 L. Thus, flow is directed into the solid organs and not into the intestine. Free egress of blood and solution is provided by opening the inferior vena caval cannula, which is drained dependently, or alternatively, by simply dividing the atriocaval junction or distal abdominal cava. At the completion of hepatic flush, Kocher clamps are placed on the aorta below the level of the celiac axis but above the takeoff of the renal arteries. A cuff of aorta is formed by dividing the aorta above and below the celiac axis, as indicated by the *broken lines,* unless a replaced right hepatic artery is present (see Fig. 10). Posterior attachments to the aorta and hepatic artery are divided. The superior mesenteric vein is divided as shown so that the portal vein and the splenic vein cannula are free.

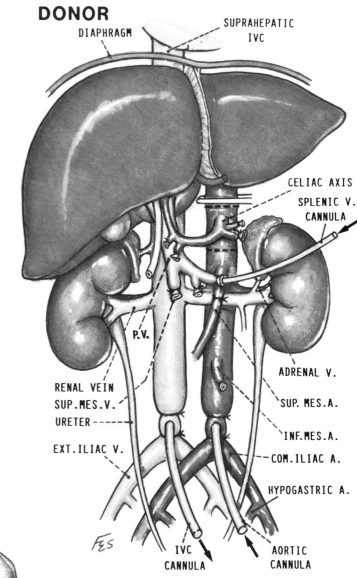

DONOR

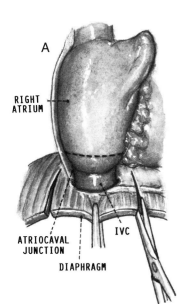

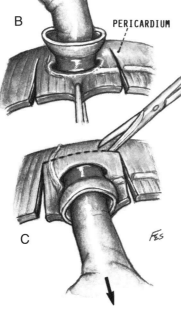

14. DIVISION OF DIAPHRAGM AND MOBILIZATION OF SUPRAHEPATIC INFERIOR VENA CAVA

▼

A to *C,* The atriocaval junction is divided sharply intrapericardially. The diaphragm directly anterior to the inferior vena caval foramen is grasped with a Kocher clamp. With a finger from the surgeon's left hand inside the inferior vena cava, the diaphragm is divided laterally on either side of the inferior vena cava, and with anterior retraction on the inferior vena cava, the diaphragm and pericardium posterior to the inferior vena cava are divided.

15. MOBILIZATION OF RIGHT LOBE OF LIVER AND DIVISION OF ADRENAL VEIN

▼

A and B, With the assistant retracting the right lobe of the liver to the patient's left, the right triangular ligament is divided sharply. This dissection extends posterior to the inferior vena cava. The adrenal vein will become apparent and must be ligated and divided. The remaining soft tissue attachments are divided posterior to the inferior vena cava. The inferior vena cava is divided just below the liver, taking caution to spare a cuff adjacent to the takeoff of the left and right renal veins.

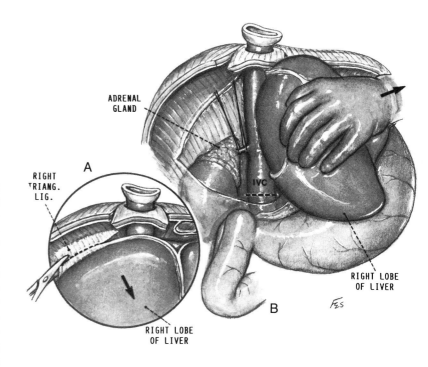

16. EXCISED GRAFT ON THE BACK TABLE

▼

It is now possible to remove the graft with an attached cuff of aorta at the celiac axis, with attached splenic vein cannula, and with attached diaphragm around the suprahepatic inferior vena cava as shown. It is placed on the back table inside two Lahey bags. The portal vein is irrigated with approximately 750 ml of preservation solution. With the two bags tightly secured, the graft is placed in ice. Finally, the iliac vessels are dissected from the donor from the level of the aortic bifurcation to the level of the bilateral inguinal ligaments, dividing the hypogastric branches. This V-shaped graft of iliac artery and iliac vein can be used in a complicated vascular reconstruction in the recipient. In addition, spleen and lymph node tissue are harvested for future cross-matching purposes.

Recipient Hepatectomy

17. POSITIONING AND INCISION

▼

The patient is positioned on the table with both arms extending at 90 degrees. A pulmonary artery catheter for cardiac monitoring and a triple-lumen catheter for infusion of vasoactive medications are both placed into the right internal jugular vein. Two or even three lines are introduced into the right subclavian, right antecubital, and right internal jugular veins to provide inflow for a rapid infusion device. Careful padding of the patient's buttocks, lower extremities, and heels is necessary. Incisions are made initially in the left axillary and left inguinal regions, through which the axillary vein and most proximal portion of the left saphenous vein will be mobilized and encircled with Rumel tourniquets. A subcostal abdominal incision is made, extending from the right flank to the

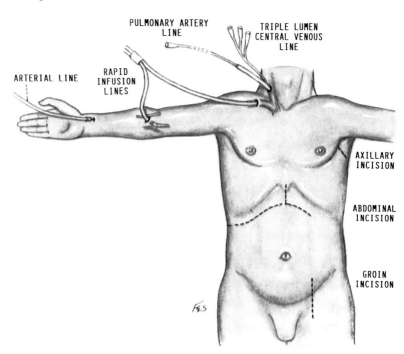

left lateral rectus border. This incision is extended in the midline to the xiphoid process, which is excised. A fixed table retractor is placed to elevate the costal margins.

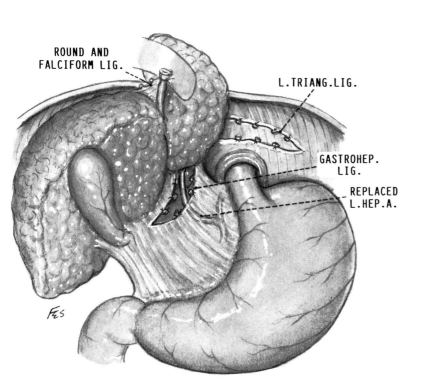

18. DIVISION OF FALCIFORM, LEFT TRIANGULAR, AND HEPATOGASTRIC LIGAMENTS

▼

The round ligament is divided between heavy silk sutures. The falciform ligament is divided in stepwise fashion between sutures. Simple electrocautery can eventually result in excessive hemorrhage. In a similar way, the left triangular ligament is divided in stepwise fashion between silk sutures. The left lateral lobe of the liver is rotated cephalad to expose the hepatogastric ligament, which is incised adjacent to the hepatoduodenal ligament in a thin area. This dissection is carried superiorly in stepwise fashion to the diaphragm just to the left of the inferior vena cava. Caution should be taken to identify and not yet divide a replaced left hepatic artery, when present.

19. DISSECTION OF HEPATODUODENAL LIGAMENT

▼

The peritoneum overlying the cystic duct and the cystic artery is divided between sutures. The cystic duct and cystic artery are identified and divided between sutures, thus providing better exposure to the portal triad. The peritoneum overlying the portal triad adjacent to the liver is divided between sutures. The common hepatic duct is identified in the right lateral aspect and without excessive skeletonization is divided between silk sutures near the bifurcation. Caution is advised in this area not to divide a replaced right hepatic artery, when present. The proper hepatic artery on its anterior surface is dissected 1 or 2 cm onto the left and right branches and inferiorly 1 or 2 cm onto the gastroduodenal artery. The dissection of the artery is carefully extended circumferentially. Soft tissues between the artery and

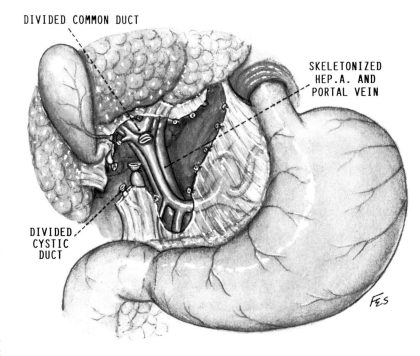

DIVIDED COMMON DUCT

SKELETONIZED HEP.A. AND PORTAL VEIN

DIVIDED CYSTIC DUCT

FES

the portal vein are divided between sutures. Soft tissues posterior to the portal vein are divided between sutures. Thus, the portal vein and hepatic artery are completely skeletonized in the region of their bifurcation as shown.

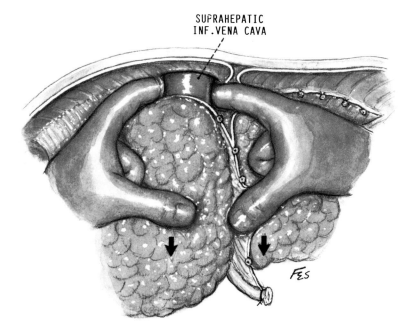

SUPRAHEPATIC INF.VENA CAVA

FES

20. MOBILIZATION OF INFRAHEPATIC AND SUPRAHEPATIC INFERIOR VENA CAVA

▼

The peritoneum overlying the inferior vena cava just below the liver and adjacent to the portal vein is divided for a distance of approximately 3 cm between silk sutures. The surgeon bluntly encircles the inferior vena cava with a finger as shown in Figure 11B of the donor operation.

Attention is turned to the inferior vena cava above the level of the liver where the surgeon institutes blunt finger dissection of soft tissues on the lateral and posterior aspects of the inferior vena cava while at the same time providing downward traction on the liver away from the diaphragm.

21. VENOVENOUS BYPASS

▼

A cannula is inserted in the left saphenous vein up to the iliac vein and held in place with a Rumel tourniquet. A second cannula is inserted into the left axillary vein up to the left subclavian vein, again held in place with a Rumel tourniquet. This peripheral venous bypass circuit is completed with a centrifugal force pump. The left and right hepatic arteries are carefully ligated and divided. The left and right branches of the portal veins are ligated and divided, with a clamp on the portal vein just above the pancreas. The portal vein cannula of the venovenous bypass circuit is inserted as the portal clamp is removed and held in place with umbilical tapes. Caution should be taken throughout the insertion process of the venovenous bypass to exclude air from the circuit.

MOBILIZATION OF RIGHT LOBE OF LIVER

▼

With the assistant providing traction on the liver, the right triangular ligament is divided. This dissection is carried posterior to the inferior vena cava where the adrenal vein will be encountered, dissected, ligated with silk sutures, and divided in a manner similar to that shown in the donor operation (Fig. 15*B*).

22. DISSECTION OF LIVER, HEPATIC VEINS, AND INFERIOR VENA CAVA

▼

A and *B*, Vascular clamps are placed on the previously mobilized inferior vena cava above and below the liver. An incision is made in the substance of the liver overlying the inferior vena cava for a distance of 4 to 5 cm. With use of blunt and sharp dissection, the right, middle, and left hepatic veins are dissected and divided 3 cm before their confluence with the inferior vena cava. Further dissection

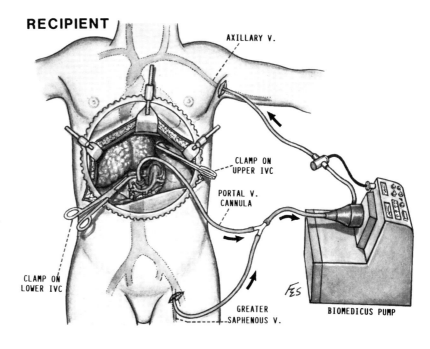

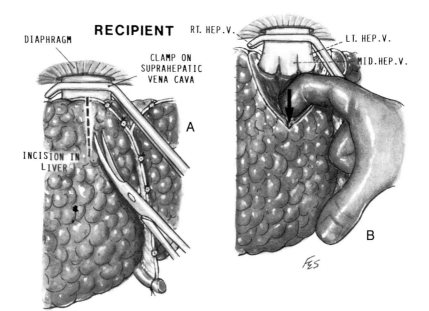

through the hepatic substance will reveal the inferior vena cava, which is also divided at this level. The inferior vena cava is divided where it enters the liver substance just below the liver, making it possible to remove the diseased organ.

23. CONTROL OF RETROPERITONEAL HEMORRHAGE

The appearance of the surgical field with the liver resected is shown. Points of hemorrhage in the retroperitoneum are easily visualized. With use of a monofilament suture, the edges of the peritoneum on either side of the bare area can be approximated. Other points of hemorrhage are controlled with figure-of-eight sutures. Alternatively, an electrocautery can be used extensively on the bare area.

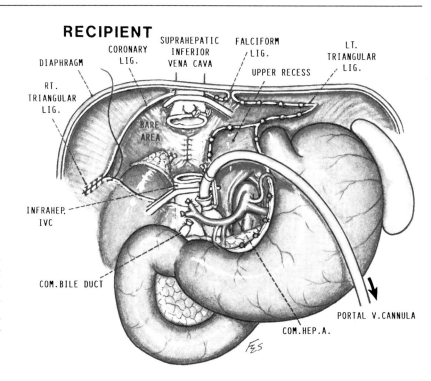

RECIPIENT

Implantation of the Graft

24. TAILORING AND ANASTOMOSIS OF SUPRAHEPATIC INFERIOR VENA CAVA

Soft tissues posterior to the vena cava are divided up to the previously placed vascular clamp. The middle and left hepatic veins are ligated with heavy silk sutures. Phrenic branches are ligated. The crotch between the right hepatic vein and the inferior vena cava is opened, providing a large single channel. Ragged margins are trimmed. The final product is shown in *A*.

Stay sutures of 3-0 polypropylene (Prolene) are placed on each lateral aspect of the donor and recipient suprahepatic inferior vena cava and are held taut. The left suture is tied, and the needle is passed from outside to inside the vena cava. The posterior wall is constructed from left to right using a continuous vertical mattress suture technique as shown in *B*. At the right lateral aspect of the anastomosis, the suture is again brought from inside to outside of the inferior vena cava and the anterior wall con-

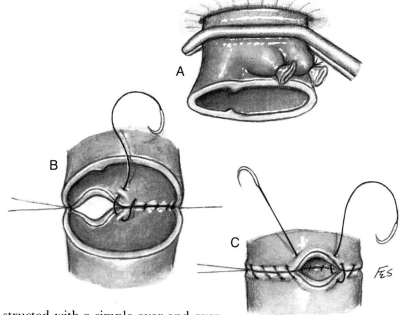

structed with a simple over-and-over suture technique. *C*, When the suture has reached the midline of the anterior wall of the inferior vena cava, the other needle of the double-arm suture on the left lateral aspect of the inferior vena cava is brought from left to right, and the two ends are tied in the anterior midline of the inferior vena cava.

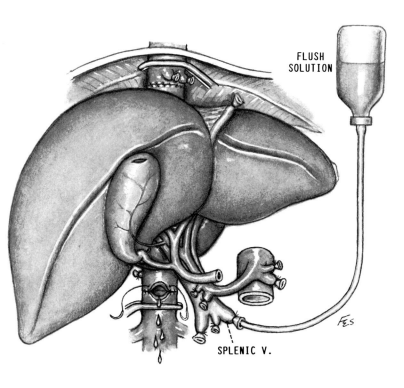

FLUSH SOLUTION

SPLENIC V.

25. INFRAHEPATIC INFERIOR VENA CAVAL ANASTOMOSIS

▼

The suture technique for this anastomosis is exactly the same as for the supracaval inferior vena caval anastomosis except that 4-0 polypropylene is the suture material. Near the completion of this anastomosis, before tying down the sutures, the portal vein must be irrigated through the splenic vein cannula with 500 ml of cold balanced saline solution to remove the high potassium preservation solution and any air in the liver and inferior vena cava.

26. PORTAL VEIN ANASTOMOSIS

▼

A and B, The recipient portal vein cannula is removed, but peripheral venovenous bypass is maintained. A vascular clamp is placed just above the level of the pancreas to control inflow. The donor and recipient portal veins are tailored to the appropriate length with one or two packs placed above the right lobe of the liver. This anastomotic technique is similar to the inferior vena caval technique, although the suture material is 5-0 polypropylene and the technique is more delicate. The portal, suprahepatic, and infrahepatic vas-

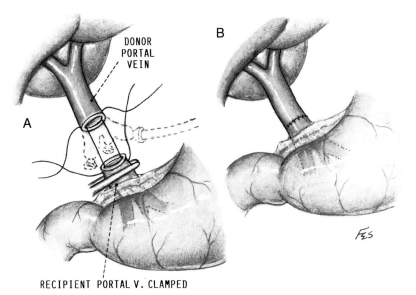

DONOR PORTAL VEIN

B

A

RECIPIENT PORTAL V. CLAMPED

cular clamps are removed to perfuse the graft. The axillary and saphenous vein cannulas are removed, taking the patient off bypass.

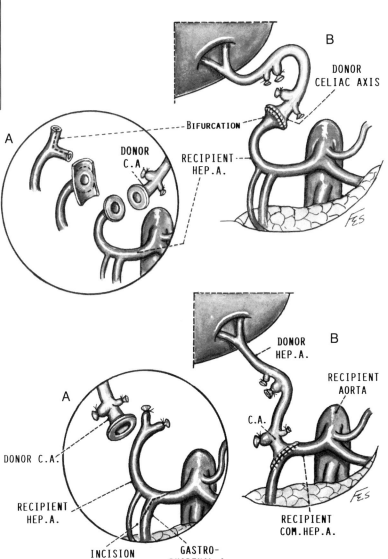

27. STANDARD ARTERIAL RECONSTRUCTION

▼

A and B, When the donor hepatic artery is of reasonable caliber and the celiac axis is not excessively diseased, a Carrel patch is formed out of the adjacent aorta. When the recipient proper hepatic artery and proximal left and right hepatic branches are of good quality, the crotch between these two branches is opened, and a second Carrel patch is created. These two Carrel patches are anastomosed to one another in continuous fashion using 6-0 polypropylene.

28. ALTERNATIVE ARTERIAL RECONSTRUCTION

▼

A and B, When the proper hepatic artery and its branches are unsuitable for anastomosis, the proper hepatic artery is amputated at the level of the gastroduodenal artery, and the donor Carrel patch is anastomosed in lateral fashion.

29. ALTERNATIVE RECONSTRUCTION OF HEPATIC ARTERY

▼

A and B, The common hepatic artery and gastroduodenal artery of the donor can be fashioned into a Carrel patch when the celiac axis or common hepatic artery is unsatisfactory. Additionally, it is possible to form a Carrel patch in the recipient at the level of the gastroduodenal artery by dividing the gastroduodenal artery and the proper hepatic artery.

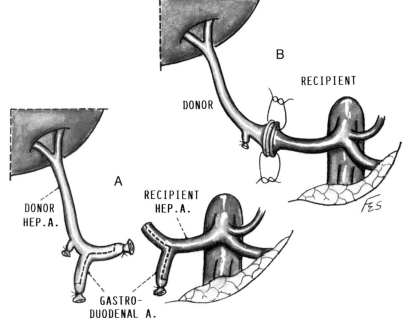

30. ALTERNATIVE ARTERIAL RECONSTRUCTION

▼

A and *B,* When the recipient hepatic arterial system is unsatisfactory all the way to the level of the splenic artery, the arterial inflow to the graft can be reconstructed by using donor iliac vessels. The recipient aorta is controlled below the level of the renal vessels, and the iliac conduit is sewn into the anterior surface. This iliac conduit is placed through a retroperitoneal tunnel behind the pancreas and to the right of the portal vein. At this location in the right upper quadrant, the donor hepatic artery is anastomosed to the donor external iliac artery conduit. Alternatively, when necessary, this conduit can be brought off the aorta above the level of the celiac axis. Although it is not

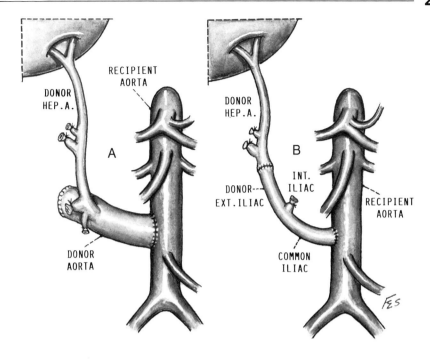

used frequently, in infants sometimes a piece of donor aorta is left attached to the celiac axis, and reconstruction of the arterial inflow is by aortoaortic anastomosis.

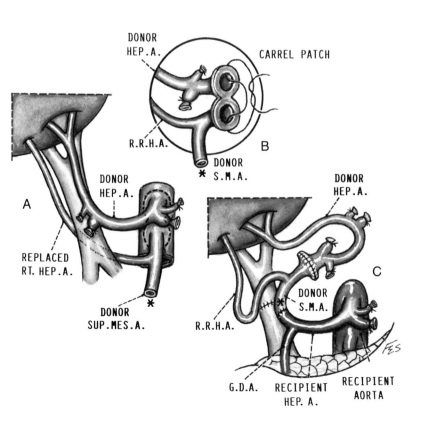

31. ALTERNATIVE ARTERIAL RECONSTRUCTION FOR DONOR REPLACED RIGHT HEPATIC ARTERY

▼

A to *C,* The donor mesenteric artery is ligated and divided 2 cm distal to the takeoff of the replaced right hepatic artery. The previously described patch of the aorta, which is taken around the celiac axis, is larger in these circumstances and includes the origin of the superior mesenteric artery. A figure-of-eight–shaped Carrel patch of aorta extends around the orifices of these two vessels. This Carrel patch is folded over and anastomosed with a running suture of 6-0 polypropylene. Inflow into both hepatic arteries is reconstituted in retrograde fashion through the donor superior mesenteric artery. Alternatively, the replaced right hepatic artery can be anastomosed to the stump of the splenic artery of the donor and the celiac axis used for reconstruction as previously described.

32. CHOLECYSTECTOMY AND RECONSTRUCTION OF BILIARY DRAINAGE

▼

A and *B*, When adequate hemostasis is ensured, cholecystectomy is performed. When the native recipient common duct is not diseased and is of good quality, it can be used for reconstruction of the biliary drainage by a straightforward choledochocholedochostomy. A T tube is brought out through the distal duct just above the duodenum, and a lateral suture in the duct ensures a watertight exit site. A posterior row of interrupted sutures of 5-0 absorbable material is placed and tied down. The T tube is placed into the donor common duct. The anterior portion of the anastomosis is completed with interrupted absorbable sutures.

When the recipient duct is unsuitable for reconstruction, such as in the presence of sclerosing cholangitis or with prior hepaticojejunostomy, a Roux-en-Y choledochojejunostomy reconstruction is performed. The posterior aspect consists of interrupted absorbable sutures. A stent,

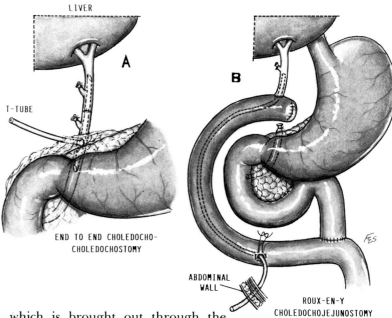

END TO END CHOLEDOCHO-CHOLEDOCHOSTOMY

ROUX-EN-Y CHOLEDOCHOJEJUNOSTOMY

which is brought out through the lateral aspect of the Roux-en-Y limb, is placed through the anastomosis and held at the level of the anastomosis with a single absorbable suture. Finally, the anterior aspect of the anastomosis is completed with absorbable sutures. The jejunum at the exit site of the stent is attached to the abdominal wall.

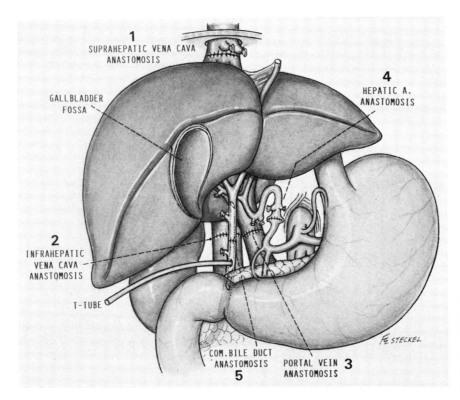

1 SUPRAHEPATIC VENA CAVA ANASTOMOSIS

GALLBLADDER FOSSA

4 HEPATIC A. ANASTOMOSIS

2 INFRAHEPATIC VENA CAVA ANASTOMOSIS

T-TUBE

COM. BILE DUCT ANASTOMOSIS 5

PORTAL VEIN 3 ANASTOMOSIS

33. APPEARANCE AFTER COMPLETED IMPLANTATION

▼

Note that the arterial reconstruction will be redundant in length. Flow through the arterial, portal, and inferior vena caval reconstruction is assessed using Doppler ultrasonography and a flow meter.

34. CLOSURE OF ABDOMEN AND PLACEMENT OF DRAINS

▼

A to *C*, The T tube or stent exits through the abdominal wall below the level of the incision. An extra length of the T tube is left in the abdominal cavity to avoid its dislodgment in the postoperative period. Three Jackson-Pratt drains exit through the abdominal wall. The right lateral Jackson-Pratt drain courses under the right lobe of the liver adjacent to the inferior vena cava and drains both inferior vena caval anastomoses and the subphrenic space. The left lateral drain is placed over the left lateral segment of the liver and again drains the suprahepatic inferior vena caval anastomosis and the left subphrenic space. The middle drain is placed just to the right of the porta hepatis and drains the bile duct anastomoses as well as the subhepatic space. The fascia is closed with buried interrupted permanent monofilament sutures. The upper midline extension of the incision is not closed entirely at the fascial level, although the entire skin incision is closed. By removing a few skin staples over the fascial opening in the upper midline exten-

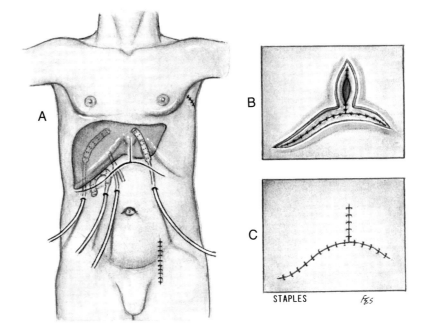

sion, it is possible to expose the liver graft for Doppler evaluation and biopsy purposes.

The axillary vein is reconstructed using a running 6-0 polypropylene venorrhaphy. The saphenous vein is ligated proximally and distally. Soft tissues are approximated with absorbable sutures, and the skin is closed with staples.

Placement of Hepatic Artery Catheter for Infusion Chemotherapy

J. LAWRENCE MUNSON, M.D.

▼ IMPORTANT FEATURES

Preoperative Knowledge of Hepatic Arterial Anatomy by
  Angiography
With Unusual Arterial Supply, Single Catheters Require Arterial
  Anastomoses or Ligations of Major Celiac Branches
Search for Extrahepatic Metastatic Disease
Concomitant Cholecystectomy
Placement of Infusion Port Over the Rigid Structure of the Chest
  Wall
Ligation of Collateral Vessels to the Stomach and Duodenum

▼ STEPS OR PLANS

Marking Incision for Infusion Port Placement
Search for Extrahepatic Metastatic Disease
Identification and Control of the Common Hepatic, Gastroduodenal,
  and Proper Hepatic Arteries
Placement of the Arterial Infusion Catheter Through the
  Gastroduodenal Artery into the Proper Hepatic Artery
Confirmation of Bilobar Infusion by Fluorescein Study
Secure Attachment of Arterial Cannula to the Gastroduodenal Artery
Extrapleural Catheter Exits from the Abdomen and Subcutaneous
  Course to the Infusion Port
Creation of Subcutaneous Pocket for the Arterial Port
Secure Attachment of the Infusion Port to the Chest Wall

1. SITE MARKED FOR INFUSION PORT AND INCISION

▼

The pocket for the infusion port is marked out on the chest wall so that the port will overlie a bony prominence to permit easy access. The abdominal incision is planned appropriately as a long right subcostal incision, which can be extended to a bilateral subcostal incision. Alternatively, an upper abdominal vertical incision can be used.

The pocket for the infusion port is not created at the outset of the operation because disseminated disease can force abandonment of the procedure. Exploratory laparotomy is undertaken, and a meticulous search is made for extrahepatic metastatic disease. Attention is paid to the pelvic cul-de-sac, the periaortic and celiac nodes, and the mesenteric lymph nodes. Any enlarged or palpably sus-

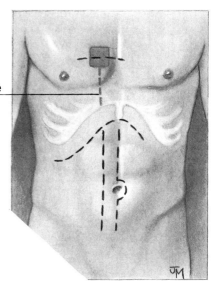

Subcutaneous course of catheter

picious nodes and any suspicious nodules in the pelvis are submitted for biopsy. Finding metastatic extrahepatic disease argues against placement of a hepatic artery infusion catheter.

2. INFUSION EQUIPMENT

▼

The arterial infusion port comes in several designs. However, we favor a high-profile port with sites for secure suture attachment to the chest wall. The arterial catheter is noteworthy for its thick wall, small inside diameter, and a beaded end for placement within the gastroduodenal artery. The catheter has a self-locking hub for attachment to the infusion port.

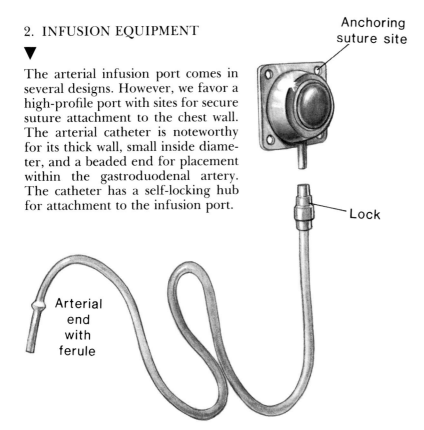

Anchoring suture site

Lock

Arterial end with ferule

3. CHOLECYSTECTOMY AND DISSECTION OF HEPATIC AND GASTRODUODENAL ARTERIES *(opposite page)*

▼

Cholecystectomy is performed to avoid cholecystitis as a complication of infusion therapy or arterial thrombosis; this procedure will also aid in the identification of the structures of the porta hepatis for further dissection. Arterial anatomy is defined by incising the hepatoduodenal ligament and skeletonizing the proper hepatic artery. The peritoneal coverings of the first portion of the duodenum, pylorus, and antrum are cleared, which also helps to eliminate the collateral flow from the hepatic artery that could lead to infusion gastritis and duodenitis. After the proper hepatic artery is identified, it is encircled with a loop for vascular control. Careful dissection is performed retrograde on the anterior surface of the proper hepatic artery

Figure 3 *Continued*
    to identify the gastroduodenal artery and the common hepatic arteries.

Commonly, the junction of these three major vessels forms a Y, with the gastroduodenal artery running inferiorly as the vertical limb of the Y. Other smaller vessels may be encountered branching off the proper hepatic artery running toward the pylorus or duodenum; these should be ligated in continuity to prevent duodenitis or gastritis from collateral infusion by chemotherapeutic agents.

4. PLACEMENT OF ARTERIAL CATHETER

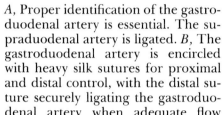

A, Proper identification of the gastroduodenal artery is essential. The supraduodenal artery is ligated. *B,* The gastroduodenal artery is encircled with heavy silk sutures for proximal and distal control, with the distal suture securely ligating the gastroduodenal artery when adequate flow through the common hepatic artery has been verified after temporary occlusion of the gastroduodenal artery.

An anterior arteriotomy is made on the gastroduodenal artery, and the beaded end of the infusion catheter is inserted with the aid of a catheter introducer or fine hemostat into the gastroduodenal artery and advanced into the proper hepatic artery. Occluding the common hepatic artery immediately proximal to the takeoff of the gastroduodenal artery will aid in the placement of the catheter in its proper position. Care must be taken not to advance the catheter close to the right or left hepatic arteries or unilobar perfusion will result.

A fluorescein solution is then injected through the hepatic artery catheter, and a Wood's light is used to examine the distribution of the infusate to the liver. Fluorescence at the liver surface should be rapid and equally distributed to both lobes of the liver. Should only one half of the liver be fluoresced with intensity, the arterial catheter must be withdrawn to lie proximal to the takeoff of the right and left hepatic arteries. Alternatively, the tip of the catheter can be placed in the common hepatic

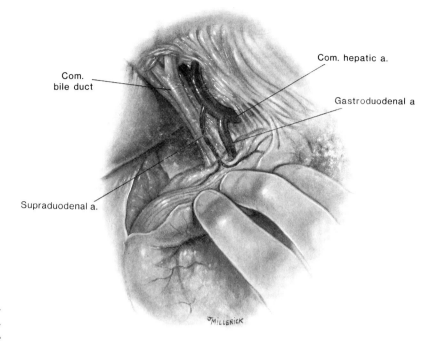

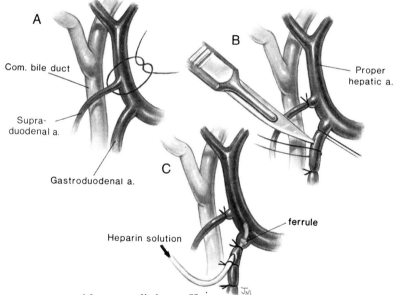

artery to avoid streamlining effects perfusing one lobe.

C, When the position is confirmed, the proximal suture on the gastroduodenal artery is secured immediately proximal to the ferrule on the cannula. The third ligature on the gastroduodenal artery encircles both artery and catheter to fix the arterial catheter within the vessel. At all times, while these securing ligatures are being tied, a steady infusion through the catheter is performed to verify flow. With adequate liver perfusion realized, the catheter is irrigated with a heparin-saline solution and capped.

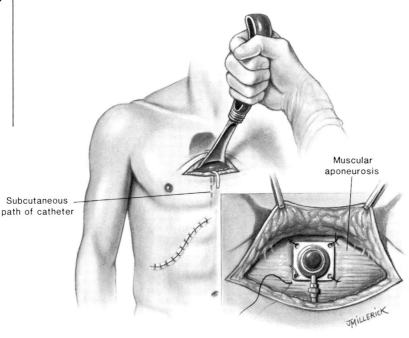

Subcutaneous path of catheter

Muscular aponeurosis

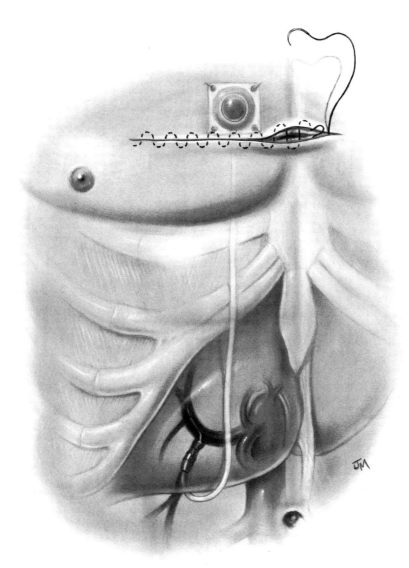

5 and 6. PLACEMENT OF INFUSING PORT AND CATHETER

▼

The subcutaneous pocket for the infusing port is now fashioned with a transverse incision overlying the chest wall as previously marked. The incision is carried down vertically to the aponeurosis of the pectoralis major muscle without violating the aponeurosis. Dissection is carried cephalad with the aid of a small right-angle retractor, dissecting only enough of a pocket to permit easy insertion of the port. Hemostasis must be meticulous in the construction of the pocket because hematoma formation around the implantable device will heighten the risk of postoperative infection. The pocket is irrigated with an antibiotic solution and packed with a moistened gauze sponge. The catheter is brought up anterior to the liver over the rib cage to pass subcutaneously into the pocket. This maneuver is facilitated by the use of alligator biopsy forceps passed inferiorly from the pocket through the subcutaneous tissue and into the abdominal cavity above the abdominal wound. The anesthesiologist is instructed to administer maximum insufflation of the lungs, bringing the diaphragm inferior. This permits accurate measurement of the length of the catheter, which should lie without tension when the patient assumes full inspiration. With an adequate distance to attach the catheter to the port within the pocket, the catheter is divided and affixed to the previously heparinized infusion port. It is important to verify that the specially designed locking hub on the port securely attaches the catheter to prevent postoperative separation. The port is sutured to the aponeurosis of the pectoralis major muscle with interrupted sutures of nylon. With the specially designed noncoring needle that comes with the infusion port, the system is aspirated to verify blood return, and a heparinized solution (100 units/dl of heparin) is administered.

Figures 5 and 6. *Continued*

The pocket for the infusion port is irrigated a final time, reassessed for hemostasis, and closed in layers with plain catgut. A subcuticular closure to the skin incision is performed, and the site is covered with a sterile dressing. The abdominal incision is closed in routine fashion. Care must be taken to avoid incorporating a catheter in the fascial closure. Administration of chemotherapeutic agents through the port may be started after full wound healing has occurred.

7. PROXIMAL TAKEOFF OF LEFT HEPATIC ARTERY

The variations in hepatic arterial anatomy are numerous and may force changes in operative placement. At times, more than one catheter may need to be placed, and dual infusion ports are now available. Other variations may necessitate arterial anastomosis, cannulation of the splenic artery, or placement of a smaller diameter polyethylene catheter fed from an externally placed portable pump.

When a proximal takeoff of the left hepatic artery is present, the right gastric artery is ligated in continuity, and the infusion catheter is placed with its tip upstream in the common hepatic artery to perfuse both left and right hepatic arteries evenly.

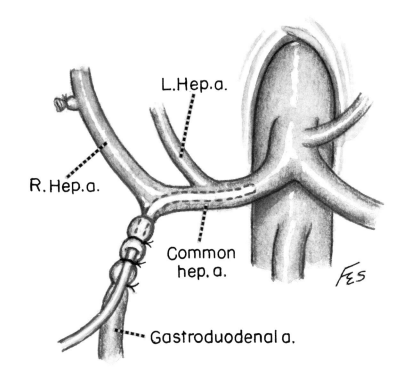

8. LEFT HEPATIC ARTERY FROM GASTROHEPATIC TRUNK

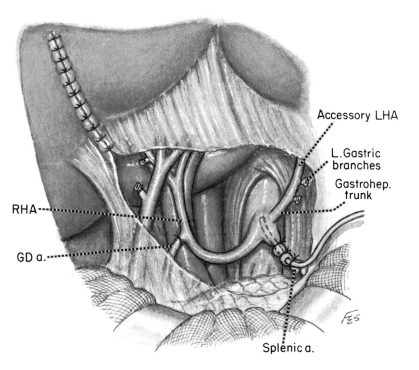

When a replaced left hepatic artery is present, the left hepatic and left gastric arteries arise from a gastrohepatic trunk off the celiac artery. The gastric vessels are ligated in continuity. The catheter can then be placed in the gastroduodenal artery and advanced upstream to the celiac artery or it can be placed in the splenic artery and advanced proximally. Alternatives include dividing the gastrohepatic trunk and anastomosing it to the hepatic artery, particularly when preservation of the splenic arterial flow is desired.

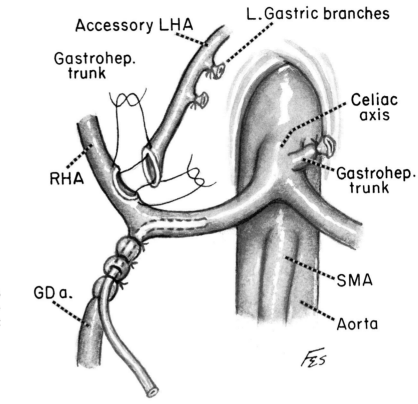

9. REPLACED LEFT HEPATIC ARTERY

▼

Another alternative is anastomosis of the gastrohepatic trunk to the hepatic artery with ligation of gastric branches.

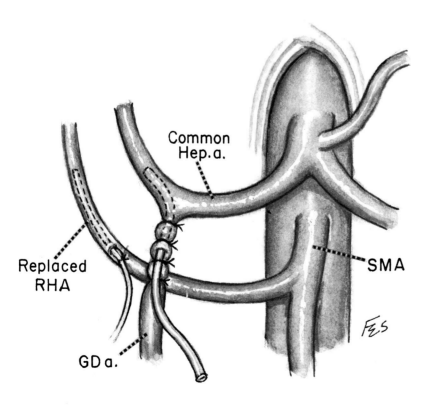

10. REPLACED RIGHT HEPATIC ARTERY

▼

When a replaced right hepatic artery (off the superior mesenteric artery) is present, the patient may require placement of two catheters or anastomosis of the right hepatic artery to the proper hepatic artery.

11. REPLACED RIGHT HEPATIC ARTERY *(Continued)*

▼

Alternatively, the variant right hepatic artery can be anastomosed to the stump of the divided gastroduodenal artery. This requires placement of the infusion catheter in the splenic artery.

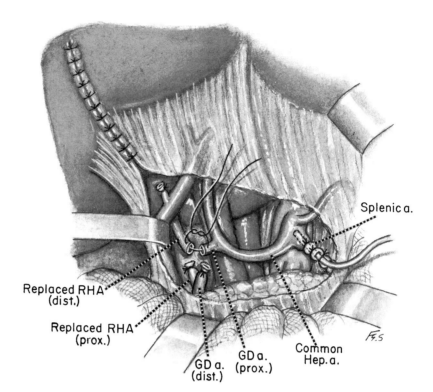

Splenic a.

Replaced RHA
(dist.)

Replaced RHA
(prox.)

GD a.
(dist.)

GD a.
(prox.)

Common
Hep. a.

37 Portosystemic Venous Shunting Procedures

RICARDO L. ROSSI, M.D.

▼ IMPORTANT FEATURES

Recognize Importance of Prograde Portal Flow

Choice of Shunt Depends on Multiple Factors (Anatomy of Portal System, Patency of Vessels, Degree of Ascites, Presence of Encephalopathy, Previous Operation, Degree of Urgency, Technical Expertise)

Adequate Exposure

Careful Hemostasis

Optimal Mobilization of Venous Structures Used In Anastomosis

Maintain Short Gastric Venous Circulation In Distal Splenorenal Shunt

Avoid Angulation, Rotation, Kinking, and Tension of Vessels Anastomosed

Accurate Venous Anastomosis Avoiding Narrowing of Anastomosis

Watertight Abdominal Closure to Avoid Leakage of Ascites

▼ STEPS OR PLANS

Portacaval Shunt

    Incision
    Mobilization of Hepatic Flexure and Kocher Maneuver
    Dissection of Inferior Vena Cava
    Dissection of Areolar Tissue of Hepatoduodenal Ligament
    Mobilization of Portal Vein
    End-to-Side Shunt
    Side-to-Side Anastomosis
    Graft Interposition Portacaval Shunt

Mesocaval Shunt

    Incision
    Exposure of Superior Mesenteric Vein
    Mobilization of Superior Mesenteric Vein
    Exposure of Second and Third Portions of the Duodenum
    Alternative Exposure Through Rent In the Mesentery
    Placement of Graft

Central Splenorenal Shunt

    Incision
    Disconnection of Gastrocolic Omentum, Short Gastric Vessels, and Splenocolic Ligament

Portacaval Shunt

1. INCISION

▼

Patient is positioned in 30 degrees of rotation of the thorax and abdomen, and an extended right subcostal incision is made.

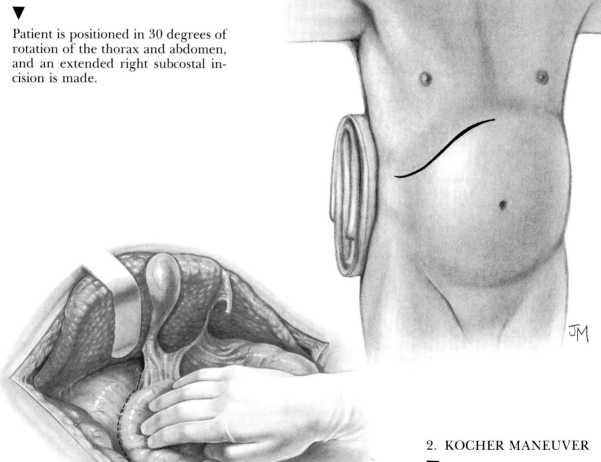

2. KOCHER MANEUVER

▼

The hepatic flexure of the colon is mobilized, and a Kocher maneuver of the duodenum is performed.

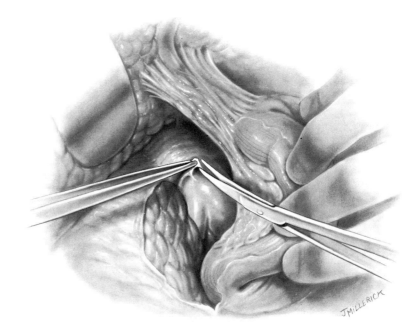

3. DISSECTION OF VENA CAVA

Elevation of the duodenum is completed, and the inferior vena cava is dissected from below the renal veins to the liver.

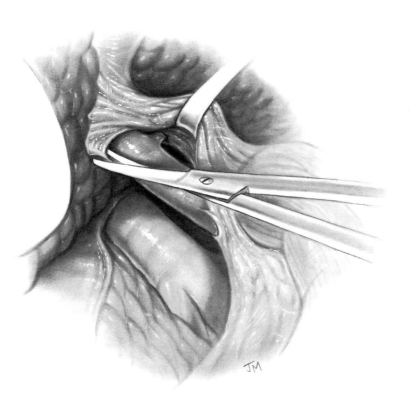

4. DISSECTION OF ANTERIOR SURFACE OF PORTAL VEIN

The areolar tissue posterior and to the right of the hepatoduodenal ligament is dissected off the portal vein.

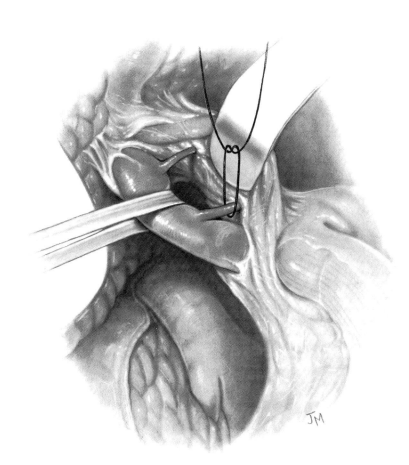

5. LIGATION OF MEDIAL BRANCHES OF PORTAL VEIN

The portal vein is mobilized, and its medial branches are ligated.

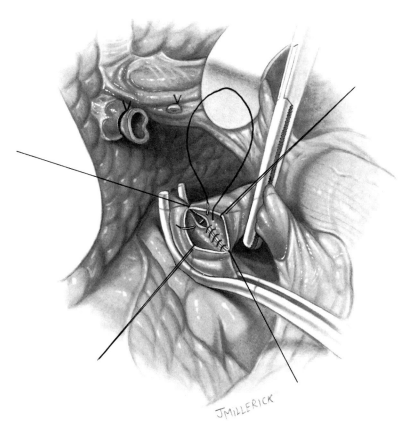

6. END-TO-SIDE PORTACAVAL ANASTOMOSIS

The portal vein is suture ligated and divided high. An ellipse of the inferior vena cava is excised, and an end-to-side anastomosis of the distal portal vein to the side of the inferior vena cava is carried out with a running suture.

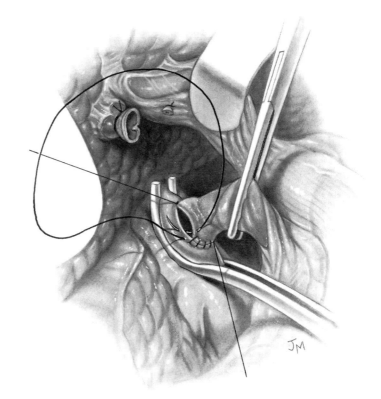

7. COMPLETED ANASTOMOSIS

▼

The portal vein is flushed, and the anastomosis is completed.

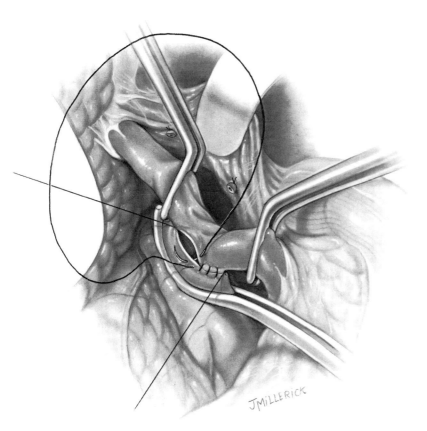

8. SIDE-TO-SIDE ANASTOMOSIS

▼

Side-to-side anastomosis is performed.

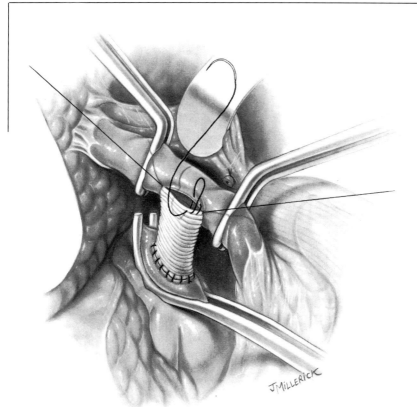

J. MILLERICK

9. GRAFT INTERPOSITION PORTACAVAL SHUNT

When portal and inferior vena cava veins can be approximated, a side-to-side anastomosis at times is preferable. When both structures cannot be approximated (that is, because of a large caudate lobe), a graft interposition portacaval shunt can be performed.

Mesocaval Shunt

10. INCISION

The incision is made upper midline to below the umbilicus.

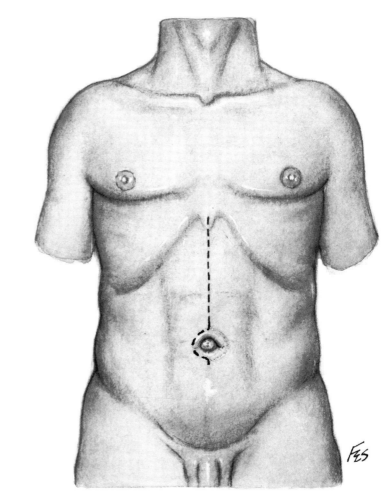

FES

11. EXPOSURE OF SUPERIOR MESENTERIC VEIN

The superior mesenteric vein is exposed through a rent in the base of the transverse mesocolon and small bowel mesentery. Mobilization of the ligament of Treitz, palpation of the superior mesenteric artery, and identification of the course of the middle colic vein can help in locating the superior mesenteric vein.

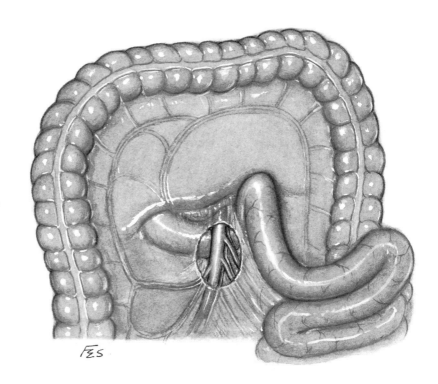

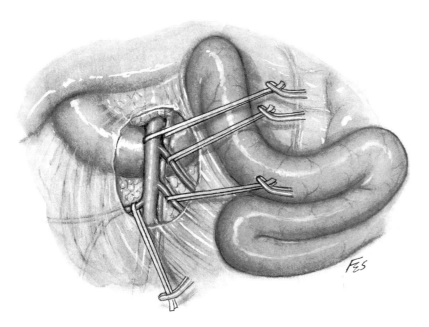

12. MOBILIZATION OF SUPERIOR MESENTERIC VEIN

The superior mesenteric vein is mobilized, and tapes are placed around a segment of the vein and its branches. Careful hemostasis of the vessels in the mesentery is required.

13. EXPOSURE OF INFERIOR VENA CAVA FROM BEHIND RIGHT COLON

▼

The inferior vena cava is exposed by extensive mobilization of the right colon to expose the second and third portions of the duodenum. Attachments of the right colon are divided between clamps and ligated. This permits mobilization of the inferior vena cava with dissection below the transverse portion of the duodenum.

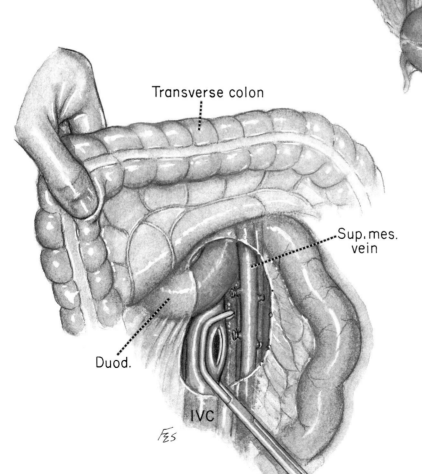

Transverse colon

Sup. mes. vein

Duod.

IVC

14. ALTERNATIVE EXPOSURE OF VENA CAVA

▼

An alternative route of exposure of the inferior vena cava is through the rent in the mesentery that exposes the superior mesenteric vein.

15. VENA CAVAL END OF GRAFT COMPLETED

▼

The anastomosis is accomplished by placing a graft between the inferior vena cava (inferior to the transverse duodenum) and the superior mesenteric vein. Grafts can be of Dacron (16 to 22 mm in diameter), internal jugular vein, or polytetrafluoroethylene, preferably externally supported. A fine vascular running suture is used.

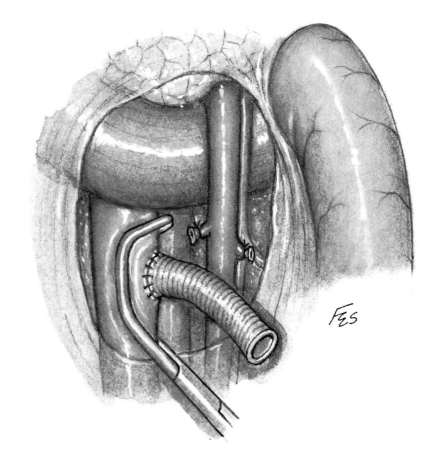

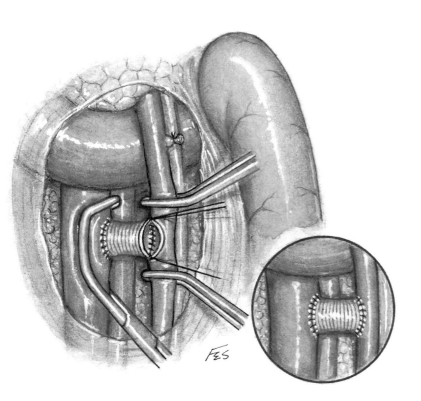

16. COMPLETED MESOCAVAL SHUNT

▼

Anastomosis to the superior mesenteric vein is partly completed. *Inset,* Completed anastomosis. An adequate length of graft and avoidance of rotation and angulation are essential.

Central Splenorenal Shunt

17. INCISION

▼

Left subcostal incision with extension to the right.

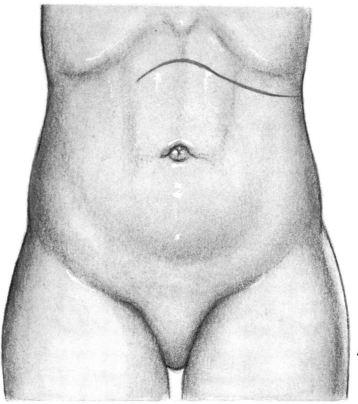

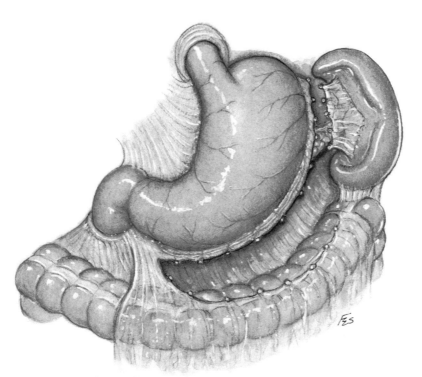

18. LESSER SAC OPENED AND SHORT GASTRIC VESSELS SEVERED

▼

The gastrocolic omentum and short gastric vessels are disconnected.

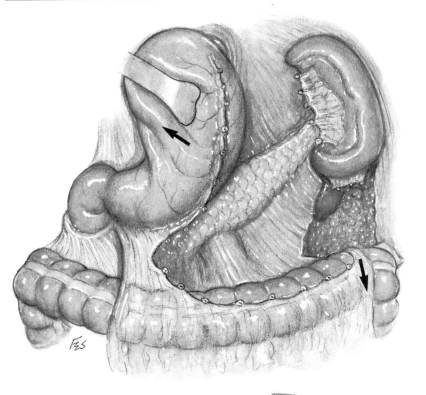

19. SPLENIC FLEXURE OF COLON LOWERED

▼

The stomach is rotated to the right, the splenocolic ligament is disconnected, and the splenic flexure of the colon is lowered to expose the pancreas.

20. MOBILIZATION OF SPLEEN AND DISTAL PANCREAS

▼

The attachments of the spleen and superior and inferior borders of the body and tail of the pancreas are freed.

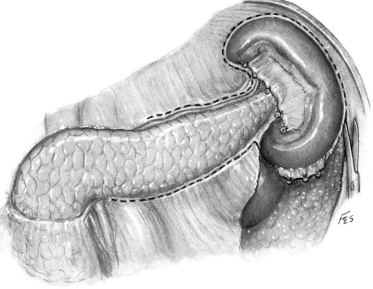

21. MOBILIZATION OF SPLEEN AND DISTAL PANCREAS
(Continued)

▼

The spleen and body and tail of the pancreas are elevated by blunt and sharp dissection. Note position of the splenic vein on the undersurface of the pancreas.

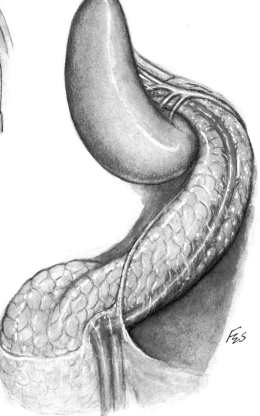

22. DISSECTION OF SPLENIC AND LEFT RENAL VEINS

▼

The splenic vein is carefully dissected from the body and tail of the pancreas. The left renal vein at the renal hilus is dissected toward the inferior vena cava, exposing the left adrenal and left gonadal veins.

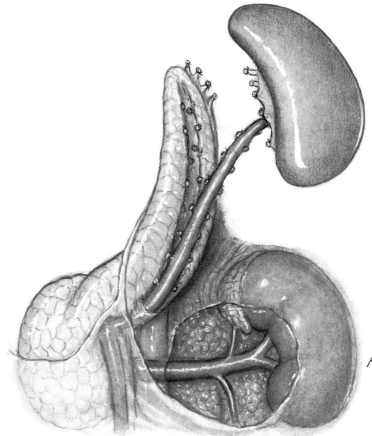

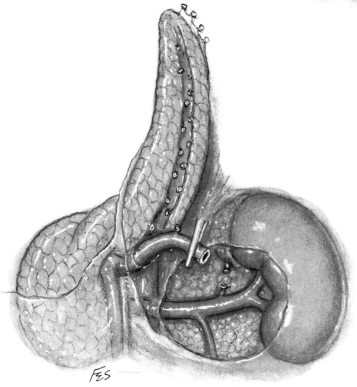

23. REMOVAL OF SPLEEN AND APPROXIMATION OF SPLENIC VEIN TO RENAL VEIN

▼

The spleen is removed, and the distal end of the splenic vein is approximated to the renal vein, avoiding acute angulation and rotation. The adrenal vein is ligated and severed.

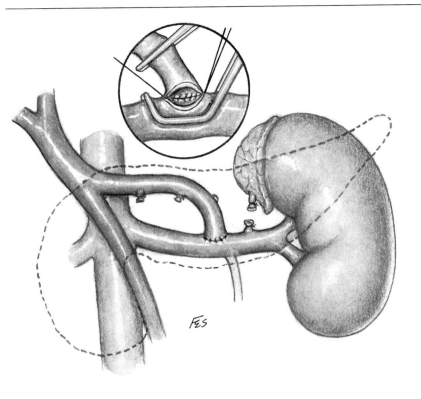

24. ANASTOMOSIS OF SPLENIC VEIN TO RENAL VEIN

▼

Anastomosis of the central end of the portal vein to the side of the left renal vein is completed using a running suture for the posterior row and interrupted sutures of fine permanent material for the anterior row.

Distal Splenorenal Shunt

25. INCISION

An extended left subcostal incision is used.

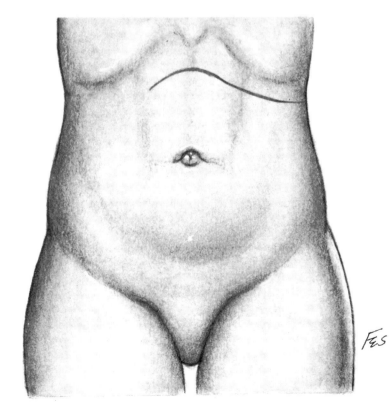

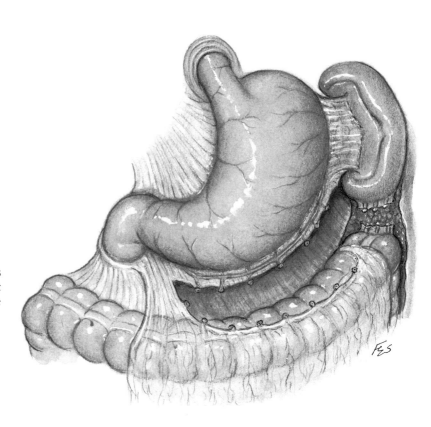

26. DIVISION OF GASTROCOLIC LIGAMENT AND PRESERVATION OF SHORT GASTRIC VESSELS

The right gastroepiploic branches are ligated and severed. The splenic flexure of the colon is mobilized. The short gastric vessels are preserved.

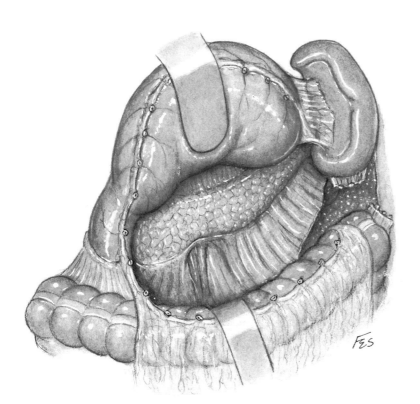

27. DISSECTION OF INFERIOR BORDER OF PANCREAS

The inferior border of the pancreas is dissected.

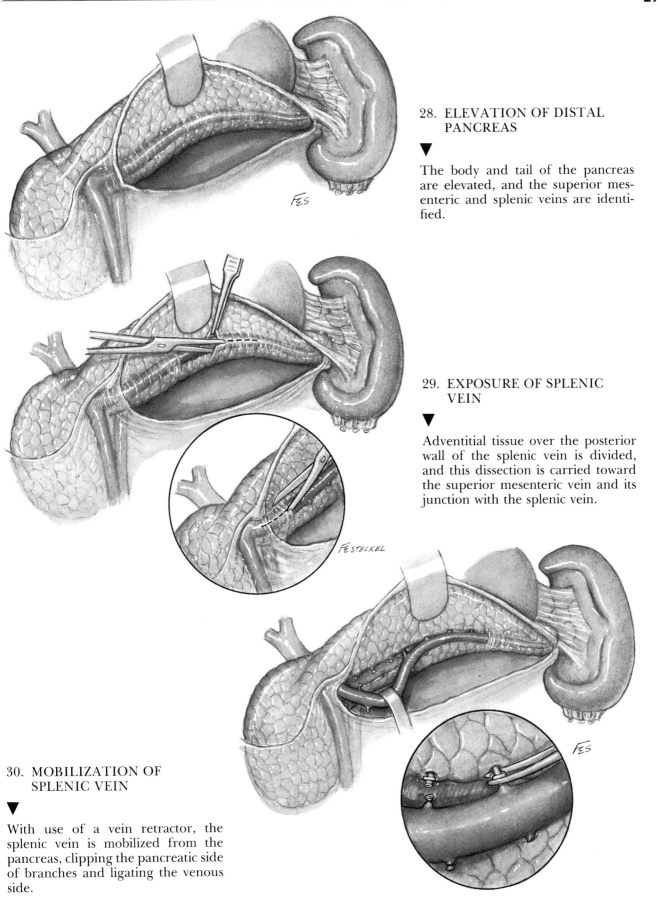

28. ELEVATION OF DISTAL PANCREAS

▼

The body and tail of the pancreas are elevated, and the superior mesenteric and splenic veins are identified.

29. EXPOSURE OF SPLENIC VEIN

▼

Adventitial tissue over the posterior wall of the splenic vein is divided, and this dissection is carried toward the superior mesenteric vein and its junction with the splenic vein.

30. MOBILIZATION OF SPLENIC VEIN

▼

With use of a vein retractor, the splenic vein is mobilized from the pancreas, clipping the pancreatic side of branches and ligating the venous side.

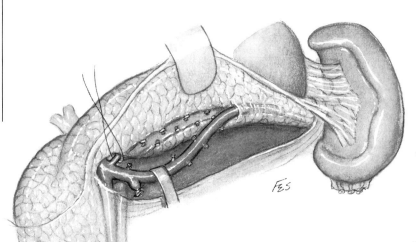

31. LIGATION OF CORONARY VEIN

▼

The junction of the splenic vein and superior mesenteric vein is further dissected to reveal the coronary vein joining the superior mesenteric vein. This branch is ligated either from below or from above the pancreas.

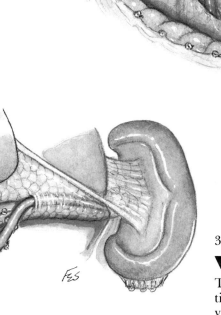

32. DISSECTION OF LEFT RENAL VEIN

▼

The left renal vein is dissected to free a suitable length together with the left adrenal and left gonadal branches.

33. SPLENIC VEIN SEVERED

▼

The splenic vein is divided at its junction with the superior mesenteric vein with oversewing of the proximal stump. The splenic vein is freed distally sufficiently to permit its end to reach the renal vein without rotation or kinking.

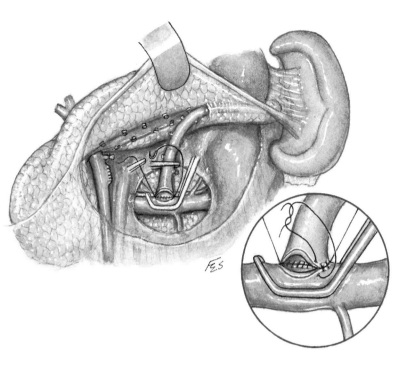

34. DISTAL SPLENORENAL ANASTOMOSIS

▼

The anastomosis is accomplished with a running suture posteriorly and interrupted sutures of fine vascular material anteriorly.

35. PATHS OF PORTAL DECOMPRESSION

The mechanism of esophageal variceal decompression is shown.

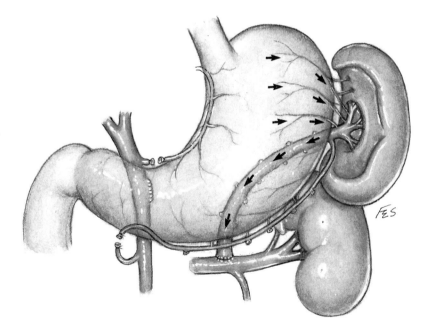

38

Cholecystectomy and Cholecystostomy

CORNELIUS E. SEDGWICK, M.D.

▼ IMPORTANT FEATURES
Adequate Incision, Good Light, Relaxation, Proper Exposure, and
    Perfect Hemostasis
Localization of the Cystic Artery Through Sentinel Node
Identification of the Cystic Duct and Common Bile Duct
Subserosal Excision of the Gallbladder

▼ STEPS OR PLANS
Incision, Including Division of the Round Ligament and Falciform
    Ligaments, and Separating the Gallbladder from the
    Surrounding Structures
Mobilization and Retraction of Adjacent Structures; Traction of
    Gallbladder into Wound
Identification of Sentinel Node for Localization of Cystic Artery
Ligation and Division of Cystic Artery and Cystic Duct

▼ SPECIAL SITUATIONS
Removal of Gallbladder from Fundus Downward
Cholecystostomy

1. INCISION

▼

A, The incision is subcostal or vertical, depending on the habitus of the patient. The subcostal incision is made 1 cm below and parallel to the costal margin, extending from the midline just below the xiphoid process laterally to the costal angle. The vertical incision may be right rectus muscle-splitting or muscle-retracting from the xiphoid process to below the umbilicus. *B*, The round ligament and falciform ligaments are divided to obtain mobility of the left lobe of the liver.

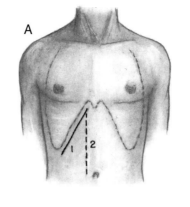

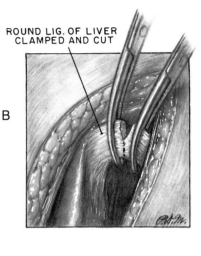

ROUND LIG. OF LIVER
CLAMPED AND CUT

B

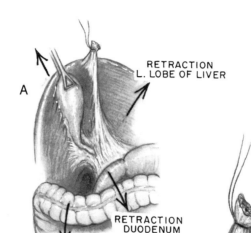

RETRACTION
L. LOBE OF LIVER

A

RETRACTION
DUODENUM

RETRACTION
HEP. FLEXURE

2. EXPOSURE

▼

A and *B*, The gallbladder is separated from the surrounding structures—stomach, duodenum, mesentery, omentum, and colon. The inferior tip of the right lobe of the liver is freed for partial mobilization of the right lobe. Air is permitted to pass under the diaphragm. A Pennington clamp is applied to the fundus of the gallbladder, and the gallbladder and partially mobilized right lobe of the liver are retracted upward and into the wound. Retractors are better for retraction than the hands of the assistants. The hepatic flexure of the colon is retracted downward. The stomach and the sweep of the duodenum are retracted downward and to the left. The proximal stomach and left lobe of the liver are retracted upward and to the left. The gallbladder and the porta hepatis are well visualized.

B

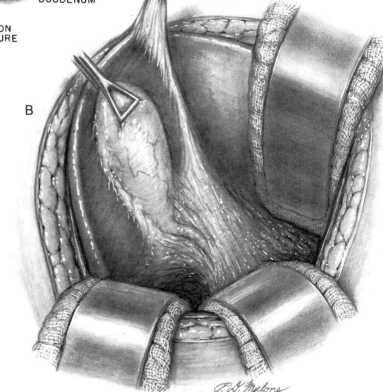

3. DISSECTION OF CALOT'S TRIANGLE

A clamp is applied to Hartmann's pouch for traction. The cystic duct lymph gland or sentinel node is the landmark for locating the cystic artery. The triangle of Calot is put on the stretch. The peritoneum of the mesentery of the neck of the gallbladder is incised both above and below so that the neck of the gallbladder is separated from its bed in the liver, and the contents of the triangle of Calot can be retracted downward into the wound for better visualization. Identification of the sentinel node locates the cystic artery, which is ligated and divided. Division of the cystic artery permits the cystic duct to be put on the stretch. The cystic duct is isolated from the surrounding tissue. Its junction with the common bile duct is visualized. Any calculi in the cystic duct are milked into the gallbladder. The cystic duct is ligated and divided 0.5 cm from its junction with the common bile duct.

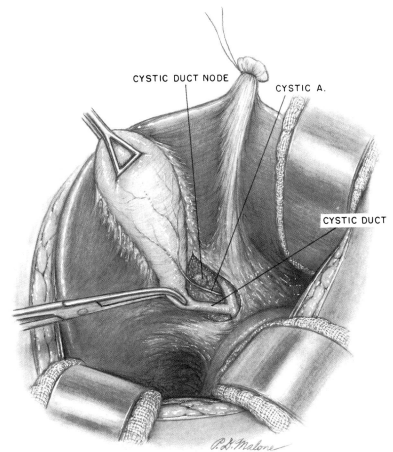

CYSTIC DUCT NODE
CYSTIC A.
CYSTIC DUCT

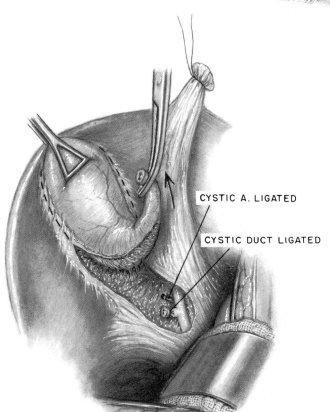

CYSTIC A. LIGATED
CYSTIC DUCT LIGATED

4. RETROGRADE EXCISION

The serosa of the gallbladder is incised, and the gallbladder is removed from its bed in the liver. Hemostasis is maintained. Careful visualization may reveal small accessory ducts, which require ligation, emerging from the bed of the liver.

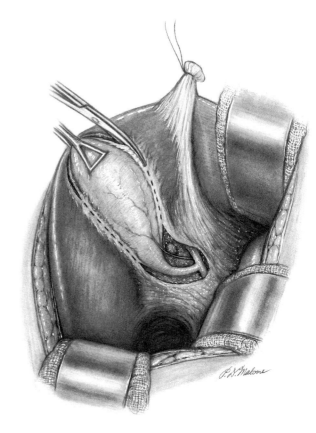

5. ALTERNATIVE EXCISION

Removal of the gallbladder is from the fundus downward. When difficulty is encountered because of unusual or obscure anatomy, it is safer to remove the gallbladder from above downward. An incision is made through the serosa of the gallbladder close to its liver margins, and the gallbladder is removed from its bed from above downward.

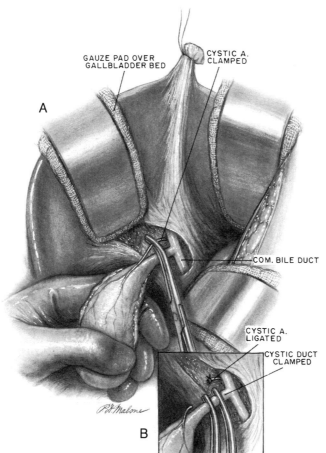

6. ALTERNATIVE EXCISION
(Continued)

A, A wet pad is placed in the gallbladder bed. A retractor is placed over the pad, and the liver is retracted upward. *B,* The gallbladder is now on a pedicle containing the cystic duct and the cystic artery, which may be isolated, ligated, and divided.

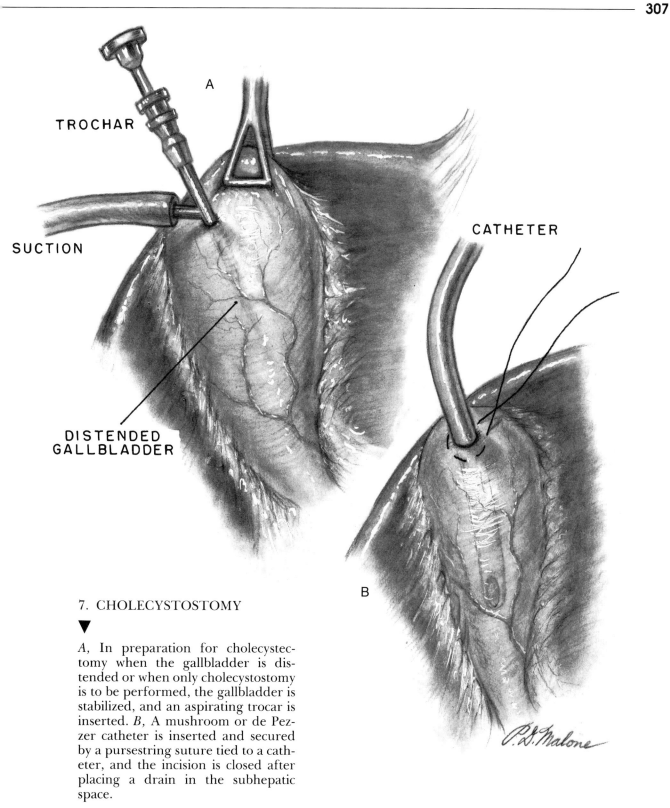

TROCHAR

SUCTION

A

DISTENDED
GALLBLADDER

CATHETER

B

P.D. Malone

7. CHOLECYSTOSTOMY

▼

A, In preparation for cholecystectomy when the gallbladder is distended or when only cholecystostomy
is to be performed, the gallbladder is
stabilized, and an aspirating trocar is
inserted. *B,* A mushroom or de Pezzer catheter is inserted and secured
by a pursestring suture tied to a catheter, and the incision is closed after
placing a drain in the subhepatic
space.

Laparoscopic Cholecystectomy

39

JONATHAN M. SACKIER, M.D.
J. LAWRENCE MUNSON, M.D.
RICARDO L. ROSSI, M.D.

▼ IMPORTANT FEATURES
Patient Selection
Teamwork
Appropriate Equipment
Safety Features
Abortion of Procedure in Unsuitable Patients
Localization of Hartmann's Pouch
Cholangiography
Localization of Cystic Artery
Excision and Extraction of Gallbladder
Inspection of Trocar Sites and Local Anesthesia

▼ STEPS OR PLANS
Preparation
Pneumoperitoneum
Position of Trocars
Retraction of Gallbladder
Definition of Junction of Gallbladder and Cystic Duct
Cholangiography
Division of Cystic Duct
Localization of Cystic Artery
Excision of Gallbladder
Hemostasis and Irrigation
Inspection of Trocar Sites and Local Anesthesia
Extraction of Gallbladder and Closure of Abdomen

▼ SPECIAL SITUATIONS
Hassan Technique of Open Laparoscopy
Dealing with Adhesions
Ligamentum Teres Sling
Insertion of Drain
Choledocholithiasis and Choledocholithotomy

1. PREPARATION

▼

It is important to select an appropriate patient. Initially, patients should be chosen who have symptomatic cholelithiasis, who are thin, and who have not had previous surgery. Obesity is a relative contraindication because insertion of the trocar is difficult. The presence of a cardiac pacemaker is a deterrent because deprogramming may occur, and during the time required to reprogram the pacemaker, uncontrollable hemorrhage may occur. Similarly, patients who are pregnant or patients with coagulopathy should not undergo laparoscopic cholecystectomy.

The preoperative work-up should include clotting studies and screening for common duct calculi. The novice surgeon should avoid patients with common duct calculi. Similarly, care should be taken to exclude the presence of an inguinal hernia because this can lead to massive inflation of the hernia sac during pneumoperitoneum if not noted and dealt with perioperatively by a truss.

The surgical team consists of primary surgeon, first assistant (ideally another surgeon), and a camera operator who is the surgeon's eyes and is vital for the expeditious completion of the operation.

The appropriate equipment should be assembled and should include high-flow insufflator (8 liters per minute), high-definition television monitors (two), color television camera, electrocautery or laser device, roller pump or other method to deliver irrigation fluid, suction pump, and video recorder to produce a permanent record of the procedure.

Because of the risk of deep venous thrombosis (caused by the position of the patient and the raised intra-abdominal pressure), prophylactic

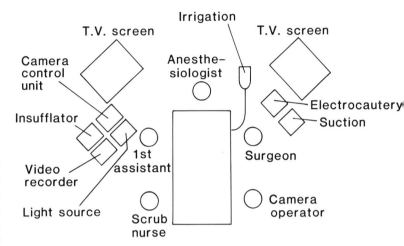

measures should be taken. We favor intermittent external pneumatic compression boots. When the electrocautery is used, the plate should be positioned on the anterior aspect of the patient's thigh. A padded footboard and thigh and body restraints prevent the patient from sliding off the table. The patient should have a Foley catheter and an orogastric tube in place, which can be removed after the operation.

The surgeon stands at the patient's left side. The first assistant is on the patient's right side; he or she controls the midclavicular and lateral trocars for manipulation of the gallbladder and cholangiography. The camera operator sits to the left of the patient, opposite the scrub nurse.

Conversion to open cholecystectomy is an option when, for instance, it is difficult to create pneumoperitoneum, adhesions are present, the cystic duct is short, Hartmann's pouch overhangs the cystic duct or is adherent to the common duct, aberrant anatomy is encountered, common duct calculi are found, or bleeding ensues.

2. PNEUMOPERITONEUM

Pneumoperitoneum allows room to maneuver in the abdominal cavity. A small stab incision is made just below the umbilicus in the midline. The Verres needle is checked for patency and to ensure that the hole in the obturator is opposite the bevel on the trocar. The assistant lifts the pannus, and the surgeon inserts and passes the needle swiftly through the abdominal wall. The operator should feel and hear a click as the obturator snaps back into the trocar as it enters the peritoneum. The disposable Verres needle, which also may be used, has a visual indicator to show the position of the obturator. Having positioned the Verres needle, the assistant should not release traction on the abdominal wall. A 10-ml syringe with 5 ml of saline solution is attached and twice aspirated and injected to be sure that it is in the peritoneal cavity. If blood is aspirated, the position of the needle is changed. If intestinal contents are retrieved, the needle is repositioned and laparoscopy is continued. After it has been assessed, an injury can be repaired immediately or treated conservatively. The "hanging drop" technique can now be applied. A drop of saline solution is placed at the top of the Verres needle, and the tap is opened. When the needle is in the peritoneal cavity, the drop will be aspirated into the abdomen.

The line from the insufflator is attached and insufflation with carbon dioxide commenced. When the needle is within the peritoneal cavity, the insufflation pressure is low (less than 4 mm Hg); the flow rate should initially be no more than 1.5 liters per minute to prevent the complications of rapid insufflation. Insufflation continues until a steady state of 15 mm Hg is reached. At this point, the Verres needle is withdrawn, and the incision is increased either circumferentially or longitudinally below the umbilicus to accommodate an 11-mm trocar. All taps are closed

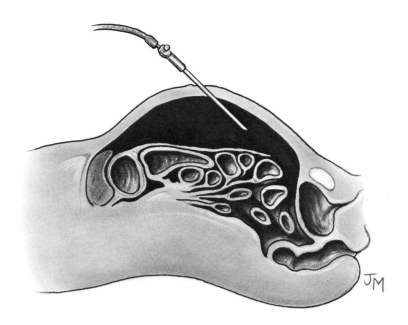

during insertion of the trocar; the operator's hand guards against accidentally introducing the trocar too far, thus avoiding damage to the aorta or iliac vessels. Disposable instruments can similarly be used. When a rush of air is heard from the top of the trocar, the stylus is withdrawn slowly (rapid withdrawal risks creation of pressure below intra-abdominal pressure and of sucking a piece of bowel into the lumen of the trocar, thus causing damage).

A 10-mm telescope, which has been warmed in warm saline solution, is introduced with television camera and light cable attached. The light must be turned down when the telescope is out of the abdomen to avert the danger of setting fire to the drapes, temporarily blinding the assistants, or damaging the television camera by "flare-out." The telescope is used to perform diagnostic laparoscopy. A 0-degree telescope is easier to use, but a 30-degree instrument permits inspection of areas that are difficult to reach.

3. POSITION OF TROCARS

▼

An additional vertical incision is made directly below the xiphoid process in the midline through which an 11-mm trocar is inserted under direct vision on the television screen. The point of the trocar should be aimed slightly to the right to avoid injury to the falciform fat pad with resultant bleeding. When the trocar has been inserted, a reducer is positioned through which an atraumatic grasping forceps is used to lift the fundus of the gallbladder to ascertain its mobility.

The best positions for the two accessory 5-mm trocars are then selected. The patient's position is changed from supine to reverse Trendelenburg, with the right side tilted up to permit the colon and stomach to drop away. As a guide, one trocar is positioned in the anterior axillary line above the iliac crest and the second below the right costal margin in the midclavicular line. When a fifth trocar is necessary to hold down the colon (four trocars and the laparoscope), the best site is the left midclavicular line just above the umbilicus.

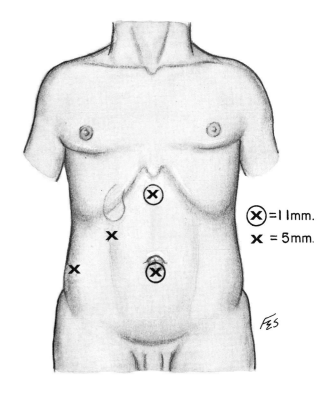

$(\times)$ = 11mm.

$\times$ = 5mm.

4. RETRACTION OF GALLBLADDER

▼

A grasping forceps with a lock is positioned through the most lateral trocar, and the gallbladder is grasped below where it is held through the subxiphoid portal. The gallbladder is retracted in a cephalic direction over the top of the liver. When an ideal position has been located, this grasping forceps is held in position with a towel clip to the drapes. Another grasping forceps introduced through the midclavicular line trocar provides mediolateral traction to Hartmann's pouch. When all four trocars are inserted, it is useful to add another insufflation line; the insufflator is set at 8 liters per minute. At any time during the procedure, if the anesthesiologist has difficulty ventilating the patient or if hypotension or hypertension or any cardiac arrhythmia occurs, pneumoperitoneum should be released.

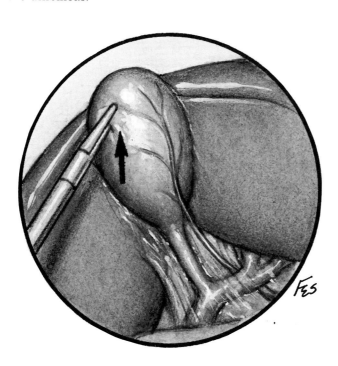

5. DEFINITION OF JUNCTION OF GALLBLADDER AND CYSTIC DUCT

▼

The hook-dissecting instrument is introduced through the subxiphoid trocar by means of a reducer. This instrument has electrocautery (usually set at 25 W of coagulation first tested on the liver) and irrigation and suction capabilities. The junction of cystic duct and gallbladder is defined, and the hook is manipulated up and down the cystic duct to create a free length. Through the subxiphoid trocar, a hemostatic clip is placed across the junction of the cystic duct and gallbladder. An attempt is made to identify the common duct before applying the clip.

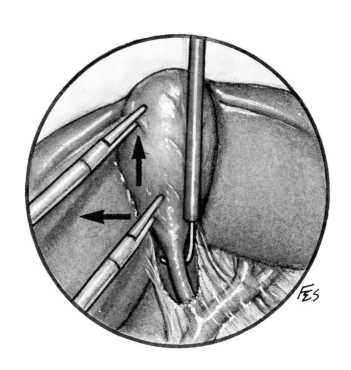

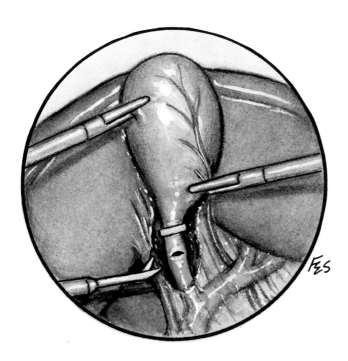

6. CHOLANGIOGRAPHY

▼

A grasping forceps introduced through the subxiphoid trocar is used to hold Hartmann's pouch. A microscissors is introduced through the midclavicular portal, and a small incision is made in the anterior aspect of the cystic duct just below the clip.

7. CHOLANGIOGRAPHY
(Continued)

▼

Through this same trocar, a grasping forceps with a No. 4 French ureteral catheter with an end-hole, having been flushed, is passed into the cystic duct and clamped to be used during cholangiography. Occasionally, it may first be necessary to pass a guide wire through the catheter should the valves of Heister impede its passage. The catheter is constantly flushed to ensure that saline solution passes easily into the catheter without leakage. The subxiphoid trocar is withdrawn over a radiolucent plastic obturator so that it does not interfere with cholangiography. Cholangiography is performed at this time. It is important to identify the entire extrahepatic ductal system, and specifically, the length of cystic duct below the clip before it enters the common hepatic, right hepatic, or common bile duct.

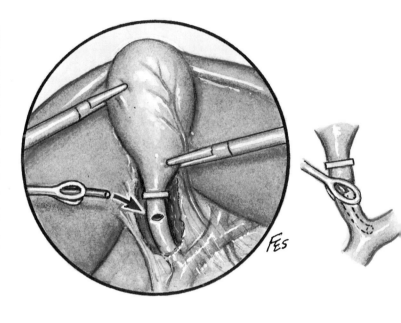

8. DIVISION OF CYSTIC DUCT

▼

Assuming that no calculi are seen, the telescope is reintroduced and the subxiphoid trocar is repositioned over the obturator, which is then removed. The cholangiographic catheter and forceps are removed and replaced with a grasping forceps. Through the subxiphoid trocar, a clip applier is introduced, and two clips are placed over the cystic duct below the incision. Through the subxiphoid trocar, the cystic duct is divided by scissors, leaving two clips in position. It is also possible to put one clip on the cystic duct and position an Endoloop on the common duct side of the cystic duct to lessen the chance of migration of the clip, which could potentially act as a nidus for formation of calculi.

9. LOCALIZATION OF CYSTIC ARTERY

A lymph node often marks the position of the cystic artery. This should be defined using the hook introduced through the subxiphoid trocar. The arterial distribution to the gallbladder is confirmed, to avoid confusing the cystic artery with the right hepatic artery. The cystic artery is doubly clipped below and singly clipped above and then divided.

10. EXCISION OF GALLBLADDER

By retracting the gallbladder in a lateral direction, the peritoneal attachments of the gallbladder to the liver can be divided on the medial side. By retracting medially, the lateral attachments can similarly be divided. The surgeon then works toward the fundus from the neck of the gallbladder, dividing attachments and sweeping the gallbladder in a cephalic direction.

HEMOSTASIS AND IRRIGATION

Before the attachments of the gallbladder to the liver have been divided completely, a careful inspection is made of the bed of the liver, and any bleeding points are localized, irrigated, and cauterized. The cystic duct and cystic artery are once again inspected to ensure that they are securely clipped or tied and that no bleeding or leakage of bile is present. Thorough irrigation is then carried out with 5000 units of heparin to each liter of saline solution so that any blood that has been spilled will not coagulate and can be aspirated easily. The final attachments of the gallbladder to the liver are divided, and a grasping forceps is positioned to hold the neck of the gallbladder.

INSPECTION OF TROCAR SITES AND LOCAL ANESTHESIA

With the telescope in the umbilical portal, insertion sites of the trocars

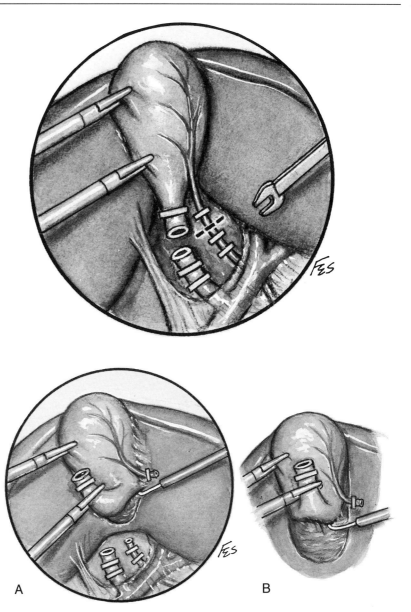

A   B

are inspected for bleeding. Because the only pain-sensitive structures in the abdominal wall are the skin and the parietal peritoneum, the latter can now be anesthetized with bupivacaine hydrochloride (Marcaine) under direct vision, raising a wheal by careful injection. This will ensure that the patient will awaken without pain. At this point in the operation, the anesthesiologist should give an antiemetic, such as domperidone, to limit postoperative nausea. The telescope is withdrawn and repositioned through the subxiphoid portal, and the subumbilical portal can now similarly be anesthetized.

11. EXTRACTION OF GALLBLADDER AND CLOSURE OF ABDOMEN

▼

A and B, Through the subumbilical trocar, a Kocher type of grasping forceps is introduced. The gallbladder is transferred to this instrument, which holds the gallbladder at its neck. The gallbladder is carefully drawn across the abdomen, and the neck is withdrawn to the surface of the abdominal wall, where a Kocher clamp is placed across the gallbladder. A small incision is made in the neck of the gallbladder, and swab specimens are sent to the laboratory for aerobic and anaerobic cultures. A neurosurgical suction cannula is introduced, and bile is aspirated. If small calculi are present, the gallbladder can be withdrawn from the abdomen by careful traction and rotation. If large calculi are found, it may be necessary to introduce a grasping forceps into the gallbladder and either withdraw each calculus individually or crush them. Occasionally, it may be necessary to stretch the subumbilical incision by passing curved Mayo scissors into the abdomen alongside the gallbladder or by passing a grooved director into the abdomen and cutting down on this.

It is now important to inspect all operative sites for bleeding and then

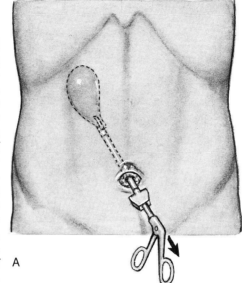

A

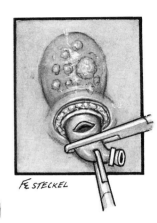

B

to release pneumoperitoneum completely. The fascia is grasped with two clamps at the umbilicus and is closed with interrupted sutures of 0 monofilament material. Subcuticular sutures of 4-0 polyglycolic acid are used to close the skin wounds, which are taped with Steri-Strips. The introduction and withdrawal of all instruments should be observed by the camera operator. To maneuver instruments blindly increases the danger of inadvertent trauma to other organs.

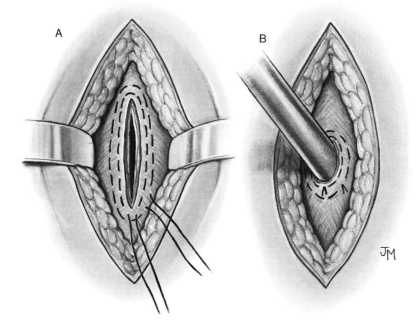

12. HASSAN TECHNIQUE OF OPEN LAPAROSCOPY

▼

A and B, In the presence of many adhesions in the abdomen from previous operations or when it is impossible to create pneumoperitoneum with a Verres needle, the technique of open laparoscopy is performed. The umbilical incision is continued down to the fascia, two pursestring sutures of 0 monofilament nylon are positioned, and a trocar sleeve minus the stylet is passed. The pursestring sutures are tightened, and insufflation commences through the trocar sleeve.

13. DEALING WITH ADHESIONS

▼

After the laparoscope has been inserted into the abdomen, the decision is made whether to continue or convert to open cholecystectomy. Adhesions to the gallbladder may be teased down with grasping forceps through the subxiphoid portal. They must be grasped close to the gallbladder and are *always* stripped toward the common bile duct—never away from this structure. Thus, the risk of cystic duct avulsion is reduced. When an adhesion appears vascular, it should be coagulated before division.

When difficulties caused by adhesions are encountered in inserting the subumbilical trocar and creating pneumoperitoneum, the surgeon can turn to the right iliac fossa, where a 5-mm trocar can be inserted through which a 5-mm 0-degree scope can be used to visualize insertion of the subumbilical trocar under direct vision.

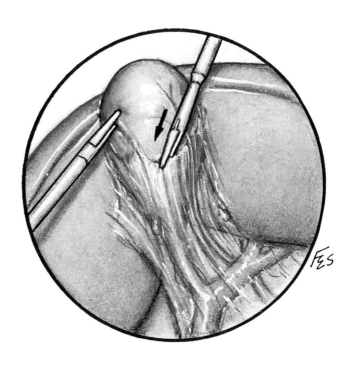

14. LIGAMENTUM TERES SLING

▼

When the falciform ligament is a fatty curtain obscuring the view and making manipulation difficult, a straight needle with strong monofilament suture material can be passed into the left side of the abdomen, grasping the needle within the abdomen and reversing the needle, passing it through the abdominal wall to the right of the falciform ligament. By tying this suture on the surface of the abdominal wall, the falciform ligament is lifted out of the way. The resultant tension on the ligamentum teres provides traction on the liver to raise the gallbladder, rendering dissection easier.

INSERTION OF DRAIN

▼

To position a drain for an oozing liver bed or spillage of bile from a tear to the gallbladder is a simple matter. After completion of the op-

Continued

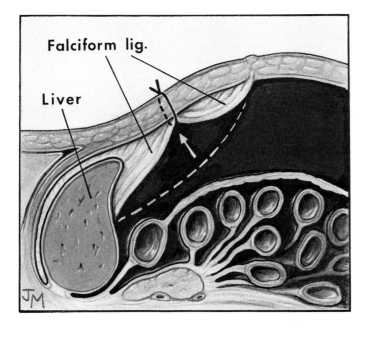

Falciform lig.

Liver

INSERTION OF DRAIN *Continued*

eration, a round closed suction drain is passed through the subumbilical incision and grasped through the anterior axillary line trocar. The drain is then positioned in the gallbladder fossa and pulled through into the abdomen. The grasping forceps through this trocar is used to pull the distal end of the drain outside through the most lateral incision, where it is secured and attached to a suction reservoir.

CHOLEDOCHOLITHIASIS AND CHOLEDOCHOLITHOTOMY

Unsuspected common bile duct calculi occur in 5 to 9 per cent of patients, and management of these calculi is controversial. In most circumstances, it is probably appropriate to convert to open surgery and choledocholithotomy with placement of a T tube. Some surgeons recommend postoperative endoscopic papillotomy, but in some instances this procedure is anatomically difficult and is associated with increased morbidity and mortality. It is occasionally possible to deal with these calculi laparoscopically. When the cystic duct is dilated, a choledochoscope, ureteroscope, or even flexible angioscope can be passed through the midclavicular line trocar under direct vision from the laparoscope. The trumpet valve on the trocar must be held open to prevent damage to these expensive and delicate instruments. The instrument is then passed into the cystic duct using the grasping forceps, and the television camera is attached to this flexible instrument, which is manipulated into the common bile duct. The calculus can be visualized and withdrawn with a basket. Obviously, it is vital to perform completion cholangiography to ensure that all calculi have been removed, after which the cystic duct is clipped and divided in the usual fashion. In only a small percentage of patients will the anatomy of the cystic and common duct junction render this technique possible. A spiral duct, for instance, will preclude this maneuver.

40

Choledochostomy and Choledocholithotomy

CORNELIUS E. SEDGWICK, M.D.

▼ IMPORTANT FEATURES

Common Duct Located by Its Relationships to the Common Duct
     Node and Pulsation of the Hepatic Artery

Possible Location of Replaced Right Hepatic Arteries Behind and
     Lateral to the Common Duct

Temporary Control of Accidental Hemorrhage by Applying Pressure
     to the Vessels with the Index Finger In the Foramen of
     Winslow Against the Thumb on the Anterior Surface of the
     Hepatoduodenal Ligament

Wide Kocher Maneuver

Exploration of the Distal Duct Is Performed with Great Care to
     Avoid Damage to the Pancreas and Postoperative Pancreatitis

Transduodenal Exploration of the Ampulla When Exploration by
     Choledochostomy Becomes Difficult

Operative Cholangiography and Choledochoscopy Are Adjuncts to
     Manual Exploration

▼ STEPS OR PLANS

Incision

Exposure of the Hepatoduodenal Ligament

Kocher Maneuver

Choledochotomy

Exploration of the Common Bile Duct

Removal of Calculi or Debris

Insertion of T Tube and Closure

▼ SPECIAL SITUATIONS

Transduodenal Exploration of Distal Bile Duct (see Transduodenal
     Sphincterotomy)

Choledochoduodenostomy (see earlier section)

Choledochojejunostomy (see earlier section)

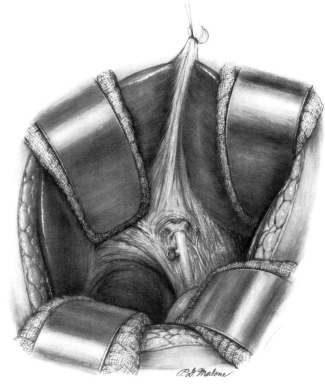

INCISION

The incision depends on the patient's habitus. The best exposure in a patient with a narrow costal arch is through a long vertical upper abdominal muscle-splitting or muscle-retracting incision. In thin patients, a midline incision is excellent. All vertical incisions should extend from the tip of the xiphoid process to below the umbilicus. In patients with a wide costal arch, a generous high right subcostal incision from left of the midline to the twelfth rib laterally affords excellent exposure.

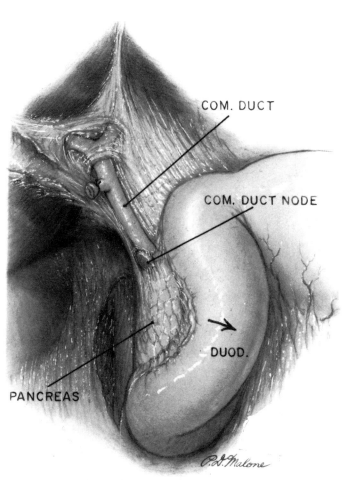

COM. DUCT

COM. DUCT NODE

DUOD.

PANCREAS

1. EXPOSURE

Exposure of the hepatoduodenal ligament and the common bile duct is performed the same way as described for cholecystectomy. The round ligament is divided to mobilize partially the left lobe of the liver, which may be retracted upward. The hepatic flexure of the colon is freed from adhesions to the undersurface of the liver and is retracted downward. The right lobe of the liver is retracted upward to provide countertraction to the partially mobilized sweep of duodenum. Thus, the hepatoduodenal ligament and its contents are put on the stretch and mobilized downward from the undersurface and hilum of the liver.

2. KOCHER MANEUVER

Before exploration of the common duct, a wide Kocher maneuver should be performed to permit accurate palpation of the distal duct and ampulla of Vater during exploration.

3. CHOLEDOCHOTOMY

▼

A and B, The common bile duct within the hepatoduodenal ligament is usually anterior to the portal vein and to the right of the hepatic artery. A finger in the foramen of Winslow may help define these structures. A longitudinal split in the peritoneum covering the structures in the hepatoduodenal ligament frequently permits the bile duct to bulge into the field, exposing its typical appearance. The visualized common bile duct should always be aspirated with a fine-gauge needle to be absolutely certain of its identity. The bile aspirate is sent for culture. Fine silk guide sutures are placed into the wall of the common duct, which is then tented for a small incision. The opening is further enlarged using scissors and a right-angle clamp in the duct as a guide.

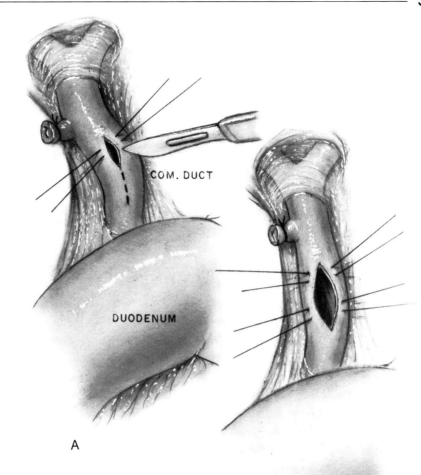

COM. DUCT

DUODENUM

A

B

P.D. Malone

4. EXPLORATION OF COMMON DUCT

▼

The common bile duct is first probed with a uterine probe, which is easily bent to the desired curve. First, it is passed proximal in the direction of the liver to identify the right and left hepatic ducts and their junction. Any possible obstructing calculi or debris is noted.

P.D. Malone

5. EXPLORATION OF DISTAL DUCT

▼

The uterine probe is passed distally and, when possible, through the ampulla of Vater into the duodenum. Extreme care must be used to avoid trauma and the possibility of establishing a false passage through the pancreas. The fingers of the operator's left hand around the ampulla can guide instruments through this structure. A right-handed surgeon may find it easier to probe the distal common bile duct from the left side of the patient. When the duodenum cannot be entered by the probe with gentle maneuvering, it is wise to perform operative cholangiography. When free passage of opaque material without evidence of obstruction is noted, further manipulation is not indicated. When the distal duct is

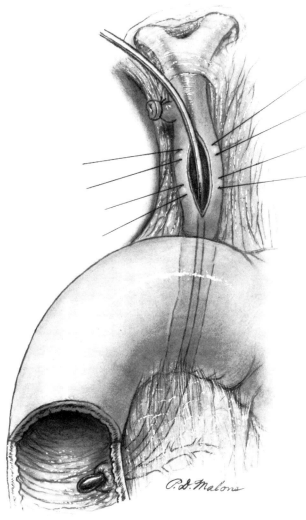

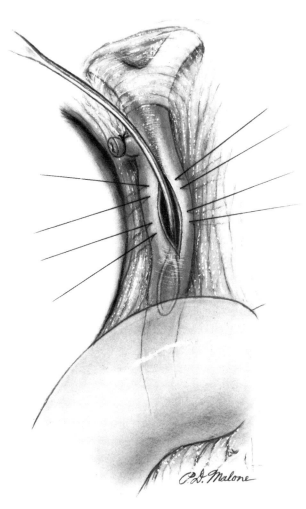

obstructed as observed on dye study, intravenously administered glucagon may relax the sphincteric muscles. When the history, laboratory findings, or palpation suggests an organic obstruction at the ampulla, transduodenal exploration of the ampulla must be carried out.

6 and 7. CHOLEDOCHO-LITHOTOMY

▼

Scoops, common duct forceps, and vigorous irrigation are used to remove all calculi and debris. For irrigation, an ordinary urinary catheter attached to a bulb syringe is used to produce pressure to flush out small calculi. On occasion, a Fogarty catheter is helpful.

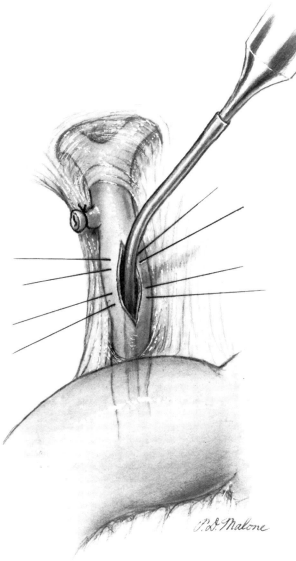

FIGURE 7.

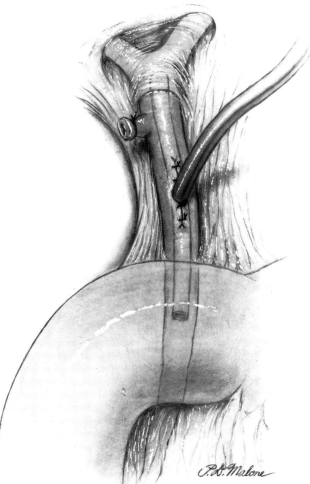

8. CHOLEDOCHOLITHOTOMY
(Continued)

A T tube with short horizontal limbs is inserted. A relatively large-caliber vertical limb is used for possible postoperative manipulation. The vertical limb of the T tube is brought through the center of the opening in the bile duct. The wall of the bile duct is closed with fine sutures of catgut. The T tube is irrigated to remove air bubbles, to detect possible leakage, and to ensure flow into the duodenum. Operative cholangiography is performed through the T tube. A small sump drain is placed in Morison's pouch, and the abdomen is closed.

41 Choledochoduodenostomy

CORNELIUS E. SEDGWICK, M.D.

▼ IMPORTANT FEATURES
Exposure of Common Duct as for Choledochostomy
Kocher Maneuver
Large Anastomosis with Interrupted Suture Technique

▼ STEPS OR PLANS
Exposure of Common Duct
Kocher Maneuver
Matching Common Duct and Duodenal Incisions
Interrupted Suture Technique
T–Tube Stent

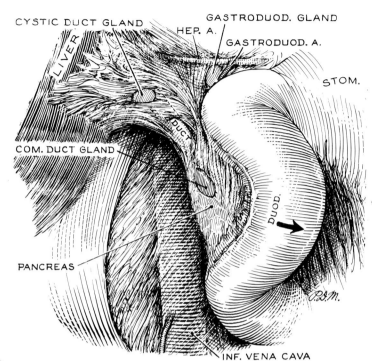

1. EXPOSURE AND MOBILIZATION

Exposure of the common bile duct for choledochoduodenostomy is the same as described for choledochostomy. The sweep of the duodenum usually requires mobilization as in the Kocher maneuver.

2. ANASTOMOSIS

▼

A to *C*, The length of the incision through the walls of the duodenum and the common bile duct depends on the diameter of the bile duct. Usually, the largest possible anastomosis is best. Interrupted through-and-through (all layers) sutures are placed through the posterior walls for a one-layer anastomosis. A large T tube is placed through a stab incision in the proximal common bile duct, and the distal transverse limb is placed over the posterior part of the anastomosis into the duodenum. This permits easier closure of the anterior wall of the anastomosis over the tube with interrupted inverting mattress sutures. Sutures are placed around the T tube, emerging from the common duct to establish a watertight closure.

42 | Choledochojejunostomy

CORNELIUS E. SEDGWICK, M.D.

▼ IMPORTANT FEATURES

End of Common Duct or Side of Duct May Be Anastomosed to a Simple or Roux-en-Y Loop of Jejunum Brought Either Anterior to the Omentum and Transverse Colon or Through the Mesocolon

In General, an End of Duct Gives a Larger Lumen for the Anastomosis and Affords Better Drainage for the Biliary System When the Duct Is Large

A Roux-en-Y Loop of Jejunum Brought Through the Mesocolon Reaches the Liver Hilum More Easily Than the Other Choices

When a Simple Jejunal Loop Is Used, Enteroenteroanastomosis at Its Base Is Advised

All Biliary Anastomoses Can Be Made with the Interrupted Suture Technique

▼ STEPS OR PLANS

Exposure of the Hepatoduodenal Ligament and Dissection of the Common Duct Are the Same as Described for Choledochostomy

A Section of Proximal Jejunum Is Identified Near the Ligament of Treitz, and a Loop Is Brought Up Over the Transverse Colon to Rest Comfortably Adjacent to the Common Duct

For End of Duct to Side of Jejunum Anastomosis, the Jejunal Wall Is Opened; Interrupted Sutures Through All Layers; T Tube Placed Before Final Closure

For Side-to-Side Anastomosis, Either a Single Layer or a Double Layer Is Suitable; T Tube Is Placed as with the End-to-End Anastomosis

1. END OF DUCT TO SIDE OF JEJUNUM

An incision, three-fourths the length of the diameter of the bile duct, is made through the serosa of the jejunal wall down to the mucosa. Bulging mucosa is excised flush with the jejunal wall. The posterior part of the anastomosis is made with interrupted sutures through all layers. A T tube is inserted through a stab incision in the proximal common duct, placing the distal limb into the jejunum. The anterior part of the anastomosis is also made with interrupted inverting sutures. Sutures are placed around the bile duct exit of the T tube to ensure a watertight closure.

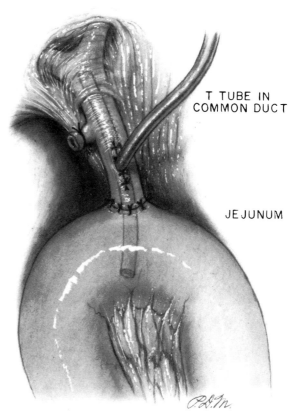

T TUBE IN COMMON DUCT

JEJUNUM

COM. DUCT

DUOD.

JEJ.

A

B

2. SIDE-TO-SIDE CHOLEDOCHOJEJUNOSTOMY

A and *B*, The antimesenteric side of the selected loop of jejunum is placed adjacent to the lateral wall of the common bile duct without tension. For a two-layer anastomosis, end guide sutures are placed in the jejunum and common bile duct to mark the extent of the anastomosis. A row of interrupted simple sutures approximating the posterior wall is placed. The bile duct and jejunum are opened, and the posterior part of the anastomosis is finished by a running locking suture, which is continued anteriorly as a Connell suture. The anterior wall is finally secured with interrupted sutures. A single-layer anastomosis using interrupted sutures is also satisfactory. Before closure, a T tube is inserted through a stab wound in the common bile duct, and the distal limb is passed into the jejunum.

Transduodenal Sphincterotomy and Sphincteroplasty

43

JOHN W. BRAASCH, M.D.

▼ IMPORTANT FEATURES
  Identification of Ampulla of Vater Before and After Duodenotomy
  Protection of Pancreatic Duct Orifice
  Adequate and Safe Division of Sphincteric Muscle

▼ STEPS OR PLANS
  Mobilization of Duodenum
  Palpation of Sphincter of Oddi
  Longitudinal Incision of Duodenum
  Recognition of Ampulla of Vater
  Elevation of Ampulla of Vater
  Dilatation of Orifice of Ampulla of Vater
  Section of Ampulla of Vater
  Location of Orifice of Duct of Wirsung
  Section of Orifice of Duct of Wirsung
  Suturing Apex of Sphincterotomy
  Optional Sphincteroplasty

INCISION

A long right upper quadrant vertical incision makes exposure of the second and third portions of the duodenum easier.

1. KOCHER MANEUVER

Beginning at the junction of the second and third portions of the duodenum, the duodenum is elevated until the aorta is bared. Especially in secondary cases, care must be taken to avoid injury to the left renal vein, which might be adherent to the posterior surface of the pancreas. The ampulla of Vater is located by pal-

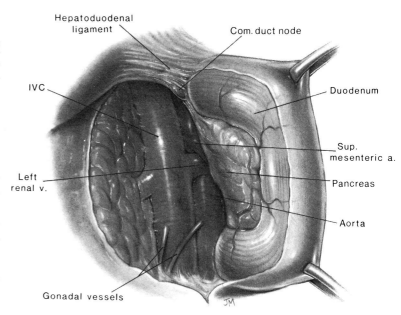

pation of its small sausage-like shape on the medial side of the duodenum. It can be found from the proximal second portion of the duodenum to the proximal third portion.

2. LOCATING AMPULLA

A longitudinal incision in the duodenum is made over the ampulla of Vater. The ampulla of Vater appears as a frenulum. Pressure on the gallbladder produces a stream of bile at its location or an instrument can be passed down the common bile duct to the duodenum for identification. Two Allis clamps grasp the duodenal mucosa superolateral and superomedial to the orifice to deliver it into the duodenotomy incision. No clamps should be placed at the 5 o'clock position, the area of the orifice of the duct of Wirsung.

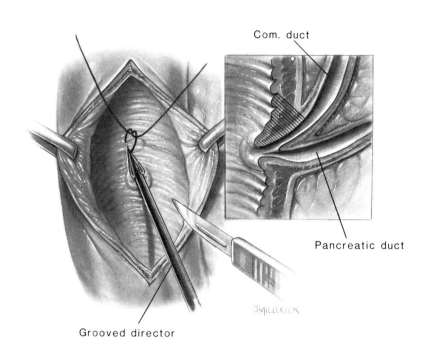

Com. duct

Pancreatic duct

Grooved director

JMILLERICK

3. SPHINCTEROTOMY

The papilla of Vater is dilated with graduated probes and a grooved director and then sectioned with Potts scissors or a knife blade for about 1.5 cm, care being taken not to penetrate the duodenal serosa with this incision. The apex of the section is sutured with interrupted simple sutures to close any gaps and to control hemorrhage. The orifice of the duct of Wirsung may be sectioned to enlarge it.

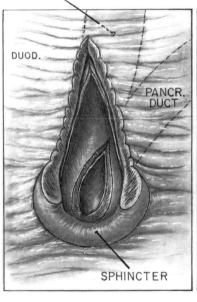

COM. DUCT

DUOD.

PANCR. DUCT

SPHINCTER

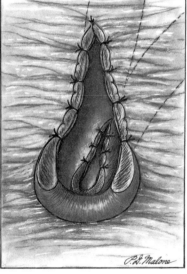

P.L. Malone

4. SPHINCTEROPLASTY

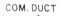

Alternatively, a pie-shaped piece may be taken out of the orifice of the ampulla of Vater at the point of section; the edges of the duodenal mucosa and the lining of the common duct are sutured. The edges of the pancreatic duct can be sutured in like manner.

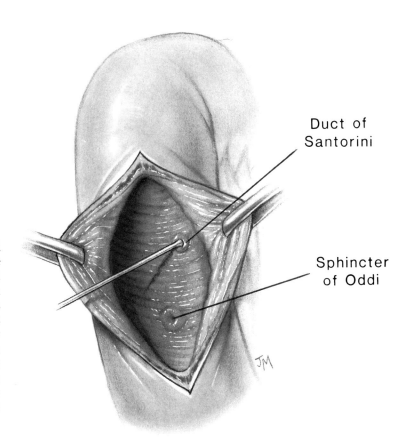

Duct of
Santorini

Sphincter
of Oddi

5. SPHINCTEROTOMY OF DUCT OF SANTORINI

The orifice of the duct of Santorini is located superior and medial to the sphincter of Oddi and may be dilated with lacrimal dilators in preparation for sphincterotomy. At times this is not possible because the opening is too small. In this case, it may simply be amputated. When its location is difficult to recognize, especially in pancreas divisum, the intravenous administration of secretin will cause a gush of pancreatic juice from the orifice for localization.

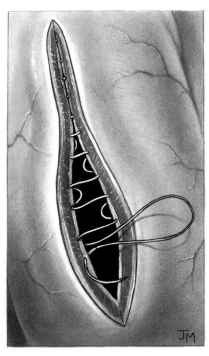

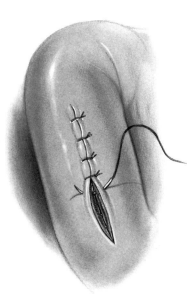

6. CLOSURE OF DUODENOTOMY

The duodenotomy is closed in two layers with an inner "table setting" running Connell chromic catgut suture for the mucosa and interrupted nonabsorbable sutures for the seromuscularis. Care must be taken to avoid inverting too much tissue, which might obstruct the duodenum.

44 Repair of Common Duct Strictures

JOHN W. BRAASCH, M.D.

▼ IMPORTANT FEATURES
Release of Adhesions
Locate Proximal Bile Duct and Confirm That All Segments of Liver
    Are Drained
Preparation of Proximal Duct, Resection of Scar, and Preservation of
    Blood Supply
Selection of Reconstruction
Stenting

▼ STEPS OR PLANS
Exposure of Right Upper Quadrant
Recognition of Proximal Bile Duct
Preserve Blood Supply of Proximal Common Duct
Preparation of Proximal Duct
Management of Strictures at Hepatic Duct Bifurcation
Choice of Repair and Technique
Alternative Repairs
Stenting

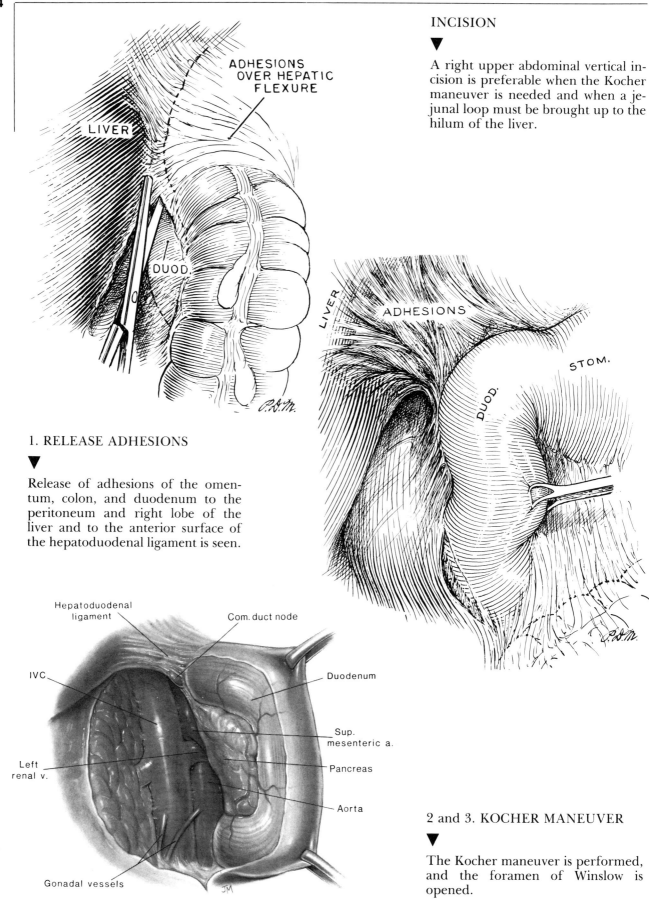

ADHESIONS
OVER HEPATIC
FLEXURE

LIVER

DUOD

1. RELEASE ADHESIONS

▼

Release of adhesions of the omentum, colon, and duodenum to the peritoneum and right lobe of the liver and to the anterior surface of the hepatoduodenal ligament is seen.

LIVER

ADHESIONS

DUOD.

STOM.

Hepatoduodenal ligament

Com. duct node

IVC

Duodenum

Sup. mesenteric a.

Left renal v.

Pancreas

Aorta

Gonadal vessels

INCISION

▼

A right upper abdominal vertical incision is preferable when the Kocher maneuver is needed and when a jejunal loop must be brought up to the hilum of the liver.

2 and 3. KOCHER MANEUVER

▼

The Kocher maneuver is performed, and the foramen of Winslow is opened.

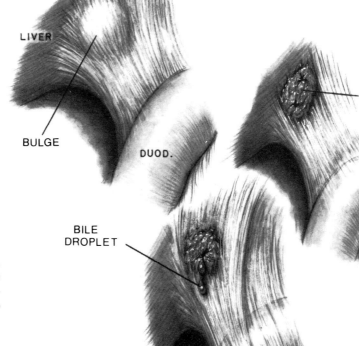

4. RECOGNITION OF OBSTRUCTED DUCT

The proximal bile duct is recognized by scar, duct bulge, suture, or bile droplet. The hepatic artery is palpated, and dissection continues into the scar at the porta hepatis.

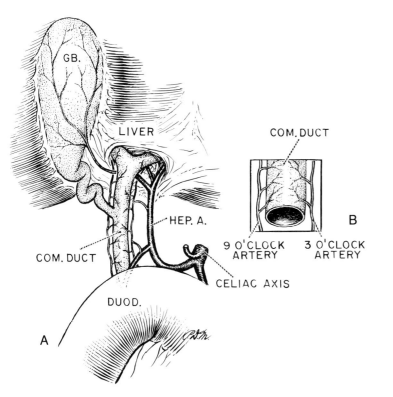

5. ARTERIAL SUPPLY OF BILE DUCT

A and *B*, Note syncytial nature of the arterial blood supply fed by twigs from two longitudinal arteries. Dissection on the proximal duct should not be extended too far beyond the point of anastomosis to preserve the blood supply to the tip of the duct.

6. PREPARATION OF PROXIMAL DUCT

A and B, Dissection continues up the proximal duct until 1 to 2 mm of duct above the scar is freed up. Failure to dissect the entire strictured segment is the most common cause of an unsuccessful operation. The stricture is excised. By probing with dilators or by cholangiography, it is proved that all liver segments are drained.

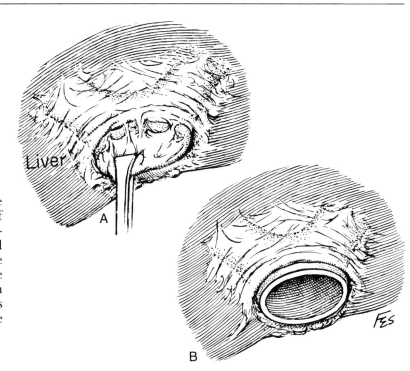

7. INCREASING DIAMETER OF DUCT *below*

With a stricture at the hepatic duct bifurcation, a plastic procedure on the orifice of the left duct can increase the diameter of the proximal duct for anastomosis.

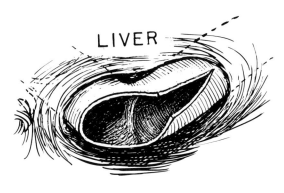

8. PROCEDURE FOR SEPARATED HEPATIC DUCTS

With partial separation of the right and left hepatic ducts, a septum can be created and incised or an existing septum can be incised to permit a single anastomosis.

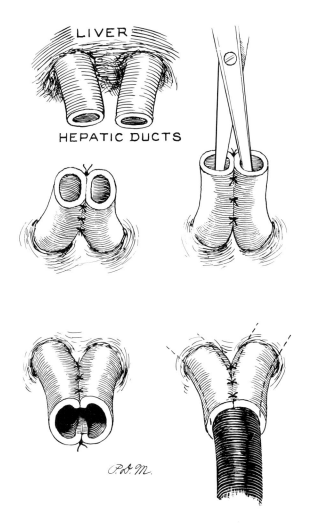

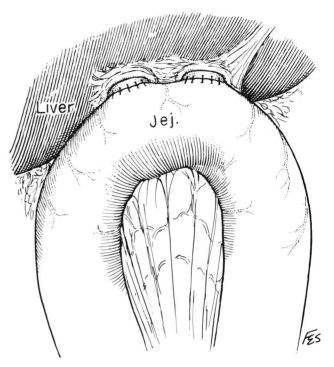

9. WIDELY SEPARATED DUCTS

▼

With too wide a separation between the two hepatic ducts, two anastomoses can be performed.

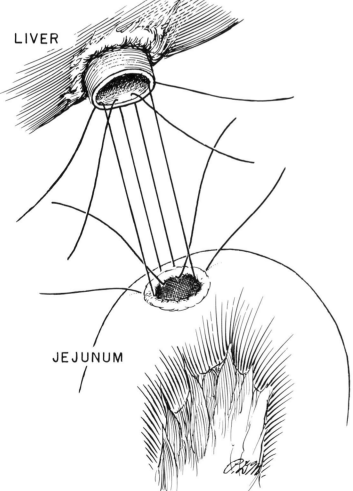

LIVER

JEJUNUM

10. ANASTOMOSIS

▼

Hepaticojejunostomy is the procedure of choice and is constructed by a single layer of full-thickness fine sutures with the posterior row placed first. The jejunum is "railroaded" down to the duct. The posterior sutures are tied. A simple jejunal loop is satisfactory unless it will not reach the duct despite passage through the mesocolon. In this situation, a Roux-en-Y loop can provide an extra 4 or 5 cm in length.

11. STENT

▼

The stent of choice is a T tube, with the vertical limb emerging from the common or left hepatic duct above the anastomosis. This is now placed, and the anterior layer of the anastomosis is accomplished. A jejunojejunal anastomosis at the base of the jejunal loop completes the operation. A Roux-en-Y loop may be used for the biliary anastomosis but is more complicated and is not necessary because reflux of small bowel contents is not harmful.

Alternative repair includes an end-to-end repair, plastic procedure, hepaticoduodenostomy, dilatation, or the Smith mucosal graft.

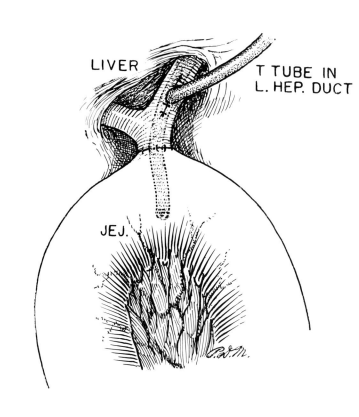

12. END-TO-END REPAIR

▼

End-to-end repair is useful only as an immediate repair of a recent injury to a large duct.

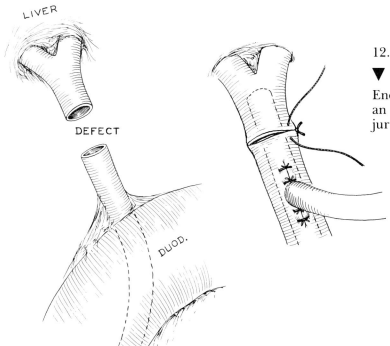

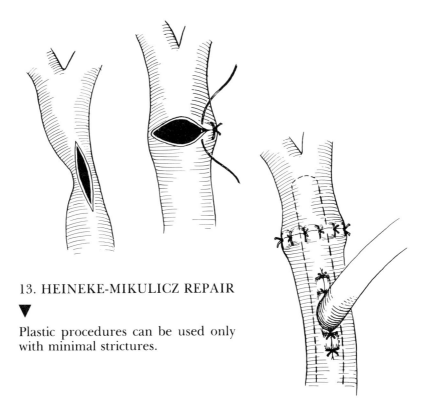

13. HEINEKE-MIKULICZ REPAIR

▼

Plastic procedures can be used only with minimal strictures.

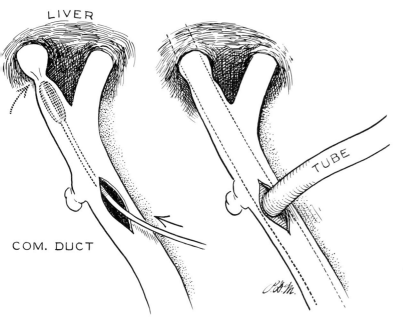

14. DILATATION

▼

Dilatation is advisable only with strictures of the right duct.

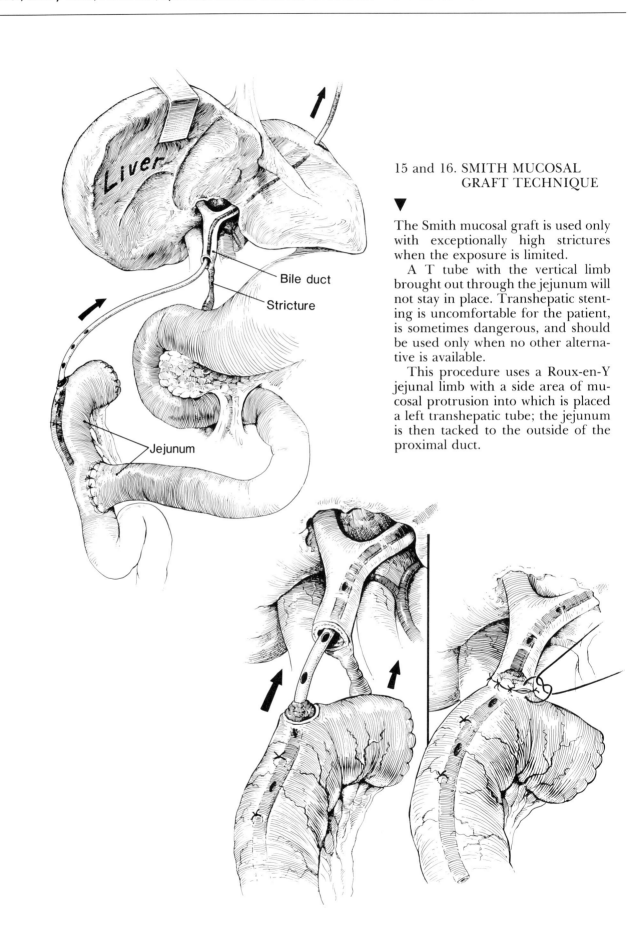

Bile duct

Stricture

Jejunum

15 and 16. SMITH MUCOSAL GRAFT TECHNIQUE

▼

The Smith mucosal graft is used only with exceptionally high strictures when the exposure is limited.

A T tube with the vertical limb brought out through the jejunum will not stay in place. Transhepatic stenting is uncomfortable for the patient, is sometimes dangerous, and should be used only when no other alternative is available.

This procedure uses a Roux-en-Y jejunal limb with a side area of mucosal protrusion into which is placed a left transhepatic tube; the jejunum is then tacked to the outside of the proximal duct.

17. INTRAHEPATIC DISSECTION OF LEFT HEPATIC DUCT

▼

When the proximal hepatic duct(s) cannot be located, dissection at the base of the round ligament may locate the left hepatic duct to the lateral segments for a decompressing jejunal anastomosis. Care must be taken with the left portal vein overlying this duct.

A sump drain placed behind the anastomosis after all procedures exits the incision at its upper angle.

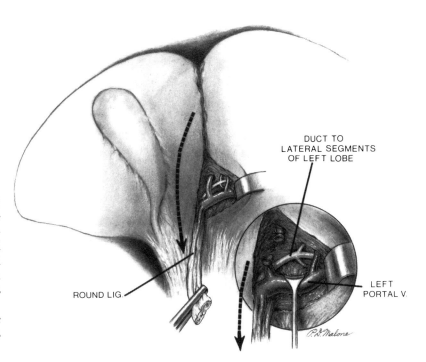

DUCT TO
LATERAL SEGMENTS
OF LEFT LOBE

ROUND LIG.

LEFT
PORTAL V.

Choledochal Cyst

RICARDO L. ROSSI, M.D.

▼ IMPORTANT FEATURES
Preferred Treatment Is Excision to Optimize Biliary Drainage and
    Prevent Carcinoma
Avoid Injury to Portal Vein and Pancreatic Duct
Pancreatic Duct Anomaly of High Juncture with the Common Duct
    Is Common
Occlude or Anastomose Distal Bile Duct to Prevent Pancreatic Fistula

▼ STEPS OR PLANS
Incision
Mobilization of Hepatic Flexure and Exposure of the Duodenum
Mobilization of the Duodenum, Head of the Pancreas, and Cyst
    (Kocher Maneuver)
Anatomic Relationships Are Defined
Dissection of Undersurface of the Liver and Cyst
Entrance to and Division of the Cyst
Identification of Openings of Right and Left Ducts
Excision of Cyst
Construction of End-to-Side Hepaticojejunostomy
Alternative Method of Removal

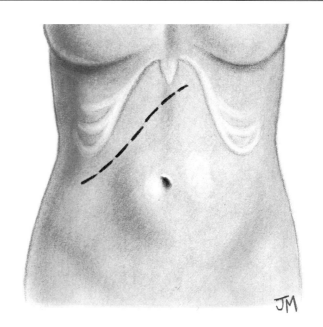

1. INCISION

An extended right subcostal incision is preferred. Alternatively, a long vertical incision can be used.

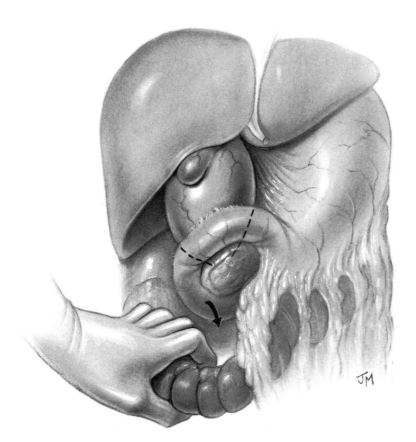

2. MOBILIZATION OF HEPATIC FLEXURE

Mobilization of the hepatic flexure of the colon and exposure of the duodenum are carried out.

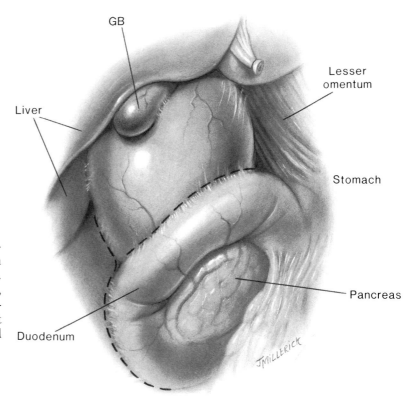

3. KOCHER MANEUVER

The duodenum, head of the pancreas, and cyst are mobilized from their retroperitoneal attachments. The peritoneum is divided sharply, and the Kocher maneuver is performed by combined sharp and blunt dissection. The cyst, duodenum, and head of the pancreas are lifted.

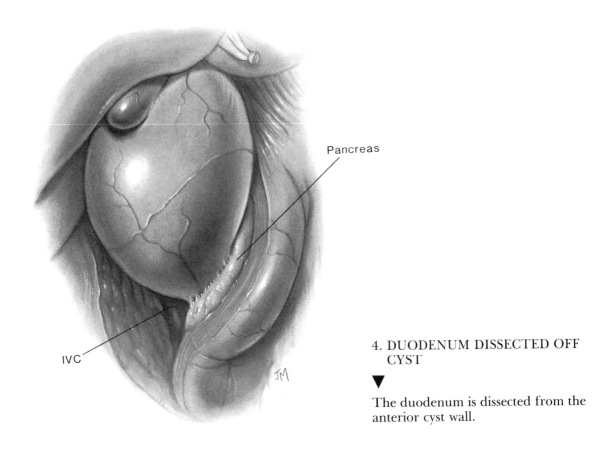

4. DUODENUM DISSECTED OFF CYST

The duodenum is dissected from the anterior cyst wall.

5. STRUCTURES POSTERIOR TO CYST

▼

Anatomic relationships of the structures posterior to the cyst are depicted.

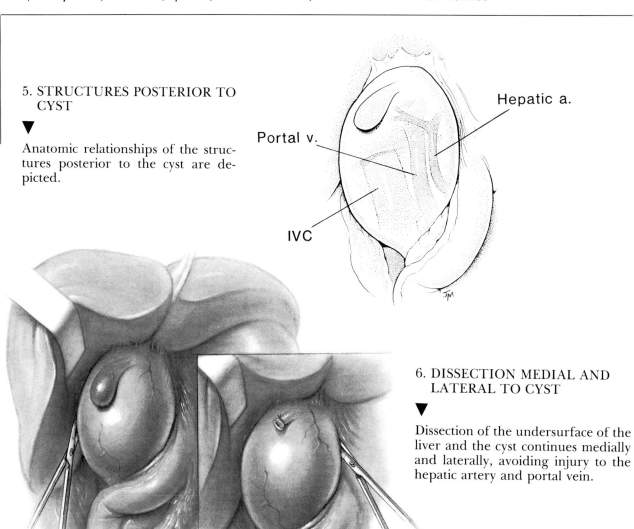

6. DISSECTION MEDIAL AND LATERAL TO CYST

▼

Dissection of the undersurface of the liver and the cyst continues medially and laterally, avoiding injury to the hepatic artery and portal vein.

7. EXCISION OF CYST

▼

Total resection is preferred. The cyst is divided distally, staying away from the pancreas and leaving a small distal cuff. The portal vein is avoided. *A*, The line of division is from right to left. *B*, The cyst is dissected proximally from the portal vein and hepatic artery. Be aware of the right hepatic artery.

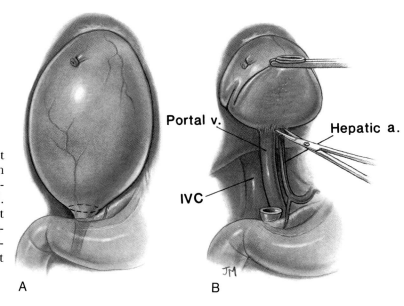

A

B

8. CYST INCISED

The cyst is incised longitudinally.

9. VISUALIZATION OF JUNCTION WITH HEPATIC DUCTS

A, The openings of the right and left ducts and of any other anomalous ducts are identified from within the lumen. B, A site for superior transection is chosen, avoiding injury to any ductal opening.

A

B

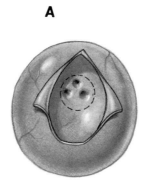

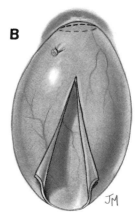

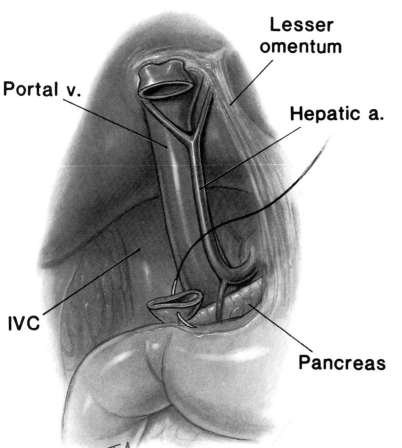

Lesser omentum

Portal v.

Hepatic a.

IVC

Pancreas

10. EXCISION OF CYST AND CLOSURE OF DISTAL DUCT

The cyst is excised. The distal cuff of the cyst is dissected to remove as much of the cyst lining as possible without endangering the pancreatic duct, which can join the common duct at a high level. This distal cuff is closed by interrupted sutures or, when it cannot be closed, it can be anastomosed to the Roux-en-Y loop of jejunum used in the proximal anastomosis.

11. HEPATICOJEJUNOSTOMY

A Roux-en-Y loop is fashioned, and an end-to-side hepaticojejunostomy is constructed. The subhepatic space is drained.

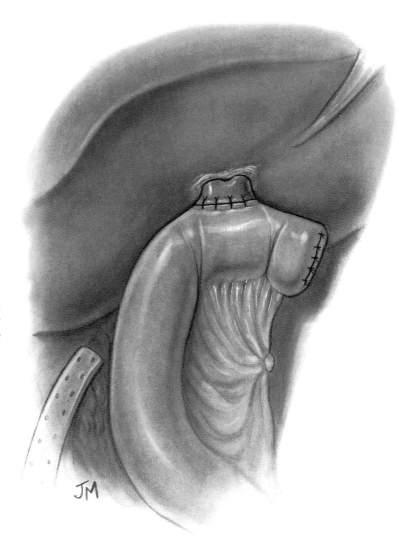

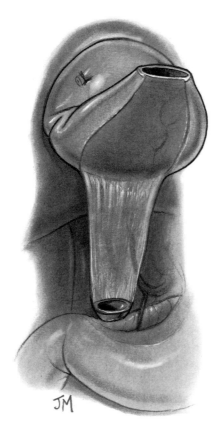

12. ALTERNATIVE EXCISION

An alternative method leaves a segment of fibrous cyst wall denuded of mucosa on the portal vein but removes all the rest of the cyst.

46 | Proximal Bile Duct Tumors

RICARDO L. ROSSI, M.D.

▼ IMPORTANT FEATURES
Some Tumors Slow Growing
Variety of Operative Procedures from Hepatectomy to Intubation
    Required for Palliation or Cure
Vascular Invasion of Hepatic Artery and Portal Vein In Some Cases
    Only Impediment to Cure
Angiography Can Be Helpful Preoperatively When Liver Resection
    Is Performed
Percutaneous Transhepatic Cholangiography Essential to Outline
    Proximal Extent of Tumor

▼ STEPS OR PLANS
Lymph Nodes Draining Porta Hepatis
Common Variations of Proximal Bile Duct Anatomy
Extent and Location of Tumor Determine Treatment
Dissection of Hepatic Duct Bifurcation
Skeletonization Resection
Transection of Right and Left Hepatic Ducts
Multiple Hepaticojejunostomies Are Performed; Alternative Types of
    Stents Can Be Used
Loop Hepaticojejunostomy with Jejunojejunostomy or Roux-en-Y
    Reconstruction
Liver Resection (see separate section)
Palliative Techniques for Proximal Tumors—Dilatation
Use of Guide Wires and Dilator with Choledochoscopy
Placement of Transhepatic Tubes
Duct and Tumor Dilatation and Stenting with T Tube
Proximal High Hepaticojejunostomy
Biliary Enteric Anastomoses to Segment III
Division and Ligation of a Branch of the Round Ligament and Portal
    Vein, When Needed
Roux-en-Y Cholangiojejunostomy Using Duct to Segment III

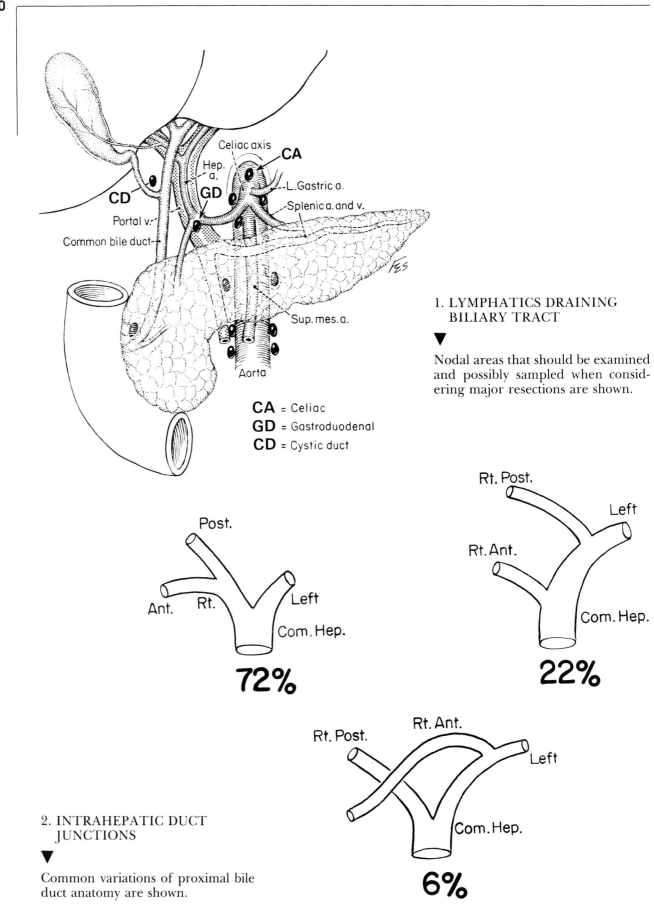

CA = Celiac
GD = Gastroduodenal
CD = Cystic duct

1. LYMPHATICS DRAINING BILIARY TRACT

▼

Nodal areas that should be examined and possibly sampled when considering major resections are shown.

72%

22%

2. INTRAHEPATIC DUCT JUNCTIONS

▼

Common variations of proximal bile duct anatomy are shown.

6%

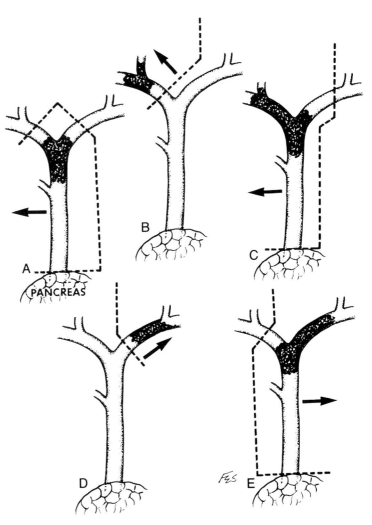

3. POSSIBLE TUMOR LOCATIONS

▼

Various extents and locations of tumor involvement that determine therapeutic options are shown. *A*, Skeletonization resection. *B* and *C*, Extended right hepatectomy. *D* and *E*, Left hepatectomy. (See section on hepatic resection.)

4. INITIAL DISSECTION AND DECISIONS

▼

Cholecystectomy is performed first to facilitate dissection. Blunt and sharp dissection of the bifurcation is carried out in the plane between the liver and the bile ducts (hilar plate) up to the segmental duct.

Depending on the apparent proximal extent of the tumor shown by cholangiography and dissection and the presence or absence of vascular invasion, a decision is made between a resective procedure (liver resection, skeletonization resection) or a palliative technique (stenting, cholangiojejunostomy). On occasion, vascular structures can be resected and reconstructed. (See section on hepatic resection.)

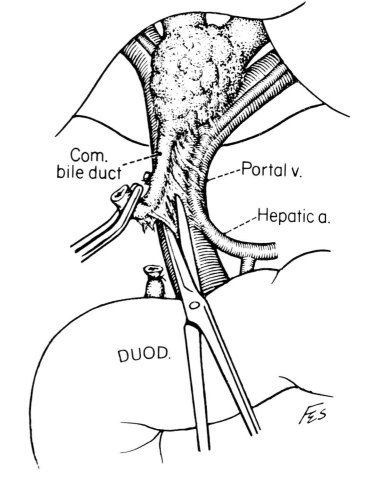

5. SKELETONIZATION RESECTION

The common duct is divided distally and dissected from the portal vein and hepatic artery.

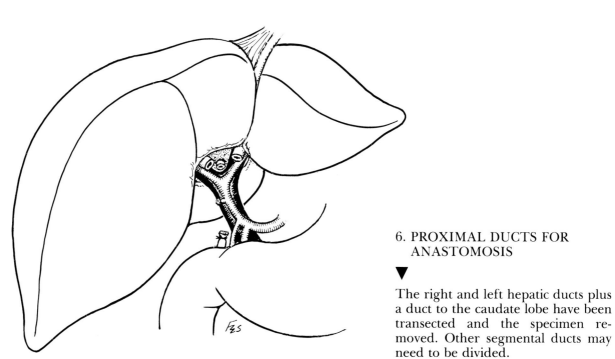

6. PROXIMAL DUCTS FOR ANASTOMOSIS

The right and left hepatic ducts plus a duct to the caudate lobe have been transected and the specimen removed. Other segmental ducts may need to be divided.

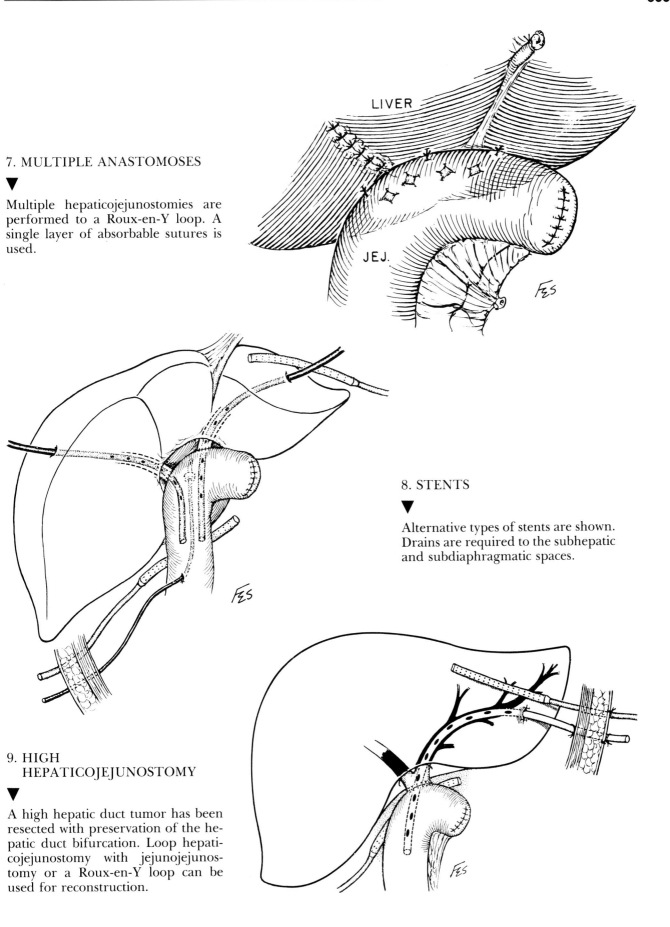

7. MULTIPLE ANASTOMOSES

▼

Multiple hepaticojejunostomies are performed to a Roux-en-Y loop. A single layer of absorbable sutures is used.

LIVER

JEJ.

8. STENTS

▼

Alternative types of stents are shown. Drains are required to the subhepatic and subdiaphragmatic spaces.

9. HIGH HEPATICOJEJUNOSTOMY

▼

A high hepatic duct tumor has been resected with preservation of the hepatic duct bifurcation. Loop hepaticojejunostomy with jejunojejunostomy or a Roux-en-Y loop can be used for reconstruction.

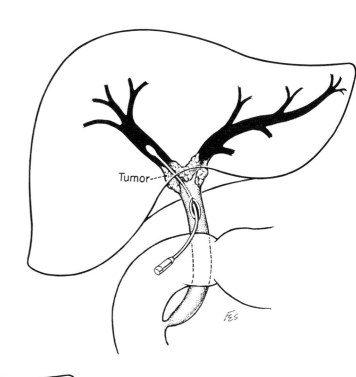

10. PALLIATIVE DILATATION

In palliative techniques for proximal tumors, dilatation is carried out using Bakes dilators.

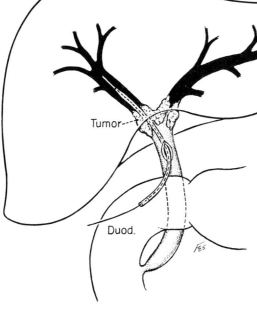

11. INDIRECT DILATATION

A guide wire and dilator are used, with or without direct visualization with choledochoscopy.

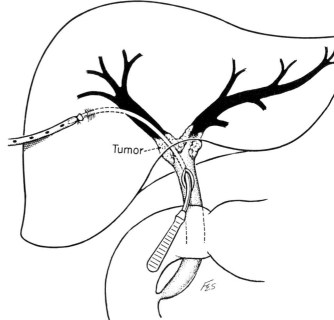

12. TRANSHEPATIC STENTING

After dilatation of one or both sides with a firm wire probe and Bakes dilator, transhepatic tubes are placed. We prefer a plastic pediatric feeding tube or a Silastic catheter, sized 8 to 10.

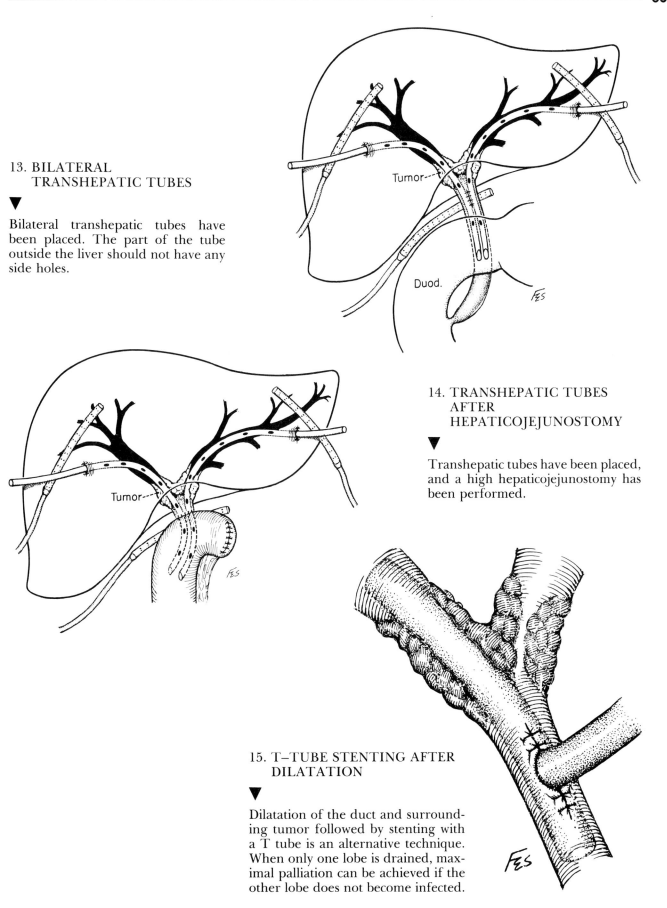

13. BILATERAL TRANSHEPATIC TUBES

▼

Bilateral transhepatic tubes have been placed. The part of the tube outside the liver should not have any side holes.

14. TRANSHEPATIC TUBES AFTER HEPATICOJEJUNOSTOMY

▼

Transhepatic tubes have been placed, and a high hepaticojejunostomy has been performed.

15. T–TUBE STENTING AFTER DILATATION

▼

Dilatation of the duct and surrounding tumor followed by stenting with a T tube is an alternative technique. When only one lobe is drained, maximal palliation can be achieved if the other lobe does not become infected.

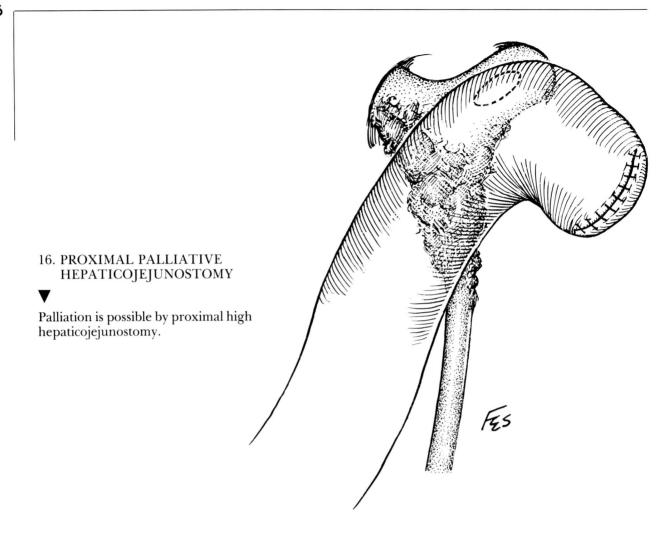

16. PROXIMAL PALLIATIVE HEPATICOJEJUNOSTOMY

▼

Palliation is possible by proximal high hepaticojejunostomy.

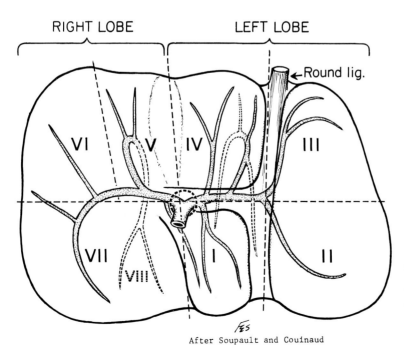

RIGHT LOBE   LEFT LOBE

←Round lig.

VI   V   IV   III

VII   I   II

VIII

After Soupault and Couinaud

17. PROXIMAL INTRAHEPATIC ANASTOMOSES

▼

The proximal segmental ducts may be used for palliative biliary enteric anastomoses. Note duct to segment III.

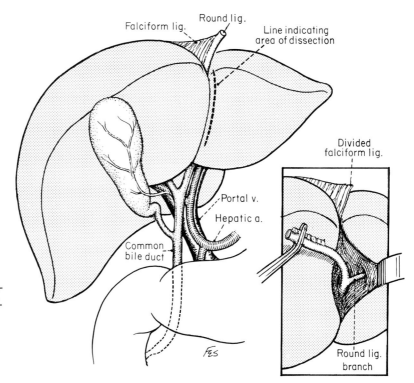

18. DISSECTION FOR SEGMENT III DUCT

▼

To reach this duct, dissection is begun to the left of the round ligament.

19. DISSECTION FOR SEGMENT III DUCT
(Continued)

▼

A, A branch of the round ligament is divided and ligated. The branch of the portal vein is ligated. *B*, The bile duct is identified by needle aspiration.

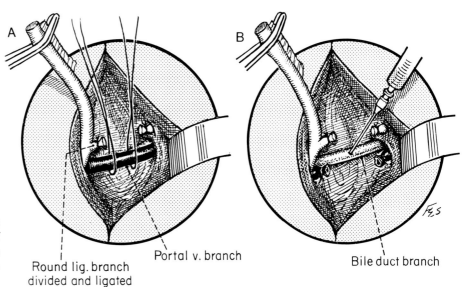

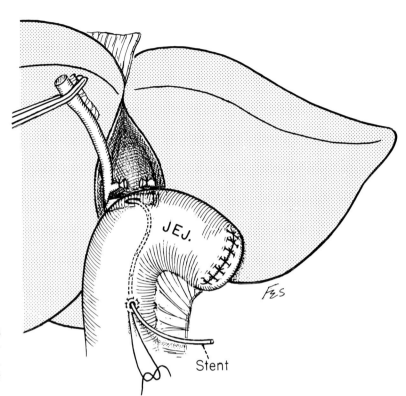

20. SEGMENT III ANASTOMOSIS TO JEJUNUM

▼

Roux-en-Y cholangiojejunostomy is performed in one layer under magnification using absorbable sutures. A small stent should be placed. The subhepatic space is drained.

47 | Annular Pancreas

STEPHEN G. ReMINE, M.D.

▼ IMPORTANT FEATURES
Recognize the Condition
Will Peptic Ulcer Need Surgical Treatment?
Avoid Injury to the Annulus
Bypass Distal to Pyloric Sphincter

▼ STEPS OR PLANS
Duodenojejunostomy Roux-en-Y Anastomosis
Duodenoduodenostomy Possible If Duodenum Is Mobilized and Is
    Flexible
Highly Selective Vagotomy In Addition If Peptic Ulcer Is Present
    (see section on gastric surgery)

1. APPEARANCE OF ANNULAR PANCREAS

Annular pancreas is found occasionally during operation for other disease. When symptomatic, it usually presents in the early pediatric age group. However, presentation of symptoms can occur at any time during adulthood, even during the later decades, especially when associated with duodenal ulcer disease. Without symptoms, the presence of an annular pancreas does not justify surgical intervention. When obstruction is present with or without peptic ulcer, surgical intervention is indicated. The appearance of annular pancreas with some dilatation of the proximal duodenum is shown.

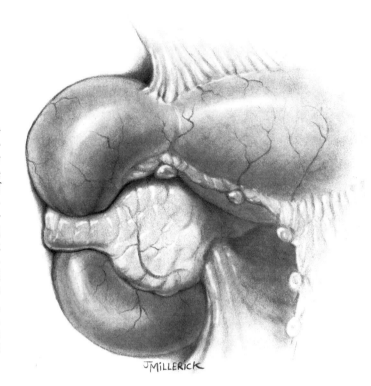

2. DUODENOJEJUNOSTOMY FOR OBSTRUCTION

The surgeon may be tempted simply to cut the annular band of pancreatic tissue to relieve the duodenal obstruction. This should be avoided because the annular band may contain a major duct from the uncinate process, and cutting this band will result in significant pancreatic leakage. In addition, cutting the pancreatic annulus probably would not relieve the obstruction because often a submucosal band of fibrous tissue underlying the pancreatic tissue is equally responsible for the obstruction.

The most effective way to treat annular pancreas with obstruction is to perform Roux-en-Y duodenojejunostomy using proximal duodenum. This is a procedure similar to that used to repair duodenal injuries from instrumentation, trauma, or chronic perforation when primary repair cannot be performed. This Roux-en-Y duodenojejunostomy is performed in a double-layer fashion using an inner layer of running 3-0 chromic catgut and an outer layer of interrupted 3-0 silk sutures. (See section on pancreaticojejunostomy for Roux-en-Y loop construction.)

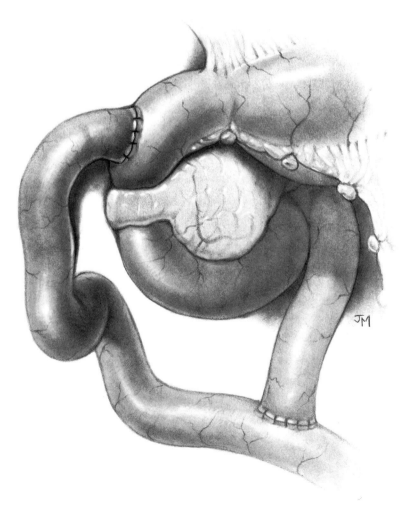

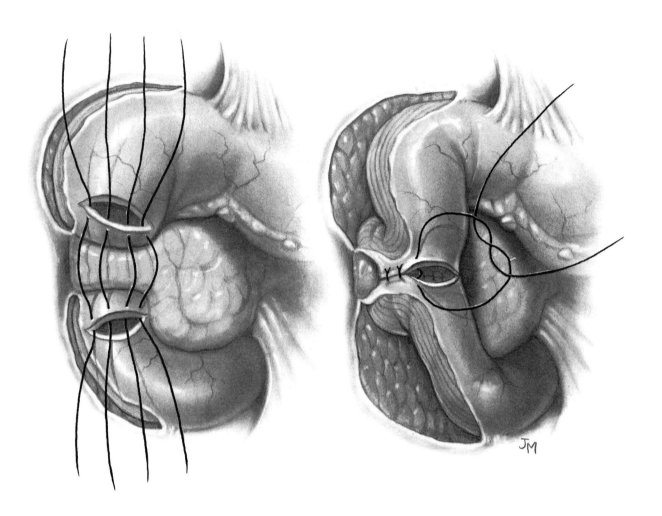

3. DUODENODUODENOSTOMY

▼

An alternative to Roux-en-Y duodenojejunostomy reconstruction is to perform side-to-side duodenoduodenostomy to bypass the annular pancreas—an accepted alternative under ideal circumstances with a mobile proximal and distal duodenum. After complete kocherization of the duodenum, permitting mobility of both the second portion of the duodenum and the third and fourth portions of the duodenum, transverse incisions can be made above and below the area of the annular pancreas. A one-layer or two-layer anastomosis can be performed with an inner layer of 3-0 chromic catgut and an outer layer of interrupted 3-0 silk sutures.

When peptic ulceration is present, a highly selective vagotomy is the ideal complement to the bypass. (See section on parietal cell vagotomy.)

Pancreatic Pseudocysts

48

STEPHEN G. ReMINE, M.D.
RICARDO L. ROSSI, M.D.

▼ IMPORTANT FEATURES
Timing of Procedure
Confirm That Cyst Is Not Neoplastic
Internal Drainage Is Procedure of Choice
Organ Used for Drainage Depends on Location of Cyst
Resection of Cyst In Tail of Pancreas
External Drainage If Not Suitable for Anastomosis
Symptoms from Pancreatitis Often Continue, So Other Procedures
    May Be Necessary

▼ STEPS OR PLANS
Cystogastrostomy
        Incise Anterior Gastric Wall
        Aspirate Cyst Through Posterior Gastric Wall
        Incise Cyst Wall, Drain, and Anastomose
        Close Anterior Gastric Wall
Duodenocystostomy
Cystojejunostomy, Roux-en-Y
External Drainage or Resection

1. GENERAL CONSIDERATIONS— ANTERIOR GASTROTOMY

In general, delay treatment of a cyst for five or six weeks after onset of symptoms because attachment of the cyst to the stomach matures, spontaneous resolution is possible, and complications are not likely during this interval.

Attempts have been made to drain pseudocysts percutaneously, either with aspiration or with an indwelling catheter. Some of these attempts have been successful, but simple aspiration usually fails. The presence of a percutaneously placed drain may convert a sterile cyst into an abscess or may result in an external pancreatic fistula, but usually these complications do not occur.

The usual location of the cyst is posterior to the body of the stomach. The first step is incision of the anterior wall of the stomach, which can be accomplished with a scalpel or the electrocautery.

2. ASPIRATION OF CYST

When the inside lumen of the stomach is visualized and the pseudocyst can be identified, needle aspiration of the cyst is performed to be sure of the location of the cyst as well as to obtain a sample of cyst fluid for culture.

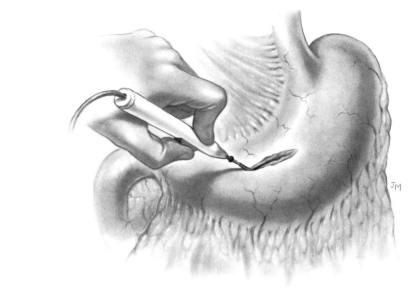

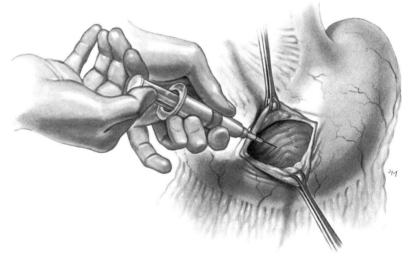

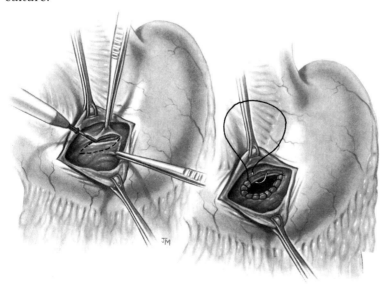

3. POSTERIOR GASTROTOMY— CYSTOGASTROSTOMY

When the cyst is clearly identified, posterior gastrotomy is performed, incising directly into the lumen of the cyst. A wedge of tissue, full thickness of the cyst wall, is sent to the laboratory for histologic review. This step is important because of the rare occurrence of a cystadenoma or cystadenocarcinoma, which may masquerade as a pseudocyst. Examination of the inside lining of the cyst is conducted delicately so as not to create further bleeding. When septations are not present and when pathologic examination of the cyst wall indicates absence of carcinoma or of epithelial lining, the cyst is evacuated completely, and cystogastrostomy can be completed by using a running suture of silk or heavy Dexon. Bleeding sites are individually suture ligated. This step ensures patency of the anastomosis, aids in hemostasis, and avoids leakage when the two walls are not completely adherent.

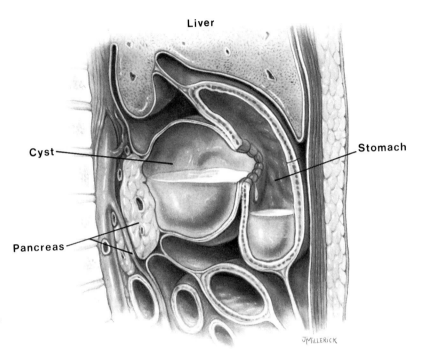

4. COMPLETED CYSTOGASTROSTOMY

Cross-sectional lateral view of the final cystogastrostomy demonstrates the anterior displaced position of the stomach and the attachment of the cyst wall to the posterior surface of the stomach.

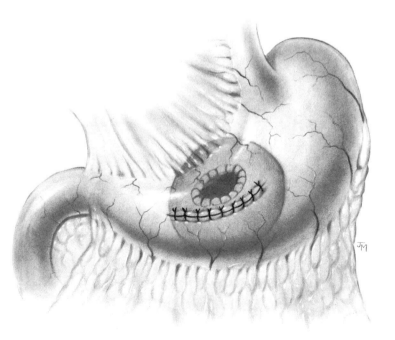

5. CLOSURE OF ANTERIOR GASTROTOMY

The anterior gastrotomy is closed in a double-layer fashion with an inner layer of running sutures of 3-0 chromic catgut and an outer layer of interrupted sutures of 3-0 silk.

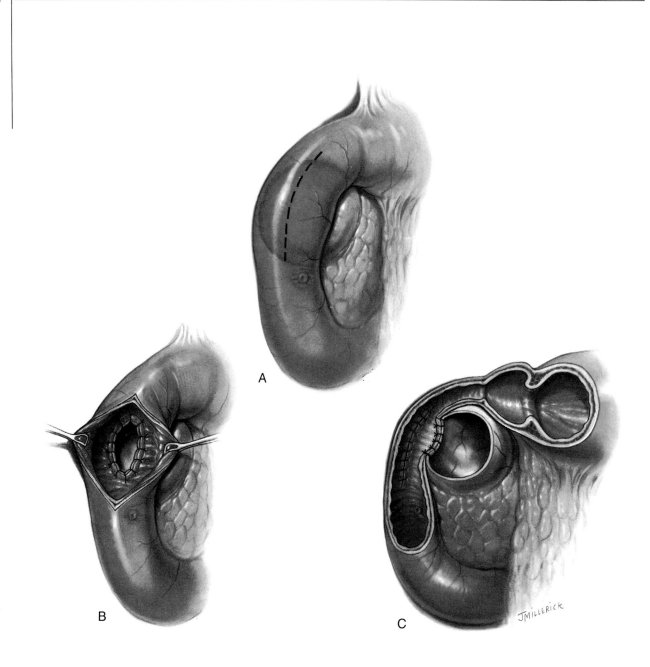

A

B

C

6. CYSTODUODENOSTOMY

▼

A cyst within the head of the pancreas can occasionally be managed by performing direct cystoduodenostomy. *A,* An anterior duodenotomy is performed in longitudinal fashion, permitting direct visualization of the duodenal displacement. The cyst is aspirated with a needle for confirmation. The ampullary area is avoided. The medial duodenal wall is incised, and the cyst is entered from within the duodenum. *B,* The cyst wall and duodenal wall are sutured. The duodenotomy is closed in a transverse or longitudinal fashion using an inner layer of running sutures of 3-0 chromic catgut and an outer layer of interrupted sutures of 3-0 silk. Care must be taken not to dissect too far posteriorly and injure the common duct or too far inferiorly and injure the ampulla of Vater. *C,* The completed procedure is seen in cross section.

7. CYSTOJEJUNOSTOMY

For lesions in the head of the pancreas that are not attached to or close to the duodenal wall or for lesions in the distal pancreas that cannot be resected, Roux-en-Y pancreatic cystojejunostomy can be performed. A defunctionalized Roux-en-Y limb is brought up either antecolic or retrocolic, and an anastomosis is made between the cyst wall and the jejunal Roux-en-Y. Pancreatic cystojejunostomy can be performed in a single layer using interrupted sutures of 3-0 silk.

EXTERNAL DRAINAGE OR RESECTION

For cysts not suitable for internal drainage because of a thin wall, general inflammation, or location, external drainage with a mushroom catheter is preferred.

Cysts of the tail of the pancreas not adherent to the stomach should, in general, be resected along with the spleen in adults because the possibility of a neoplasm is eliminated along with the cyst. (See this technique in the section on distal pancreatectomy.)

After adherence to the principles of dependent drainage, whenever possible, and selection of an appropriate operation, resolution of the pseudocyst should be obtained in more than 90 per cent of patients.

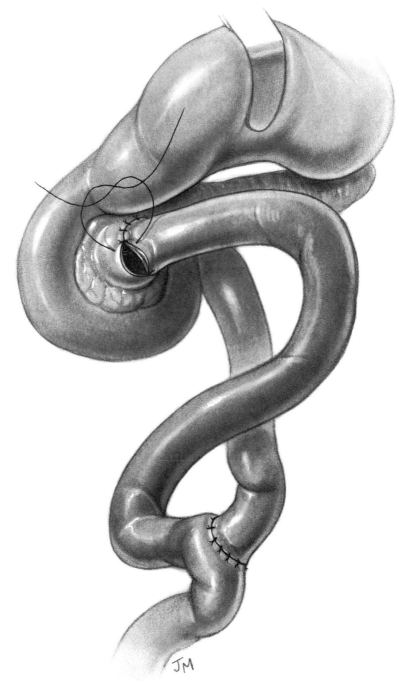

49

Decompression of Pancreatic Duct with Pancreaticojejunostomy

J. LAWRENCE MUNSON, M.D.

▼ IMPORTANT FEATURES

Preoperative Endoscopic Retrograde Pancreatography or
   Intraoperative Pancreatography Demonstrating "Chain of
   Lakes" or Dilatation of the Main Pancreatic Duct
Identification of, Incision into, and Evacuation of the Pancreatic Duct
Evaluate and Relieve Obstruction of Ducts In the Head of the Gland
Creation of Roux-en-Y Jejunal Loop
Lateral Anastomosis of the Pancreatic Capsule to the Jejunum

▼ STEPS OR PLANS

Incision and Exploration to Rule Out Associated Biliary Tract
   Disease
Opening of the Lesser Sac and Exploration of the Pancreas
Aspiration of the Pancreatic Duct and Contrast Study of the
   Pancreatic Duct When Preoperative Endoscopic Retrograde
   Cholangiopancreatography Has Not Been Performed
Incision of the Pancreatic Duct and Removal of Calculi and Debris
Exploration of the Duct; Special Attention to Ducts In the Head of
   the Gland
Creation of a Roux-en-Y Jejunal Loop Brought Up Through the
   Transverse Mesocolon
Lateral Anastomosis to the Capsule of the Pancreas
Jejunal Reanastomosis and Closure of the Mesenteric Defect

1. PANCREAS SUITABLE FOR PANCREATICOJEJUNOSTOMY

This view represents a schematic diagram of the "chain of lakes" configuration of the main pancreatic duct; subsequent fibrosis has caused stricturing and formation of calculi from debris within the pancreatic duct. With obstruction from pancreatitis in the head of the gland, the pancreatic duct may be a dilated tubular structure. Often the pancreas is considerably atrophied with a tough capsule of fibrosis created by the chronic inflammatory state. Preoperative endoscopic retrograde pancreatography may demonstrate this well; however, when the ampulla of Vater cannot be cannulated preoperatively, intraoperative pancreatography is desirable.

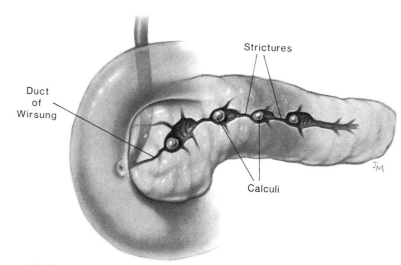

EXPOSURE

Excellent exposure for lateral pancreaticojejunostomy can be obtained through a bilateral subcostal incision, which can be extended toward the left flank. A self-retaining retractor aids in the exposure necessary for this procedure. Unless preoperative studies with ultrasonography or endoscopic retrograde cholangiopancreatography have demonstrated a normal biliary tract, the gallbladder should be evaluated and, when diseased, should be removed. Cholangiography should be performed to rule out choledocholithiasis.

2. LESSER SAC OPENED

With this accomplished, the lesser sac is opened by dividing the gastrocolic ligament from the duodenum to the splenic hilum. Often dense adhesions between the posterior aspect of the stomach and the capsule of the pancreas must be taken down to visualize the gland adequately. A Kocher maneuver is performed to permit bimanual palpation of the head of the pancreas, and the body and tail of the gland are inspected for evidence of pseudocyst or tumor. Dissection inferior and superior to the body of the gland may aid palpation.

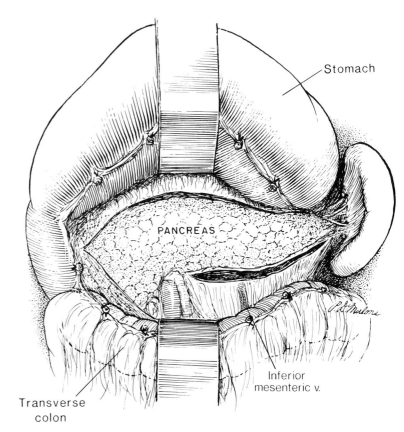

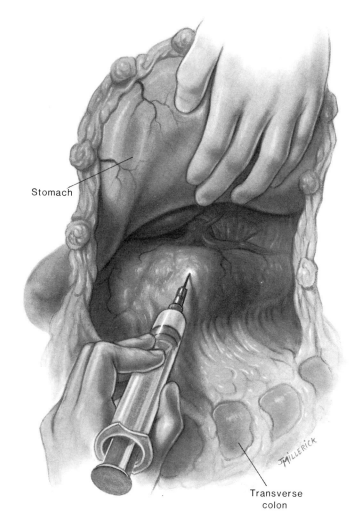

3. ASPIRATION OF PANCREATIC DUCT

▼

After appropriate exposure of the pancreas, a syringe and aspirating needle are used to locate the dilated pancreatic duct in the body of the pancreas. When the pancreatic duct has not been evaluated preoperatively, intraoperative pancreatography can be performed to delineate the configuration and drainage of the pancreatic duct.

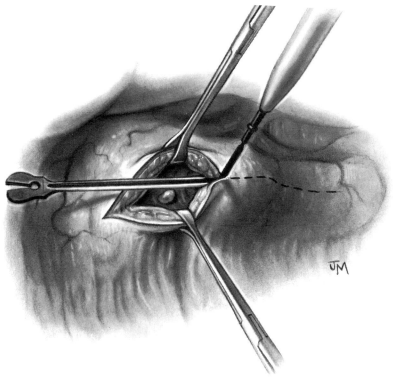

4. OPENING OF PANCREATIC DUCT

▼

After a small incision is made at the point of needle aspiration in the pancreatic duct, a right-angle clamp or grooved director can be inserted into the pancreatic duct, which is opened using the knife or Bovie electrocautery. The duct must be opened as far distally as necessary to incorporate all the dilated portions of the duct and must be opened proximally to the point of the proximal obstruction. Care is taken not to incise too close to the second portion of the duodenum. The edges of the thickened capsule of the pancreas can then be retracted with Allis forceps or traction sutures.

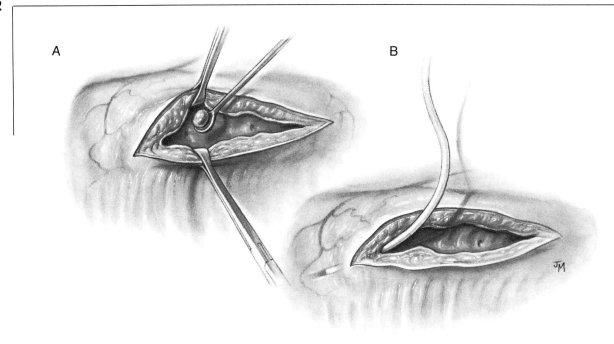

Transverse mesocolon

5. REMOVAL OF DEBRIS FROM PANCREATIC DUCT

▼

A and *B*, Stone scoops and irrigating catheters are used to remove ductal calculi and flush out any ductal debris. When the incision of the pancreatic duct has passed well out onto the head of the gland, a fine red rubber catheter can be passed through the papilla when it is unobstructed. Special efforts must be made to clean out ducts in the head of the gland and uncinate process.

6. ROUX-EN-Y JEJUNAL LOOP

▼

After the pancreatic duct has been cleaned of all debris, a Roux-en-Y loop of jejunum is created. The Roux-en-Y loop is usually taken at a point approximately 15 cm distal to the ligament of Treitz. The jejunum is divided with a gastrointestinal stapling device, and the mesenteric vessels are divided with suture ligature control.

7. JEJUNAL LOOP THROUGH MESOCOLON

▼

When adequacy of the Roux-en-Y limb of the Roux-en-Y loop has been established, it can be passed up through the transverse mesocolon to reach the lesser sac. Although classically an avascular space is usually found immediately to the left of the middle colic vessels, enough antecedent pancreatitis may be present to have fused the mesentery to the capsule of the pancreas. A dissection plane must be established to separate the mesocolon from the adherent pancreas.

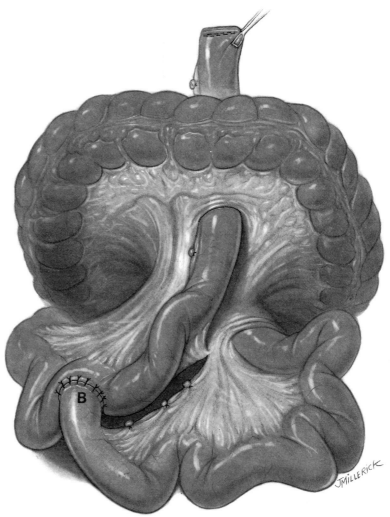

Capsule
of pancreas

8. LATERAL PANCREATICOJEJUNOSTOMY

▼

In the performance of lateral pancreaticojejunostomy, the jejunum is incised on its antimesenteric border, no closer than 2 cm from the closed end of the loop. An anastomosis is performed, placing interrupted sutures of 3-0 silk full thickness through the jejunum and through the entire fibrotic capsule of the pancreatic gland. The sutures are placed no more than 5 mm apart, and care should be taken not to attempt a direct mucosa-to-mucosa anastomosis that could close off pancreatic ductal tributaries.

Avascular space
of transverse mesocolon

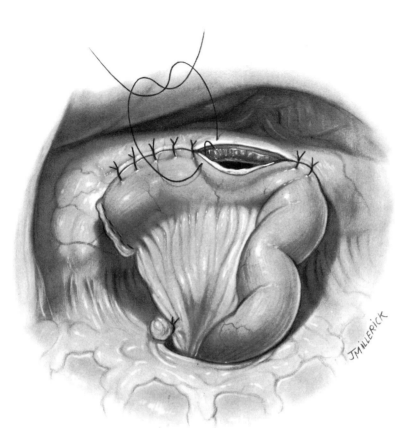

9. LATERAL PANCREATICOJEJUNOSTOMY *(Continued)*

▼

The anterior aspect of the anastomosis is completed only after the corners have been inverted securely. This anterior single layer of sutures is also carried full thickness through the small intestine but still catching only the capsule of the pancreas superiorly. With each suture, the first assistant grasps the full thickness of the jejunum at its edge and holds it in inversion against the capsule of the pancreas while the sutures are being tied.

10. ROUX-EN-Y ANASTOMOSIS

▼

Schematic diagrams show the cross section of the anastomosis permitting free drainage of pancreatic ductal tributaries into the decompressed main pancreatic duct.

A two-layer end-to-side jejunal anastomosis is created to complete the Roux-en-Y anastomosis, using an inner layer of catgut and an outer layer of 3-0 silk. Care is taken to close the mesenteric defect of the jejunum by suturing it to the distal limb of the jejunum ascending through the transverse mesocolon. The avascular space in the transverse mesocolon is approximated about the jejunal limb. Soft closed suction drains of the Jackson-Pratt type are placed above and

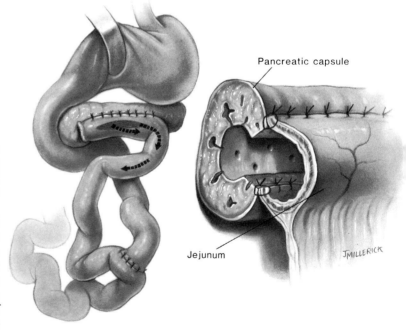

Pancreatic capsule

Jejunum

below the lateral pancreaticojejunostomy and brought out through lateral counterincisions. Closure of the subcostal incision is performed in routine fashion.

Resection of Pancreatic Adenoma

50

RICARDO L. ROSSI, M.D.

▼ IMPORTANT FEATURES

Accurate Preoperative Diagnosis

Preoperative Localization by Angiography

Adenomas Are Equally Distributed Throughout the Gland; 1 Per
Cent or Less Are In Ectopic Location, and 80 to 90 Per Cent
Are Solitary. When Multiple Adenomas Are Present, Multiple
Endocrine Neoplasia Syndrome Type I Should Be Suspected.
About 10 Per Cent of Adenomas Are Considered Malignant

▼ STEPS OR PLANS

Upper Transverse Incision or Midline Vertical Incision

Explore for Metastatic Disease; Biopsy Suspicious Nodes

Kocher Maneuver, Division of Gastrocolic Ligament, Division of
Peritoneum Inferior to Pancreas, Mobilization of Spleen and
Tail of Pancreas, Assessment of Uncinate Process; Tumor Is
Seen as Dark or Reddish Brown Lesion or Is Palpable

Explore Entire Pancreas and Peripancreatic Regions Even When One
Lesion Is Discovered Initially

Multiple or Malignant Lesions of Body and Tail Are Treated with
Distal Pancreatectomy; Small Lesions on Surface of Pancreas
Can Be Enucleated, Especially When In Head of Pancreas;
Pancreatoduodenectomy Is Indicated for Malignant Lesions of
Head of Pancreas

With Malignant Lesions, Even When Not All Disease Can Be
Removed, as Much of the Primary and Metastatic Disease as
Possible Should Be Resected

When an Adenoma Cannot Be Found After Careful Exploration,
Including Use of Ultrasonography, Alternatives Include Blind
Distal Pancreatectomy (50 Per Cent Success Rate) or a Trial of
Diazoxide and Further Evaluation with Transhepatic
Catheterization of Pancreatic Veins. Distal Pancreatectomy Can
Also Be Helpful In Some Instances of Islet Cell Hyperplasia
or Nesidioblastosis. Reexploration and Possibly Total
Pancreatectomy Is a Last Resort In Patients with Severe
Hypoglycemia and When Medical Treatment Fails

1. MOBILIZATION OF PANCREAS FOR INSPECTION

The lines of dissection shown are those that will achieve full mobilization of the pancreas for adequate assessment. The technique includes a wide Kocher maneuver to the aorta, division of the gastrocolic ligament with exposure of the body and tail of the pancreas, dissection of the colon and transverse mesocolon from the head of the pancreas, and mobilization of the spleen and body and tail of the pancreas.

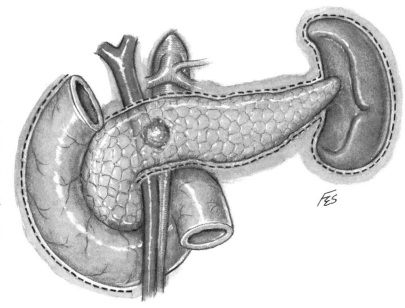

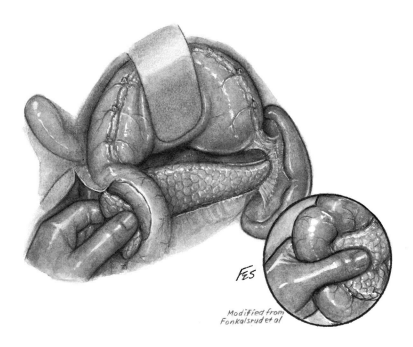

Modified from
Fonkalsrud et al

2. PALPATION OF HEAD OF PANCREAS

After a Kocher maneuver has been performed, the head of the gland and the uncinate process can be examined bimanually.

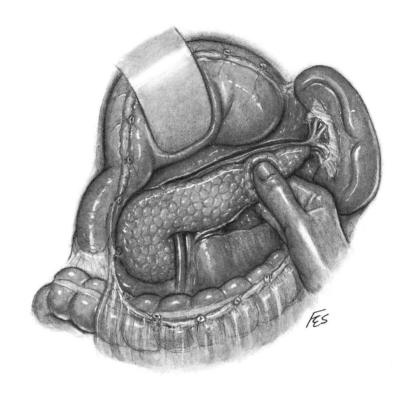

3. PALPATION OF BODY OF PANCREAS

▼

Bimanual palpation of the pancreas is essential.

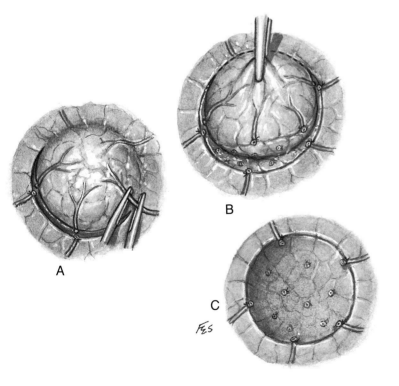

4. EXCISION OF ADENOMA

▼

A to *C*, Dissection of the adenoma using small mosquito clamps is shown. Dissection is performed close to the adenoma, clamping small vessels or ductal structures and ligating them with fine silk. The main pancreatic duct is spared and protected from the dissection. The adenoma is removed and submitted for frozen-section examination to confirm the diagnosis and to attempt to rule out carcinoma. A closed system drain is placed.

51 | Pancreatoduodenectomy (Pylorus Preserving)

JOHN W. BRAASCH, M.D.
RICARDO L. ROSSI, M.D.

▼ IMPORTANT FEATURES
Mobilization for Diagnosis
Isolate Duodenum, Distal Common Bile Duct, Head of Pancreas
Control Blood Supply: Gastroduodenal Artery, Pancreatic Veins,
     Inferior Pancreaticoduodenal Artery
Resection of Periampullary Area
Pancreas, Bile Duct, and Gastrointestinal Tract Reconstruction

▼ STEPS OR PLANS
Extensive Kocher Maneuver (Plane I)
Open Lesser Sac
Isolate First Part of Duodenum and Sever Duodenum 1 cm Distal to
     Pylorus
Sever Common Duct and Develop Plane II Down to Gastroduodenal
     Artery
Ligate and Sever Gastroduodenal Artery
Elevate Neck of Pancreas (Plane III)
Mobilize Ligament of Treitz
Sever Proximal Jejunum
Dissect Duodenojejunum to Mesenteric Vessels and Pass Bowel
     Under Vessels
Dissect to Right of Superior Mesenteric Vein (Plane IV)
Sever Pancreas at Neck
Resect Head of Pancreas
Pancreatic Anastomosis (Dunking Type)
Pancreatic Anastomosis (Two-Layer Sutured)
Biliary Tract Anastomosis
Duodenojejunostomy
Drainage

1. EXPOSURE OF PANCREAS, KOCHER MANEUVER, PLANE I

Access to the pancreas can be gained by a bilateral subcostal incision or a vertical right upper quadrant incision. To assess the problem, an extensive Kocher maneuver (plane I), which bares the aorta and is carried over to the ligament of Treitz, is essential.

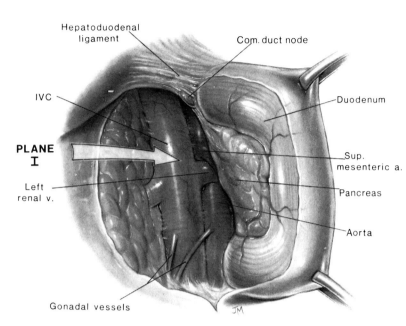

2. DISSECTION OF LESSER SAC

The lesser sac is entered, the posterior wall of the stomach is freed from the pancreas, and the fused area between the pancreatic head and the mesocolon is separated to permit bimanual palpation of lesions of the periampullary area and the head of the pancreas. The common duct gland, the gastroduodenal gland, and possibly the cystic duct gland are thus available for biopsy along with para-aortic nodes and celiac nodes.

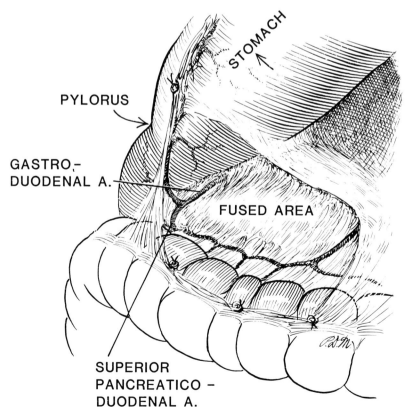

3. BLOOD SUPPLY TO HEAD OF PANCREAS AND LIVER

▼

The arterial blood supply of the head of the pancreas is provided by the gastroduodenal artery arising from the hepatic artery. The gastroduodenal artery splits promptly into anterior and posterior superior pancreaticoduodenal arteries, and subsequently the anterior artery divides into the right gastroepiploic artery and the superior pancreaticoduodenal artery. No real right gastric artery is present in most subjects; instead, a supraduodenal artery arises from the hepatic artery or the gastroduodenal artery and supplies the first portion of the duodenum. The venous drainage of the head of the pancreas is afforded by multiple small veins that

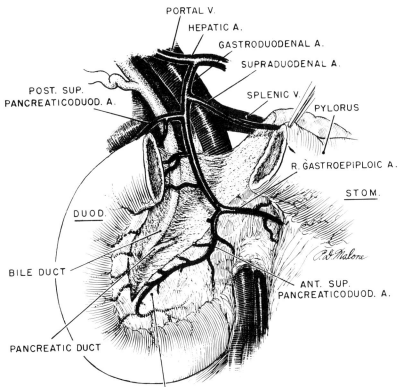

go directly to the superior mesenteric vein and portal vein. Inferiorly, a large vein goes to the superior mesenteric vein from the uncinate process.

4. REPLACED RIGHT HEPATIC ARTERY

▼

In one half of subjects, an anomalous artery goes from the superior mesenteric artery to the liver. This can be the entire hepatic artery or a segmental artery to the right lobe. More often, when present, it is the right hepatic artery.

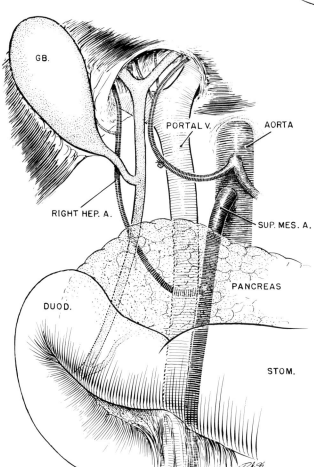

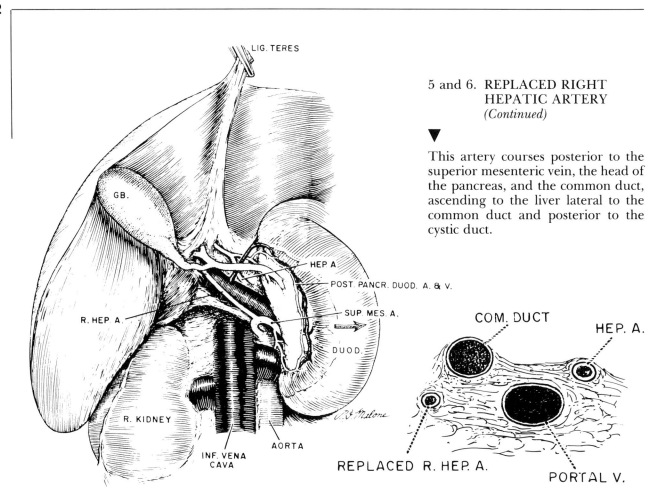

LIG. TERES

GB.

HEP. A

POST. PANCR. DUOD. A. & V.

SUP. MES. A.

R. HEP. A.

DUOD.

R. KIDNEY

AORTA

INF. VENA CAVA

COM. DUCT

HEP. A.

REPLACED R. HEP. A.

PORTAL V.

5 and 6. REPLACED RIGHT HEPATIC ARTERY *(Continued)*

▼

This artery courses posterior to the superior mesenteric vein, the head of the pancreas, and the common duct, ascending to the liver lateral to the common duct and posterior to the cystic duct.

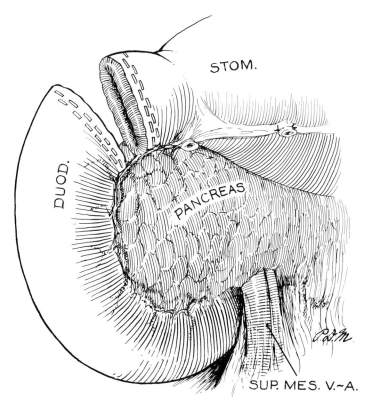

STOM.

DUOD.

PANCREAS

HEP.

SUP. MES. V.~A.

7. DUODENUM SEVERED

▼

To give access for dissection superior to the pancreatic head (plane II), the duodenum is isolated and severed with a gastrointestinal autosuture device 1 cm distal to the pylorus. An effort should be made to preserve the supraduodenal artery to the portion of the duodenum remaining adjacent to the pylorus.

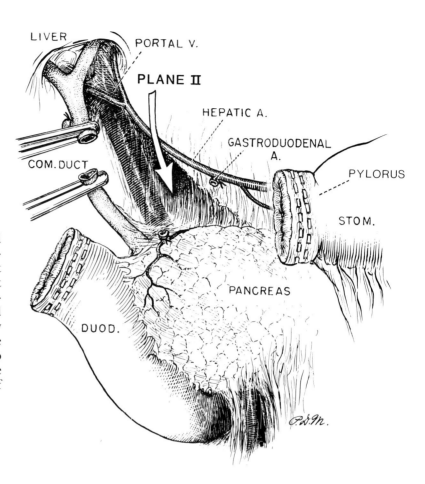

8. PLANE II SUPERIOR TO PANCREAS DEVELOPED

▼

The common bile duct is dissected and severed, usually distal to the cystic duct junction; when the cystic duct has a low insertion however it must be severed above this junction. Extreme care must be taken to avoid damage to a replaced hepatic artery at this step. The second plane to be developed then proceeds anterior to the portal vein and lateral to the hepatic artery down to the origin of the gastroduodenal artery.

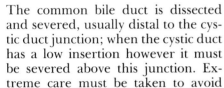

9. CONTROL OF GASTRODUODENAL ARTERY

▼

At the origin of the gastroduodenal artery from the hepatic artery is a characteristic configuration such that the hepatic artery is shaped like a V, and the gastroduodenal artery comes off inferiorly from the bottom of the V. Often the gastroduodenal artery is bifurcated so that it gives off the posterior arcade close to the hepatic artery; care must be taken in isolating, clamping, and ligating the gastroduodenal artery because of this branching.

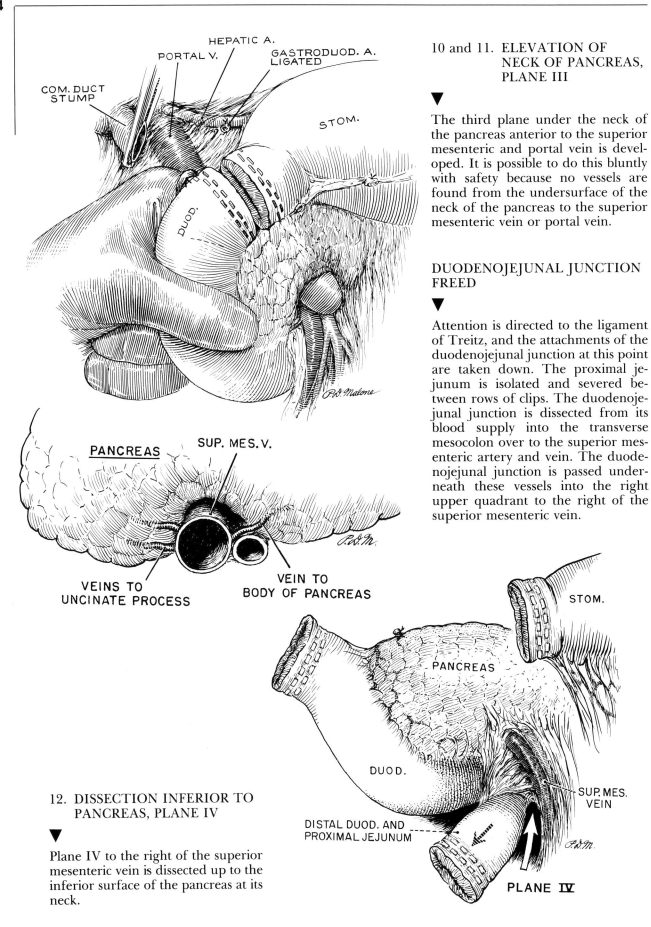

PANCREAS

SUP. MES. V.

VEINS TO
UNCINATE PROCESS

VEIN TO
BODY OF PANCREAS

10 and 11. ELEVATION OF NECK OF PANCREAS, PLANE III

▼

The third plane under the neck of the pancreas anterior to the superior mesenteric and portal vein is developed. It is possible to do this bluntly with safety because no vessels are found from the undersurface of the neck of the pancreas to the superior mesenteric vein or portal vein.

DUODENOJEJUNAL JUNCTION FREED

▼

Attention is directed to the ligament of Treitz, and the attachments of the duodenojejunal junction at this point are taken down. The proximal jejunum is isolated and severed between rows of clips. The duodenojejunal junction is dissected from its blood supply into the transverse mesocolon over to the superior mesenteric artery and vein. The duodenojejunal junction is passed underneath these vessels into the right upper quadrant to the right of the superior mesenteric vein.

12. DISSECTION INFERIOR TO PANCREAS, PLANE IV

▼

Plane IV to the right of the superior mesenteric vein is dissected up to the inferior surface of the pancreas at its neck.

PLANE IV

13. RESECTION OF HEAD OF PANCREAS

Sutures are placed through the upper and lower borders of the pancreas just distal to the neck of the pancreas to control the transverse pancreatic arteries in this area, and the neck of the pancreas is severed. The head of the pancreas, duodenum, and distal bile duct are now ready for resection. Great care must be taken in removing the pancreas from the superior mesenteric vein because the small tributaries from the head of the gland directly to this vein are easily torn. The largest vein drains the uncinate process into the superior mesenteric vein and is always present. The surgeon must be careful not to rotate the superior mesenteric artery into the field during this maneuver, which might subject it to injury. After the head of the pancreas and the duodenum have been removed, the gastrointestinal tract is readied for reconstruction.

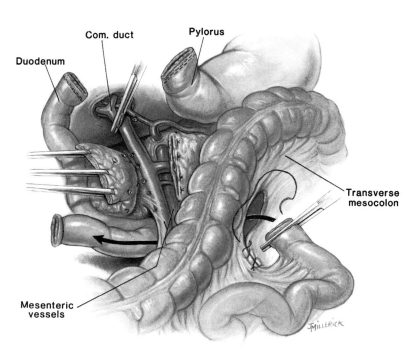

PANCREATIC ANASTOMOSIS

The pancreatic anastomosis is the most critical part of pancreatoduodenectomy. When a watertight anastomosis can be constructed, the patient should have an uncomplicated postoperative course. Leakage at this anastomosis can produce serious consequences. Basically, two types of anastomosis should be used. In patients with a soft pancreas and with a small normal pancreatic duct, a dunking type of anastomosis is safest. In the presence of carcinoma of the duodenum, benign tumors of the head of the pancreas, or carcinoma of the ampulla or distal duct in which the pancreatic duct is not obstructed, the pancreas is likely to be soft and the pancreatic duct small. In these patients, a dunking anastomosis is required. The alternative is a two-layer anastomosis that is useful in patients with a firm gland and a large pancreatic duct. In both types of anastomosis, the end of the pancreas is closed off with mattress sutures of permanent material, care being taken not to occlude the pancreatic duct. A pancreatic stent is passed through the jejunum distal to the future site of the biliary anastomosis. The stent with small ducts can be an infant feeding tube or in a larger duct, it can be as large as a No. 8 or 10 French red rubber catheter. This tube is passed up the jejunum, out the site of the anastomosis, and into the pancreatic ductal system. It is secured by a suture through the edge of the pancreatic duct and pancreatic tissue.

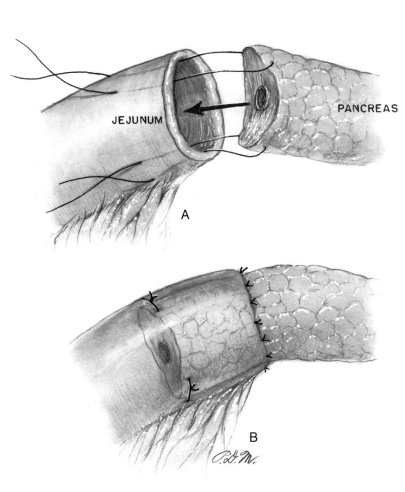

14. DUNKING PANCREATICO-JEJUNOSTOMY

▼

A and *B*, The jejunum is brought either anterior (preferably) or posterior to the transverse colon for the reconstruction. For the dunking anastomosis, traction sutures on the superior and inferior borders of the pancreas are passed into the lumen of the jejunum and through the jejunal wall, and the pancreas is dunked into the open end of the jejunum for a distance of about 1 inch. Seromuscularis sutures are placed around the circumference of the open jejunum into the capsule of the pancreas. The jejunal mucosa is inverted into the pancreatic capsule so it is not visible. The traction sutures are tied, completing the anastomosis.

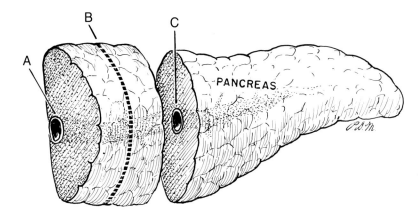

15. END-TO-SIDE TWO-LAYER PANCREATICO-JEJUNOSTOMY

▼

A to *C*, When a two-layer anastomosis is to be used with chronic pancreatitis or with an obstructed pancreatic ductal system, it is important to have the pancreatic duct in the middle of the cut edge of the pancreas. When the pancreas has been severed at its neck, often this duct is at the posterior edge of the gland, and serial sectioning of the pancreas must be carried out until the duct is located at the midportion of the gland.

16. PANCREATIC DUCT ANASTOMOSIS

▼

Fine sutures of 4-0 or 5-0 silk are placed on the posterior edge of the pancreatic duct, and the posterior capsule of the pancreas is sutured to the seromuscularis of the jejunum. A stab wound is made in the jejunum opposite the pancreatic duct, and the posterior duct sutures are continued through the posterior lip of the stab wound and tied. A stent, which has been placed down the jejunum, is pushed out through the stab wound and into the pancreatic duct. It is held in place in the duct by a suture through pancreas and ductal tissue and tied to the stent.

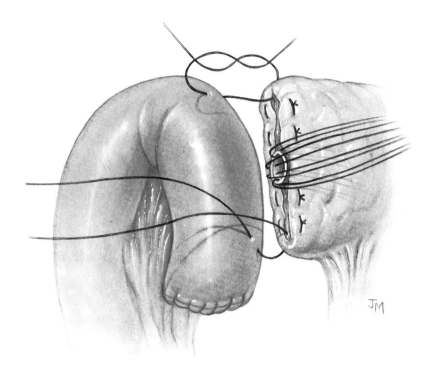

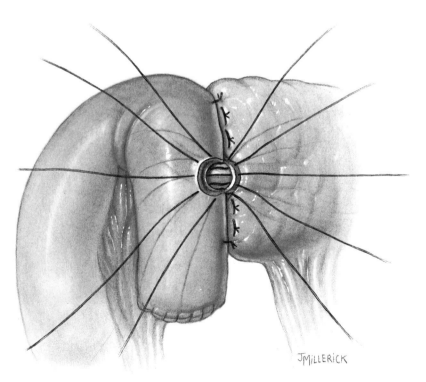

17. PANCREATIC DUCT ANASTOMOSIS *(Continued)*

▼

An anterior row of sutures is placed in the duct and tied. The seromuscularis of the jejunum is sutured to the capsule of the pancreas anteriorly to complete the anastomosis.

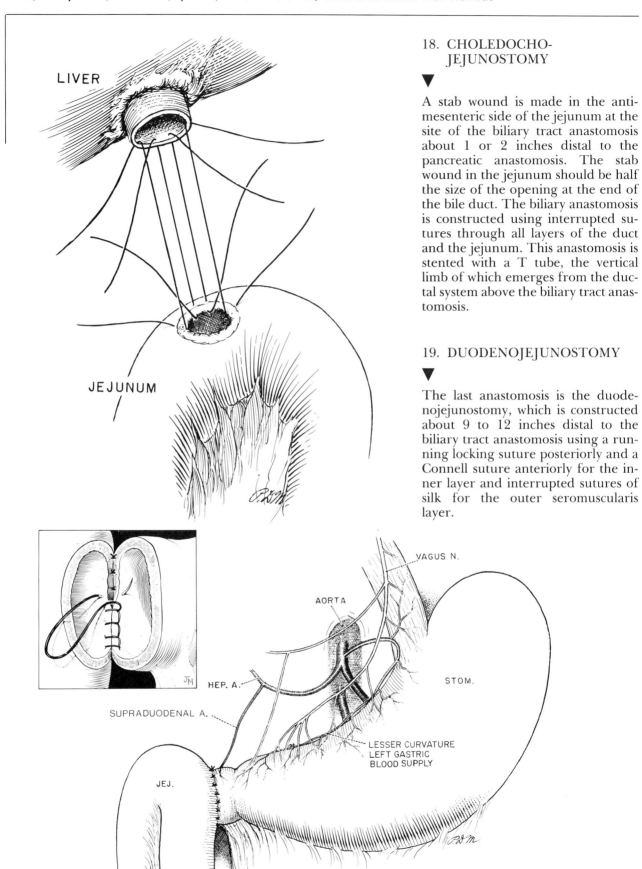

18. CHOLEDOCHO-JEJUNOSTOMY

▼

A stab wound is made in the anti-mesenteric side of the jejunum at the site of the biliary tract anastomosis about 1 or 2 inches distal to the pancreatic anastomosis. The stab wound in the jejunum should be half the size of the opening at the end of the bile duct. The biliary anastomosis is constructed using interrupted sutures through all layers of the duct and the jejunum. This anastomosis is stented with a T tube, the vertical limb of which emerges from the ductal system above the biliary tract anastomosis.

19. DUODENOJEJUNOSTOMY

▼

The last anastomosis is the duodenojejunostomy, which is constructed about 9 to 12 inches distal to the biliary tract anastomosis using a running locking suture posteriorly and a Connell suture anteriorly for the inner layer and interrupted sutures of silk for the outer seromuscularis layer.

16. PANCREATIC DUCT ANASTOMOSIS

Fine sutures of 4-0 or 5-0 silk are placed on the posterior edge of the pancreatic duct, and the posterior capsule of the pancreas is sutured to the seromuscularis of the jejunum. A stab wound is made in the jejunum opposite the pancreatic duct, and the posterior duct sutures are continued through the posterior lip of the stab wound and tied. A stent, which has been placed down the jejunum, is pushed out through the stab wound and into the pancreatic duct. It is held in place in the duct by a suture through pancreas and ductal tissue and tied to the stent.

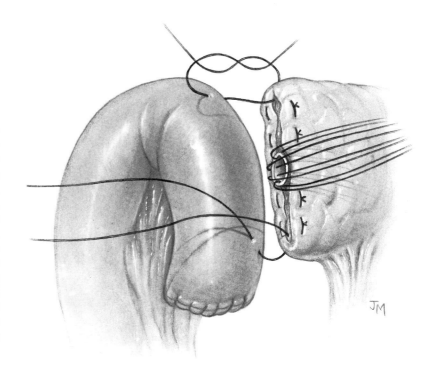

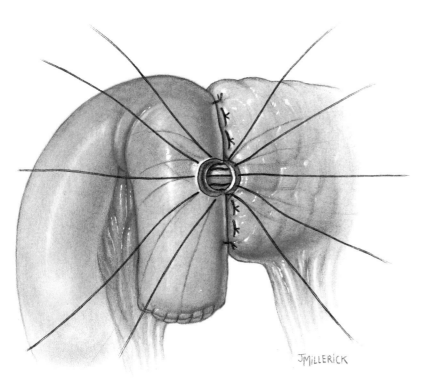

17. PANCREATIC DUCT ANASTOMOSIS *(Continued)*

An anterior row of sutures is placed in the duct and tied. The seromuscularis of the jejunum is sutured to the capsule of the pancreas anteriorly to complete the anastomosis.

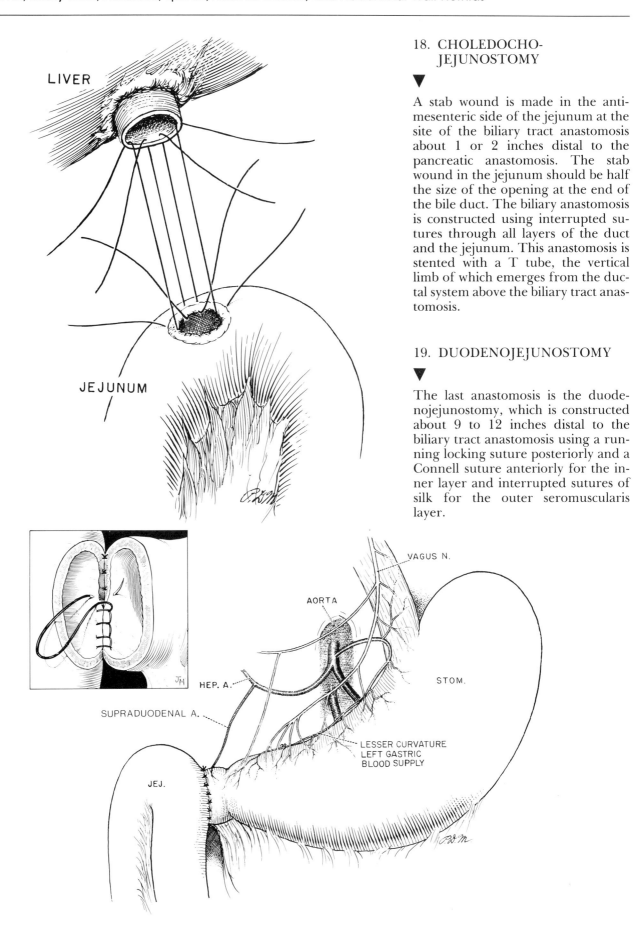

18. CHOLEDOCHO-JEJUNOSTOMY

▼

A stab wound is made in the anti-mesenteric side of the jejunum at the site of the biliary tract anastomosis about 1 or 2 inches distal to the pancreatic anastomosis. The stab wound in the jejunum should be half the size of the opening at the end of the bile duct. The biliary anastomosis is constructed using interrupted sutures through all layers of the duct and the jejunum. This anastomosis is stented with a T tube, the vertical limb of which emerges from the ductal system above the biliary tract anastomosis.

19. DUODENOJEJUNOSTOMY

▼

The last anastomosis is the duodenojejunostomy, which is constructed about 9 to 12 inches distal to the biliary tract anastomosis using a running locking suture posteriorly and a Connell suture anteriorly for the inner layer and interrupted sutures of silk for the outer seromuscularis layer.

20. COMPLETED PROCEDURE

The ligament of Treitz is closed with a running suture of chromic catgut, and when the loop of jejunum has been brought through the mesocolon, this defect must be closed around the jejunum. The pancreatic stent is brought through the abdominal wall where it emerges from the jejunum. It is fixed to the serosa of the jejunum, and the jejunum is sutured to the peritoneum around the stab wound in the abdominal wall. Four sump drains are placed behind the biliary and pancreatic anastomoses. These drains, along with the T tube, can be brought out the upper end of the incision if it is a vertical incision.

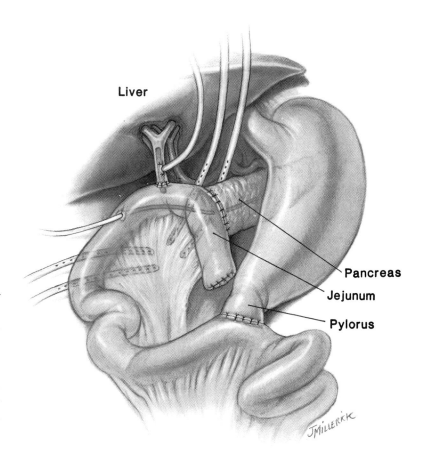

Liver

Pancreas

Jejunum

Pylorus

JMILLERKK

52 | Distal (40 to 50 Per Cent) Pancreatectomy

JOHN W. BRAASCH, M.D.
RICARDO L. ROSSI, M.D.

▼ IMPORTANT FEATURES

In Teenagers and Children, Distal Pancreatectomy Is Performed with Preservation of Splenic Artery and Vein (a Difficult Technical Procedure), Permitting Preservation of the Spleen In These Age Groups

Avascular Planes to Seek In Dissection Are Lateral to Spleen, Posterior to Spleen, Inferior and Posterior to Body and Tail of Pancreas, and Anterior to Left Kidney and Adrenal Gland

Care Must Be Taken to Preserve Splenic Flexure of Colon, Middle Colic Vessels, and Superior Mesenteric Vein and Portal Vein

In Subacute or Chronic Pancreatitis, the Avascular Planes May Be Lost, and Elevation of Pancreas and Spleen Must Proceed By Sharp Dissection with Accompanying Unavoidable Blood Loss

Closure of Severed End of Pancreas Is Crucial to Avoid Postoperative Pancreatic Fistulas

When the Duct In the Remaining Pancreas Is Not Patent into the Duodenum, a Distal Drainage Procedure to a Roux-en-Y Jejunal Loop Must Be Performed

▼ STEPS OR PLANS

Incision Is Left Upper Abdominal Vertical or Extended Left Subcostal

Short Gastric Vessels Are Dissected

Stomach Is Rotated to Right, and Splenocolic Ligaments Are Severed

Splenorenal Attachments and Peritoneum on Inferior and Superior Aspects of Spleen Are Severed

Left Adrenal Gland Must Not Be Damaged

Care Is Taken to Trace and Isolate Splenic Artery Before Its Ligation

Avascular Plane Under Neck of Pancreas Is Dissected

Splenic Vein Junction with Superior Mesenteric Vein Is Dissected, and Splenic Vein Is Severed and Ligated

Pancreas Is Severed Just Distal to Neck of Gland for 40 to 50 Per Cent Resection

Pancreatic Duct Is Suture Ligated, and Pancreas Is Closed

When the Pancreatic Duct Is Obstructed in the Head of the Pancreas, as Seen on Pancreatography or by Probing, Pancreaticojejunostomy Roux-en-Y Anastomosis Is Performed

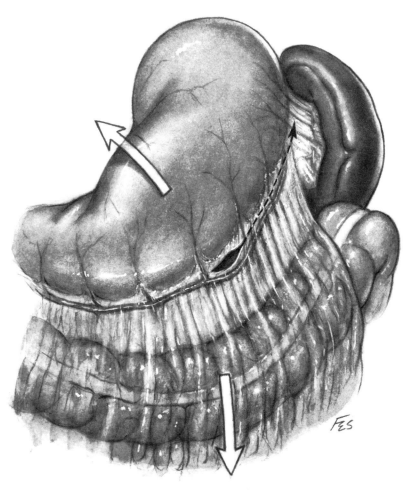

1. INCISION AND OPENING OF LESSER SAC

▼

Distal pancreatectomy can be performed through a left upper abdominal vertical incision or by an extended left subcostal incision. The lesser sac is entered by opening the gastrocolic omentum, either superior to the gastroepiploic arcade or outside this arcade.

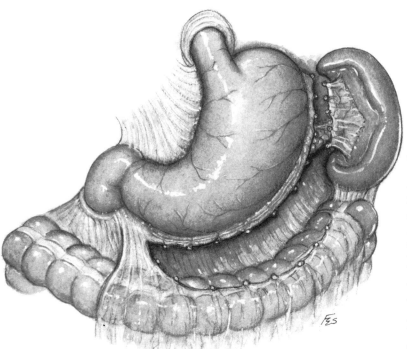

2. SHORT GASTRIC VESSELS SEVERED

▼

Dissection of the short gastric vessels is continued proximally on the stomach and distally over to the right gastroepiploic artery. With suitable subjects, the most superior short gastric artery can be severed at this time, but in others it is advisable to leave this artery until the spleen can partially be delivered into the incision. Attachments of the posterior wall of the stomach to the anterior surface of the pancreas are severed by sharp dissection.

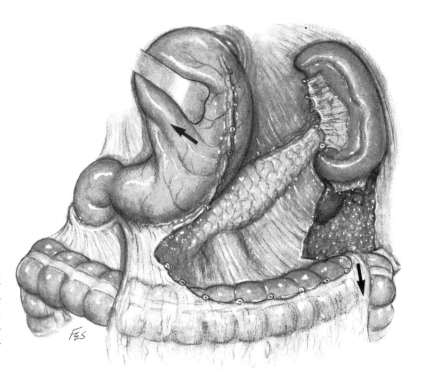

3. DISSECTION OF SPLENOCOLIC LIGAMENTS

▼

The stomach is rotated to the right, exposing the body and tail of the pancreas and the attachments of the spleen. At this time, the splenic and distal pancreatic mobilization is begun by severing the splenocolic ligaments, dropping the splenic flexure.

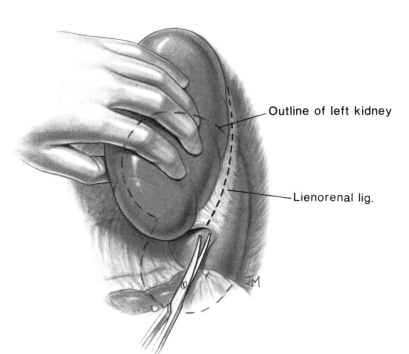

Outline of left kidney

Lienorenal lig.

4. DISSECTION OF POSTERIOR PERITONEAL ATTACHMENTS TO SPLEEN

▼

The splenorenal attachments along with the peritoneal reflections on the posterior aspect of the spleen are dissected.

5. ELEVATION OF SPLEEN, VESSELS, AND DISTAL PANCREAS

The peritoneum on the inferior aspect of the pancreas is dissected, which usually permits bloodless access to the posterior plane of the pancreas. In some instances, it is necessary to raise the spleen and pancreas from their bed by sharp dissection. Care must be taken not to enter the left adrenal gland, which lies under the distal body of the pancreas. After this dissection, the spleen, the body and tail of the pancreas, and the splenic artery and vein can be elevated by blunt and sharp dissection until the superior mesenteric vessels are approached.

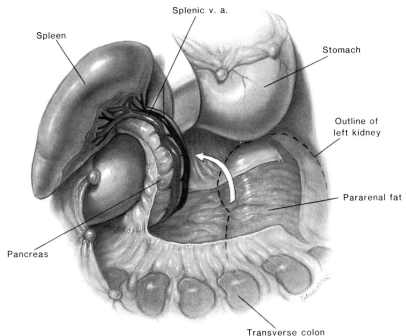

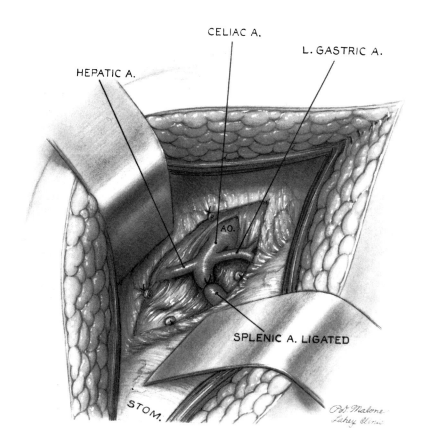

6. LIGATION OF SPLENIC ARTERY

Superior to the neck of the pancreas, the splenic artery can be traced and ligated after it is temporarily occluded, and the hepatic artery pulse is confirmed.

7. ELEVATION OF NECK OF PANCREAS

▼

The plane under the neck of the pancreas can be dissected because it is avascular. A Penrose drain is passed around the neck of the pancreas to help in identification of the junction of the splenic vein with the superior mesenteric vein. Further dissection of the posterior aspect of the pancreas permits tracing of the splenic vein to this junction and its ligation and section there.

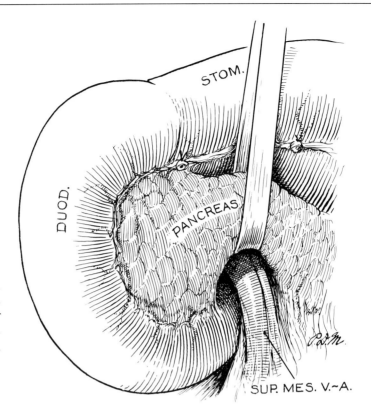

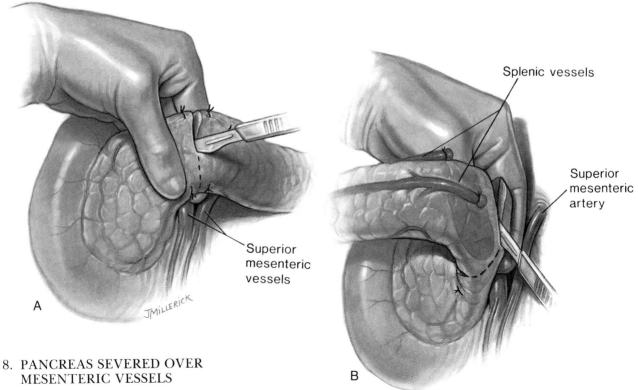

8. PANCREAS SEVERED OVER MESENTERIC VESSELS

▼

Sutures are placed into the superior and inferior borders of the pancreas. *A*, Anterior view. *B*, Posterior view. With the left hand controlling the neck of the pancreas, it is severed by a fishmouth incision just over the superior mesenteric vessels.

A

B

9. END OF PANCREAS CLOSED

▼

A and *B*, After patency of the pancreatic duct to the duodenum is determined, this duct can be suture ligated with silk and the pancreas closed with interrupted sutures of silk.

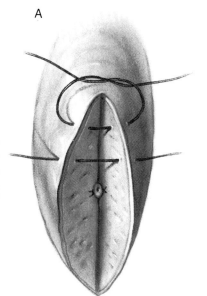
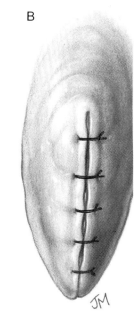

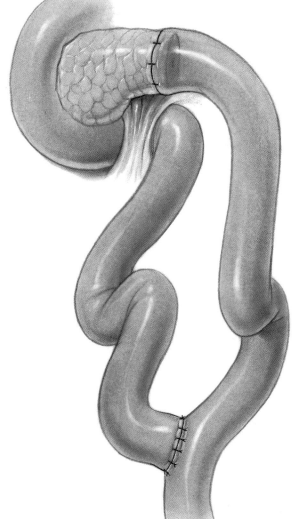

10. OPTIONAL ROUX-EN-Y ANASTOMOSIS TO PANCREAS

▼

When it is difficult to close the end of the pancreas or when an obstruction is present in the pancreatic duct at its entrance to the duodenum, a Roux-en-Y anastomosis of the stump of the pancreas to a loop of jejunum should be carried out. A sump drain is placed next to the remaining pancreas, and the incision is closed.

53

Distal (90 to 95 Per Cent) Pancreatectomy

JOHN W. BRAASCH, M.D.
RICARDO L. ROSSI, M.D.

▼ IMPORTANT FEATURES

Procedure for 90 to 95 Per Cent Distal Pancreatectomy Is an Extension of 40 to 50 Per Cent Distal Pancreatectomy

Dissection Is Carried into the Head of the Pancreas, Implying Mobilization of Head and Ligation of Some of the Blood Supply to That Portion of the Pancreas

▼ STEPS OR PLANS

Follow 40 to 50 Per Cent Pancreatectomy

Kocher Maneuver

Gastroduodenal Artery Is Dissected from Hepatic Artery and Ligated

Traction Permits Partial Dissection

T Tube Is Placed, and Fishmouth Incision into the Pancreatic Head Is Made to Remove 90 to 95 Per Cent of Pancreas

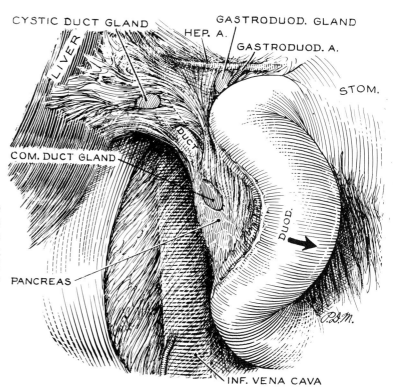

1. KOCHER MANEUVER

The procedure as outlined for 40 to 50 per cent distal pancreatectomy is carried out except that the pancreas is not severed to the left of the neck of the gland. Elevation of the head of the pancreas is accomplished by an extended Kocher maneuver.

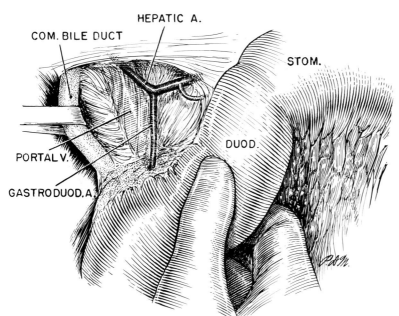

2. GASTRODUODENAL ARTERY LIGATED

The origin of the gastroduodenal artery from the hepatic artery is dissected and ligated. The inferior pancreaticoduodenal arcade must be preserved.

3. FISHMOUTH INCISION INTO PANCREATIC HEAD

The posterior attachments of the neck of the pancreas to the superior mesenteric vein and the portal vein are freed. The left hand of the surgeon is posterior to the head of the gland. After a T tube has been placed in the common duct and the distal limb led down into the duodenum to enable identification of the intrapancreatic portion of the common duct, a fishmouth incision is made into the head and uncinate process to remove approximately 90 to 95 per cent of the pancreas. Hemostasis is by suture.

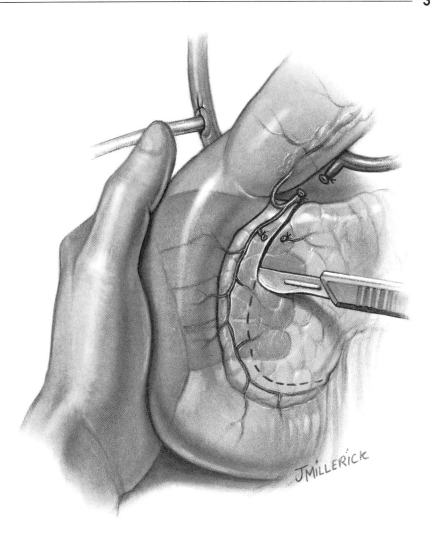

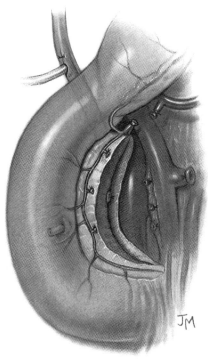

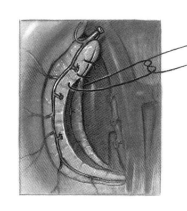

4. PANCREATIC REMNANT CLOSED

The remaining pancreas is sutured with permanent sutures in an interrupted fashion after suture ligation of the stump of the pancreatic duct. Sump drains are placed, and the incision is closed.

Total Pancreatectomy (Pylorus Preserving)

JOHN W. BRAASCH, M.D.
RICARDO L. ROSSI, M.D.

▼ IMPORTANT FEATURES
Technique for Total Pancreatectomy Is a Combination of Distal Pancreatectomy and Pancreatoduodenectomy (see previous sections)
Procedure Is Facilitated by Dissection of the Planes for Pancreatoduodenectomy as a First Step
Procedure Should Be at a Lesser Risk Than Pancreatoduodenectomy Because No Pancreatic Anastomosis Is Performed

▼ STEPS OR PLANS
Dissect the Four Planes for Pancreatoduodenectomy (as noted in that section)
Mobilize the Spleen and Body and Tail of the Pancreas as In Distal Pancreatectomy
Elevate the Neck of the Pancreas with a Penrose Drain Before Severing the Splenic Vein Near the Superior Mesenteric Vein
Dissect Head of Pancreas and Uncinate Process Off Superior Mesenteric and Portal Veins

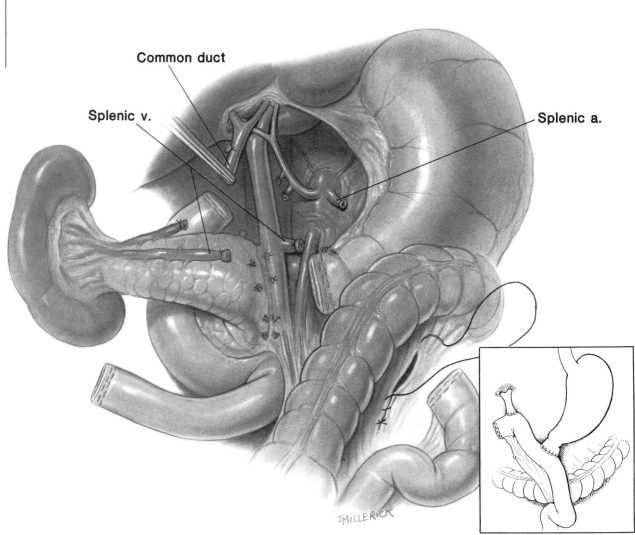

Common duct

Splenic v.

Splenic a.

1. FINAL STAGE OF RESECTION OF PANCREAS

▼

In the final stage for total pancreatectomy, the attachments of the uncinate process of the pancreas are about to be severed from the superior mesenteric vein and the portal vein. At times, the fourth portion and part of the third portion of the duodenum can be preserved, and the upper small bowel can be closed at the point of section in the third portion of the duodenum just to the right of the superior mesenteric vein. This technique avoids the necessity for tunneling the duodenojejunal junction back underneath the mesenteric vessel. Reconstruction of the upper gastrointestinal tract is by choledochojejunostomy proximal to the duodenojejunostomy.

Splenectomy and Splenorrhaphy

JOHN W. BRAASCH, M.D.

▼ IMPORTANT FEATURES
Early Ligation of Splenic Artery
Appropriate Sequential Mobilization
Avoid Damage to Pancreas and Stomach
Impeccable Hemostasis
Consider Splenorrhaphy for Trauma

▼ STEPS OR PLANS
Extended Left Subcostal or Left Rectus Incision
Open Lesser Sac
Ligate and Sever Short Gastric Vessels
Ligation of Splenic Artery In Continuity
Free Posterior Peritoneal Splenic Attachments
Elevation of Spleen Off Kidney Posteriorly and from Splenic Flexure
 Inferiorly
Deliver Spleen Partially into Wound and Sever Highest Short Gastric
 Vessels
Dissection and Ligation of Vessels at Splenic Hilum
Splenic Trauma—Evaluate Possibility of Preservation of the Spleen
 and Attempt Reconstruction, Especially In Children
Possible Partial Splenectomy or Closure of Splenic Laceration

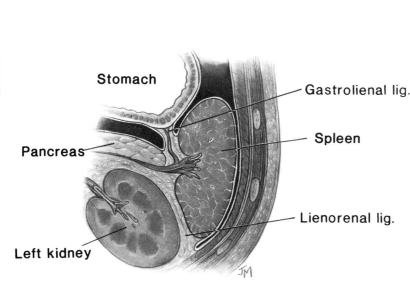

Stomach

Pancreas

Left kidney

Gastrolienal lig.

Spleen

Lienorenal lig.

1. INCISION AND SPLENIC RELATIONSHIPS

With a small spleen, the best exposure is by a left subcostal incision. With a large spleen, a left upper abdominal vertical incision is best because the splenic hilum is more accessible and more room is needed for removal of the spleen. The figure shows the attachments of the spleen, which must be released for splenic mobilization, and the proximity of the pancreatic tail, which could be injured.

In the presence of a major, life-threatening splenic hemorrhage, expeditious mobilization of the spleen and vascular control at the hilum are best carried out with steps 5, 6, and 7.

2. LESSER SAC OPENED

For elective splenectomy, the initial dissection is just distal to the gastro-epiploic arcade in the gastrocolic omentum.

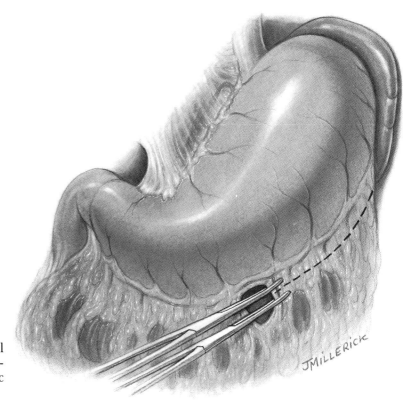

3. SHORT GASTRIC VESSELS SEVERED

▼

This dissection continues to the left, clamping and cutting the left gastro-epiploic artery and the short gastric vessels. The dissection proceeds as far as practical toward the most ceph-alad short gastric artery, which should be dissected later, after partial mobilization of the spleen.

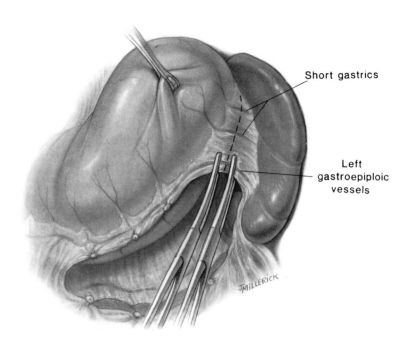

Short gastrics

Left gastroepiploic vessels

Splenic a.

Short gastrics

Left gastro-epiploic a. & v.

4. SPLENIC ARTERY LIGATED

▼

The splenic artery can be dissected and ligated in continuity after the hepatic artery pulse has been proved after temporary occlusion of the splenic artery.

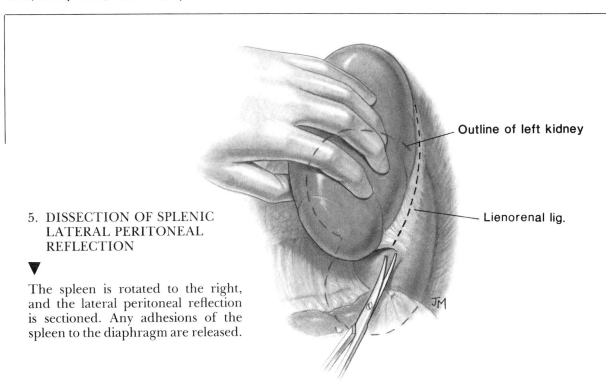

Outline of left kidney

Lienorenal lig.

5. DISSECTION OF SPLENIC LATERAL PERITONEAL REFLECTION

▼

The spleen is rotated to the right, and the lateral peritoneal reflection is sectioned. Any adhesions of the spleen to the diaphragm are released.

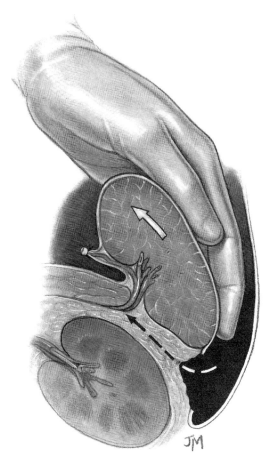

6. SPLENOCOLIC LIGAMENT SEVERED AND SPLEEN AND PANCREATIC TAIL ELEVATED

▼

The spleen is elevated off the anterior surface of Gerota's fascia, and the lienocolic ligament is dissected. This plane is continued anterior to the adrenal gland, elevating the tail and distal body of the pancreas.

7. FURTHER ELEVATION OF SPLEEN

▼

The spleen can now partially be delivered from the abdomen and the highest short gastric vessels dealt with.

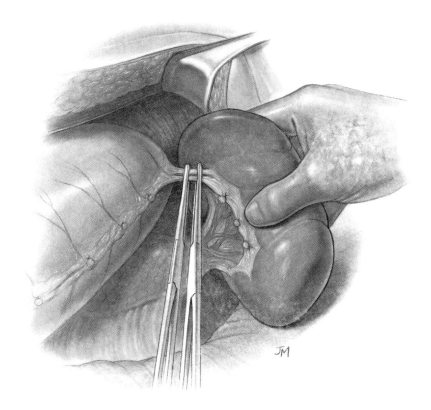

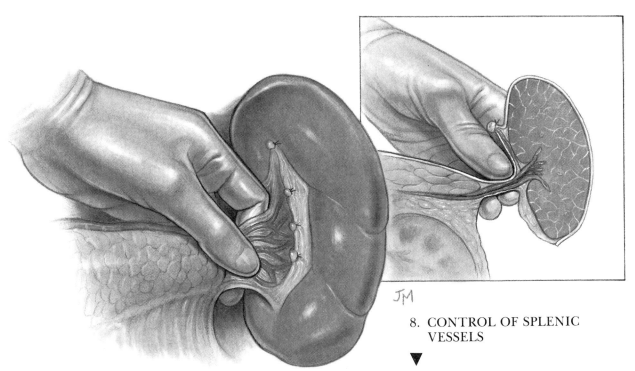

8. CONTROL OF SPLENIC VESSELS

▼

With the surgeon's left hand grasping the splenic pedicle to protect the tail of the pancreas, the splenic vessels are dissected, clamped, and severed at the hilum.

9. REMOVAL OF SPLEEN AND HEMOSTASIS

▼

The last splenic vessel is dealt with, completing splenectomy. After this maneuver, extensive efforts at accurate hemostasis in the right upper quadrant are most important. Whether a drain is necessary or not is controversial. A sump drain is left in the subphrenic space for 24 hours or longer when appreciable drainage is encountered.

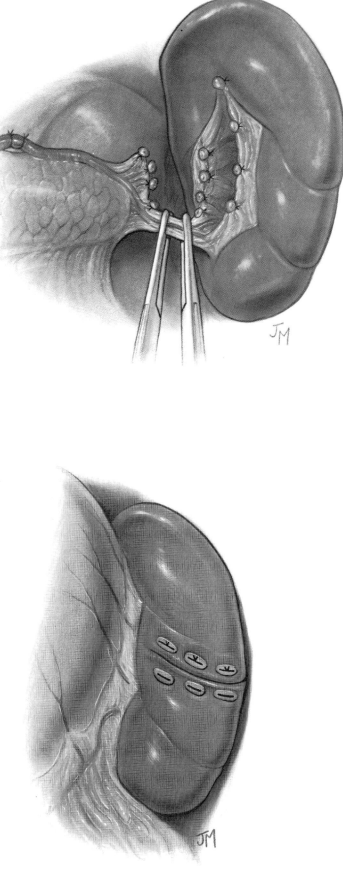

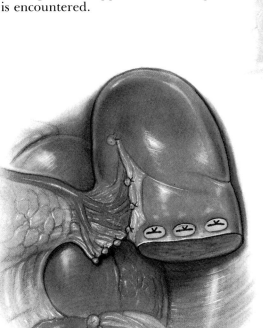

10. SPLENORRHAPHY AFTER TRAUMA

▼

Splenorrhaphy for trauma should seriously be considered in children. Illustrated is partial splenectomy with hilar ligation and closure for hemostasis of the lower pole of the spleen by bolstered mattress sutures. Extensive mobilization of the spleen is required for splenorrhaphy.

11. SPLENORRHAPHY (*Continued*)

▼

For a laceration, the same basic technique is used to stop lateral hemorrhage.

56 Adrenalectomy

JOHN A. LIBERTINO, M.D.

▼ IMPORTANT FEATURES

Diagnosis, Size of the Lesion, and Body Habitus of the Patient
Determine Incision to Be Used

With Pheochromocytoma, Early Ligation of the Adrenal Vein Is
Desirable

With Adrenal Carcinoma, There Must Be the Capacity for En Bloc
Resection of Spleen, Kidney, and Pancreas

Preservation of Renal Attachments to the Adrenal Gland Permits
Downward Traction on the Kidney to Bring the Adrenal
Gland into the Field for Dissection Superiorly

▼ STEPS OR PLANS

Surgical Anatomy
Anterior Approach
Left Adrenalectomy—Initial Dissection of Splenic Flexure
Elevation of the Pancreas and Spleen
Lateral Dissection of the Left Adrenal Gland
Control of the Inferior Phrenic Vessels
Rotation of the Left Adrenal Gland
Complete Devascularization
Left Adrenal Gland Pheochromocytoma
Right Adrenalectomy—Initial Exposure
Mobilization of the Adrenal Gland
Control of the Medial Vessels
Supracostal Incision
Thoracoabdominal Incision
Bilateral Posterior Incisions

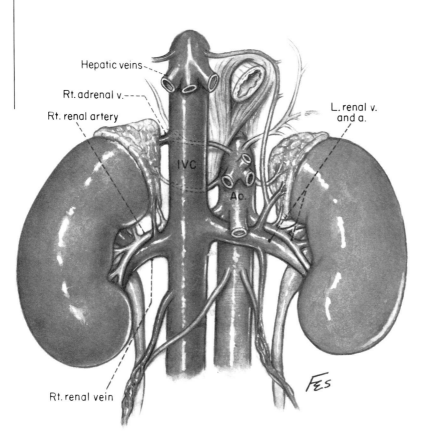

1. SURGICAL ANATOMY

▼

The position of the adrenal glands in the retroperitoneum adjacent to the upper pole of the kidneys is constant. The arterial supply arises from the inferior phrenic artery above, the aorta medially, and the renal artery inferiorly. The venous drainage is more variable. The right adrenal vein is short and enters the inferior vena cava on its posterolateral aspect. Visualization of this vein may be obscured at its origin from the inferior vena cava by an enlarged adrenal gland. On the left side, the adrenal vein is prominent and exits from the anteroinferior aspect of the adrenal gland and drains into the left renal vein.

The three major routes to the adrenal gland are the anterior transabdominal approach, the flank or thoracoabdominal approach, and the posterior approach.

2. ANTERIOR CHEVRON INCISION

▼

The anterior approach is preferred in most patients with bilateral hyperplasia when pituitary surgery is not appropriate and in patients with pheochromocytoma or an adrenal neoplasm when exploration of the extra-adrenal organs is essential. In obese patients or whenever bilateral exposure of the adrenal gland is required, a chevron incision is preferred.

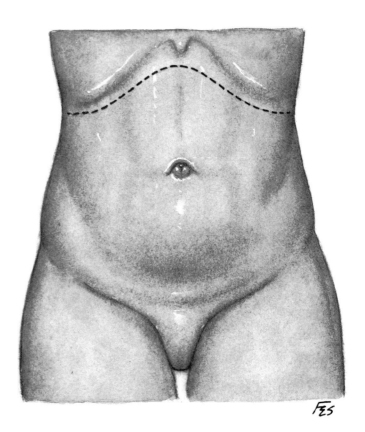

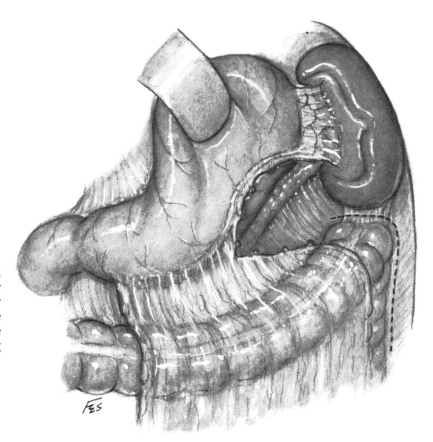

3. LEFT ADRENALECTOMY AND INITIAL DISSECTION OF SPLENIC FLEXURE

▼

After the peritoneal cavity has been entered and explored, the posterior peritoneum lateral to the left upper colon is incised vertically, and the incision is carried upward to divide the splenocolic ligament, mobilizing the splenic flexure.

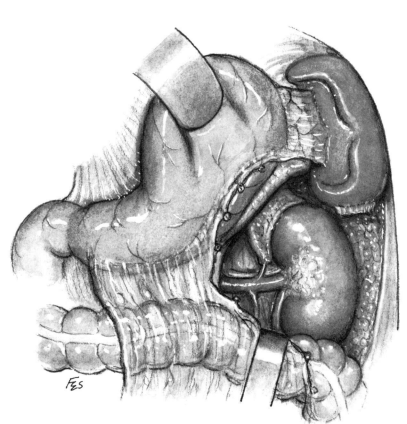

4. RETROPERITONEAL EXPOSURE OF LEFT ADRENAL GLAND

▼

The plane between the kidney and adrenal gland posteriorly and the pancreas and spleen anteriorly is developed by sharp dissection. The splenic flexure and duodenum are reflected medially and inferiorly and the pancreas and the spleen cephalad, care being taken not to injure the spleen or pancreas at this point.

5. INITIAL DISSECTION

▼

The dissection is started infralaterally on the adrenal gland and is carried laterally in an upward direction as shown by the *small arrow*. The kidney is retracted downward as shown by the *large arrow*, and the fascial attachments between the kidney and the adrenal gland are preserved. This will aid in gaining exposure to the upper pole of the adrenal gland. Strands of adventitia are preserved laterally to serve as a handle for manipulating and repositioning the adrenal gland. The gland itself should not be grasped with forceps, and meticulous hemostasis is maintained by the use of silver clips or the electrocautery.

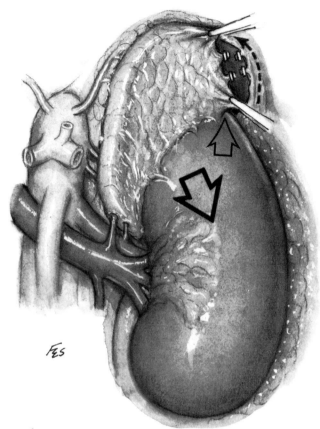

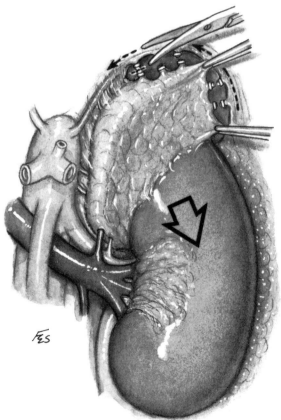

6. CONTROL OF INFERIOR PHRENIC VESSELS

▼

The inferior phrenic artery and vein are brought into view (*arrow*) by downward traction on the kidney. These are clipped with silver clips or ligated.

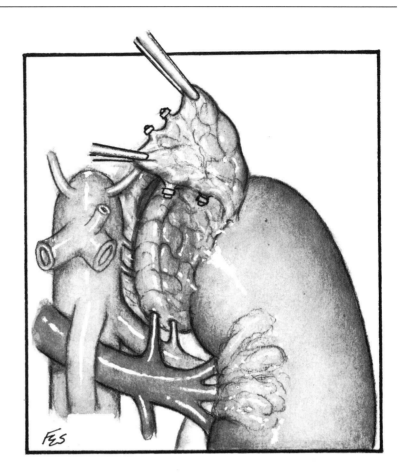

7. ROTATION OF GLAND MEDIALLY

▼

The gland can now be rotated medially and the posterior surface completely exposed. The adrenal vein is seen ascending from the left renal vein, and two or three arteries enter from the aorta.

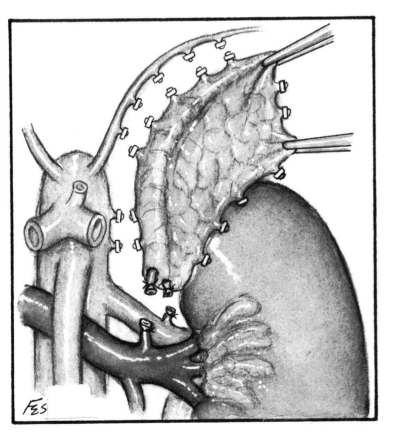

8. CONTROL OF AORTIC AND RENAL VESSELS AND REMOVAL OF ADRENAL GLAND

▼

When the medial blood supply from the aorta is completely controlled with silver clips, the inferior adrenal artery and vein emanating from the left renal artery and left renal vein are identified, isolated, ligated, and divided in continuity. The left adrenal gland can now be removed.

9. TECHNIQUE FOR LEFT PHEOCHROMOCYTOMA

When a pheochromocytoma is in the left adrenal gland, the approach to the gland is different. After the abdomen has been entered and the left adrenal gland exposed, the left adrenal vein is ligated and divided in continuity with sutures of 2-0 silk. The suture on the adrenal side may be left long to serve as a retractor during subsequent mobilization of the left adrenal gland. After the major adrenal venous drainage has been secured in this fashion, left adrenalectomy is accomplished as previously described.

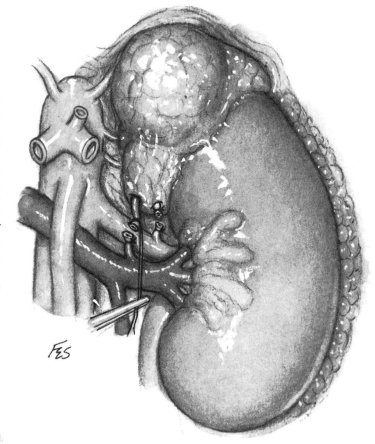

10. RIGHT ADRENALECTOMY, INITIAL EXPOSURE

After the abdomen has been entered, the posterior peritoneum lateral to the right colon is incised vertically, and the incision is carried up along the inferior vena cava (IVC) to the level of the hepatic veins. The colon is reflected medially, and the liver and gallbladder are retracted upward. The kidney is gently retracted inferiorly to bring the anterior surface of the right adrenal gland into view. Care must be taken to avoid trauma to the minor hepatic veins, which may enter the inferior vena cava at this level.

11. CONTROL OF SUPERIOR AND LATERAL VESSELS

▼

After all fatty and areolar tissue has been dissected from the anterior surface of the gland, the lower pole fascial attachments to the kidney are preserved and used as a handle to retract the adrenal gland downward by inferior traction on the right kidney. The adrenal gland is mobilized as described for left adrenalectomy. The lateral border of the right adrenal gland and the superior pole of the right adrenal gland are mobilized, and the vessels are ligated securely.

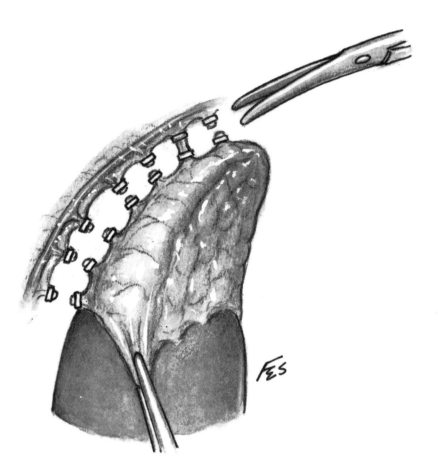

12. MEDIAL BLOOD SUPPLY

▼

A and B, Attention is directed to the medial blood supply to the right adrenal gland. The smaller arteries and veins are controlled with silver clips. The large central right adrenal vein is doubly ligated with sutures of 2-0 silk and divided. A silver clip should not be placed on this large central adrenal vein because it frequently becomes dislodged. The right adrenal vein is always higher than anticipated. Adequate inferior vena caval retraction and downward traction on the adrenal gland are essential for adequate exposure. When a pheochromocytoma is found in the right adrenal gland, the approach is altered in that the right central adrenal vein is ligated before the adrenal gland is manipulated.

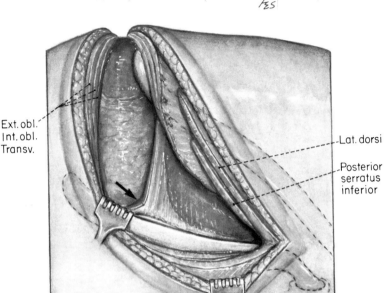

13. FLANK SUPRACOSTAL INCISION

▼

In patients with unilateral adrenal endocrinopathy, a supracostal eleventh or twelfth rib approach to the adrenal gland is used, depending on the site of the lesion. A flank approach is usually appropriate for the patient with an aldosteronoma, a small adrenal adenoma, or a small adrenal carcinoma.

The patient is positioned for a flank approach supracostal incision. The incision is made at the tip of either the eleventh or the twelfth rib and carried posteriorly along the upper border of the rib.

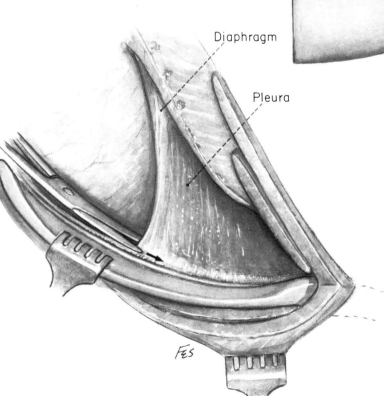

14 and 15. FLANK SUPRACOSTAL INCISION *(Continued)*

▼

The latissimus dorsi, external oblique, internal oblique, and transversus abdominis muscles as well as the intercostal muscles are divided along the upper border of the rib. The course of the intercostal nerve is followed to dissect the pleura from the inner aspect of the rib. The investing fascia, which surrounds the intercostal nerve, is divided. This protects the integrity of the pleura and maintains consistent extrapleural mobilization of the diaphragm and pleura.

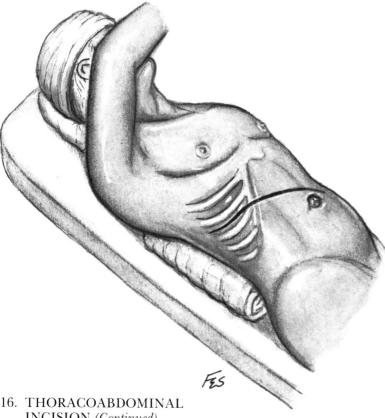

16 to 19. THORACO-ABDOMINAL INCISION

▼

The thoracoabdominal approach is useful in a patient with a large adrenal carcinoma who might also require concomitant splenectomy, distal pancreatectomy, or radical nephrectomy. In addition, this is a reasonable approach for a patient with a large pheochromocytoma because it affords exposure and palpation of the entire retroperitoneum and abdominal viscera through a single incision.

16. THORACOABDOMINAL INCISION *(Continued)*

The patient is placed in a semioblique position, at a 45–degree angle, with a rolled sheet placed longitudinally beneath the flank. The incision is begun in the ninth intercostal space near the angle of the rib and carried across the costal margin to the midpoint of the contralateral rectus muscle just above the umbilicus. As an alternative, the incision can be made in the bed of either the ninth or the tenth rib.

17. THORACOABDOMINAL INCISION *(Continued)*

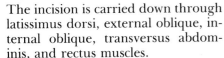

The incision is carried down through latissimus dorsi, external oblique, internal oblique, transversus abdominis, and rectus muscles.

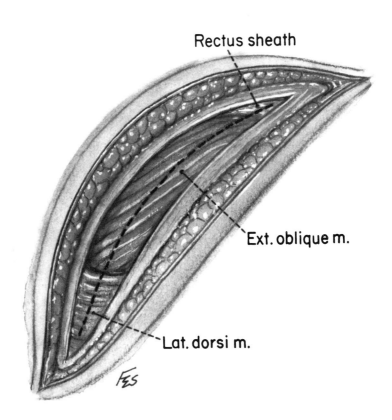

Rectus sheath

Ext. oblique m.

Lat. dorsi m.

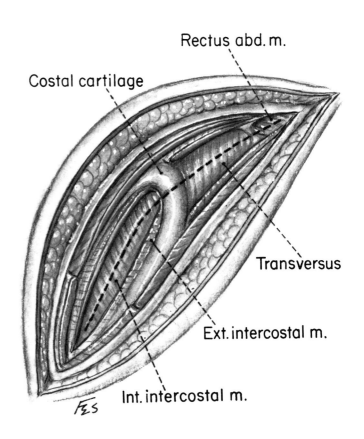

18. THORACOABDOMINAL INCISION *(Continued)*

▼

After the latissimus dorsi, external oblique, and rectus muscles have been divided, the intercostal muscles are divided in the direction of the incision. The costal cartilage between the ninth and tenth ribs is divided.

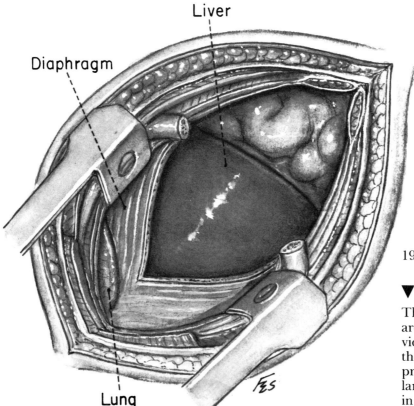

19. THORACOABDOMINAL INCISION *(Continued)*

▼

The peritoneal and pleural cavities are entered. The diaphragm is divided, taking care to avoid injury to the phrenic nerve. The lungs are protected with a Mikulicz pad, and a large Finochietto retractor is placed in the incision.

20 to 24. BILATERAL POSTERIOR INCISIONS

This is an older approach used for the removal of normal adrenal glands in a patient undergoing adrenalectomy for carcinoma of the breast as well as for the removal of a primary aldosteronoma.

20. POSITION ON TABLE

The patient is placed in the prone position on the operating table with a roll beneath the hips and the rib cage.

21. BILATERAL POSTERIOR INCISIONS

Two incisions are made over either the eleventh or twelfth rib, depending on the level of each adrenal gland, and extended medially to the paraspinal muscles. When necessary, the kidney bar can be elevated to give further flexion.

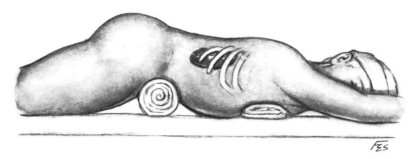

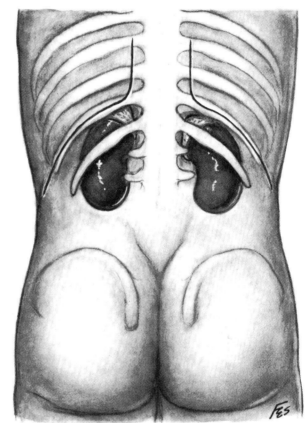

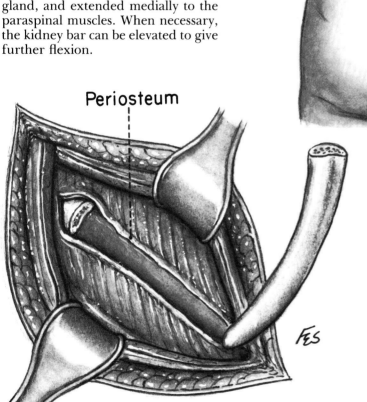

Periosteum

22. POSTERIOR APPROACH

The ribs are excised subperiosteally.

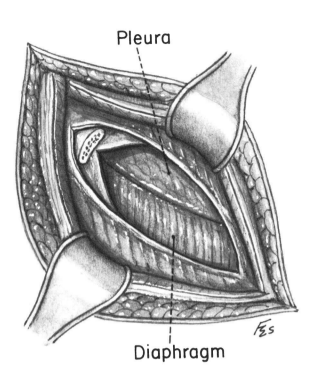

Pleura

Diaphragm

23. POSTERIOR APPROACH
(Continued)

▼

The incision is carried down through the periosteum of the ribs. After the periosteum has been divided, the pleura is mobilized superiorly.

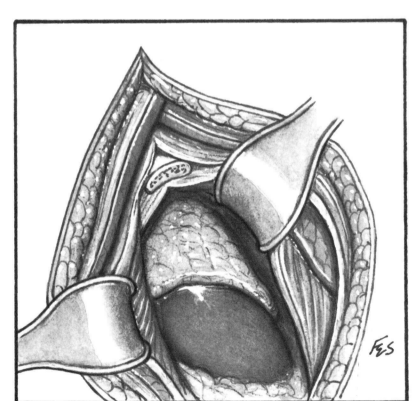

24. POSTERIOR APPROACH
(Continued)

▼

The diaphragm and pleura are retracted superiorly, and the paraspinal muscles are retracted medially, exposing the adrenal gland and the upper pole of the kidney.

Repair of Inguinal Hernia

J. LAWRENCE MUNSON, M.D.

▼ IMPORTANT FEATURES

Relaxing Incision Routinely Performed in the Deep Lamina of the
Rectus Sheath

Exploration of Cord Structures and the Inguinal Floor to Avoid
"Recurrence" by Finding Coexisting Hernias

Accurate Identification of the Transversus Abdominis Aponeurosis

Lateral Suture Incorporating Both the Iliopubic Tract and the
Shelving Edge of Poupart's Ligament

Using Cooper's Ligament for Repairs of Direct and Femoral Hernias

▼ STEPS OR PLANS

Incision

Retraction and Preservation of the Ilioinguinal Nerve

Sharp Dissection of the Cord at the Level of the Pubic Tubercle

Mobilization and Dissection of the Cord from the Inguinal Floor to
the Level of the Internal Ring

Evaluation of the Inguinal Floor and Femoral Canal Before Closure
of the Indirect Hernial Sac

Making an Adequate Relaxing Incision

Identification of the Transversus Abdominis Aponeurosis, the
Iliopubic Tract, and, If Necessary, Cooper's Ligament

An Interrupted Repair Without Tension

Reapproximation of the External Oblique Aponeurosis over the Cord
Structures and the Ilioinguinal Nerve

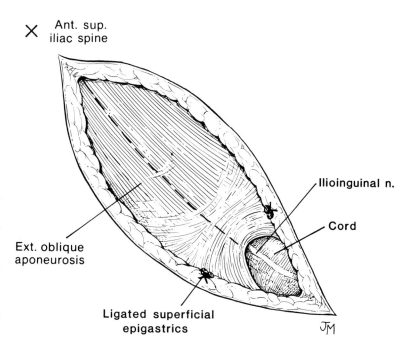

Ant. sup.
iliac spine

Ilioinguinal n.

Cord

Ext. oblique
aponeurosis

Ligated superficial
epigastrics

1. EXPOSURE OF EXTERNAL OBLIQUE APONEUROSIS

▼

The incision for the repair of most inguinal hernias is made cephalad and parallel to the inguinal ligament between the anterosuperior iliac spine and the pubic tubercle. The superficial epigastric vessels usually require suture control. However, other important vessels may be encountered laterally. Dissection through Scarpa's fascia exposes the aponeurosis of the external oblique muscle and the external ring. Frequently, the ilioinguinal nerve can be seen coursing along the cord as it exits the external ring. Self-retaining retractors are placed, and the aponeurosis of the external oblique muscle is incised in the direction of its fibers through the external ring.

2. OPENING OF EXTERNAL OBLIQUE APONEUROSIS AND DISSECTION OF ILIOINGUINAL NERVE

After the external oblique aponeurosis is opened, sharp dissection is used to elevate the aponeurosis medially and laterally to identify the inguinal ligament and the iliopubic tract laterally and the deep lamina of the rectus sheath medially. The ilioinguinal nerve is dissected off the cord structures and retracted either medially or laterally without tension for protection. Use of an Allis forceps to encircle the nerve atraumatically is helpful for countertraction on the nerve for ease of dissection. As the nerve crosses the internal oblique muscle to reach the cremaster muscle on the cord, usually a small blood vessel is present that requires control. The electrocautery should not be used for hemostasis at this point because current may track along the vessel and reach the nerve, causing damage.

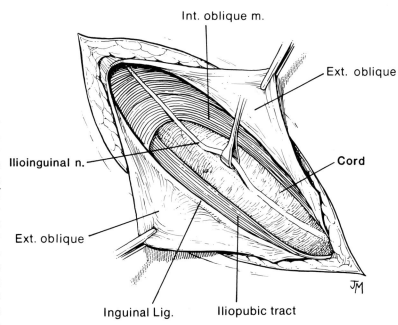

Int. oblique m.

Ext. oblique

Ilioinguinal n.

Cord

Ext. oblique

Inguinal Lig.

Iliopubic tract

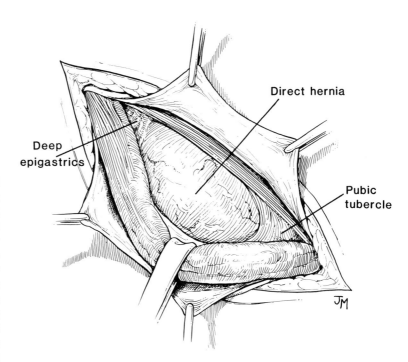

3. DISSECTION OF CORD AND DIRECT HERNIAL SAC

The cord is dissected off the inguinal floor sharply at the level of the pubic tubercle, approaching it medially and laterally until the cord has been freed. A Penrose drain is placed for traction. Dissection is carried cephalad to mobilize the cord completely from the floor up to the level of the internal ring. Two sets of vessels are identified: the deep epigastric vessels just below the level of the internal ring deep to the transversalis and the external spermatic vessels, which course in the cremaster muscle. These latter vessels provide considerable collateral flow to the testis and may help preserve viability of the testis in the event the testicular artery

is divided. Inspection of the floor of the inguinal canal should now reveal the presence or absence of a direct hernia.

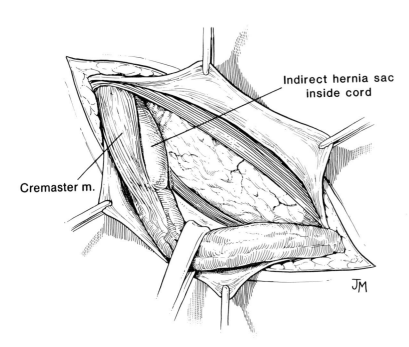

4. INDIRECT HERNIAL SAC

It is important not to neglect the cord structures. The cremaster muscle is divided circumferentially about the cord at the level of the internal ring. This division will permit accurate inspection of the cord for the presence of an indirect hernial sac, which may coexist with a direct hernia. When an indirect hernia is identified, the sac is grasped with forceps and sharply dissected from the rest of the cord structures up to the internal ring.

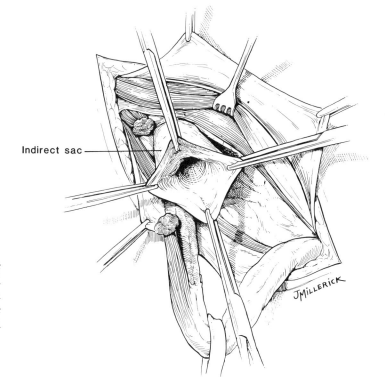

Indirect sac

5. EXPLORATION OF POSSIBLE HERNIAL SITES

The hernial sac is opened, and the sac is inspected for intra-abdominal contents. A finger inserted through the sac into the abdomen can palpate the femoral canal and the inguinal canal for strength.

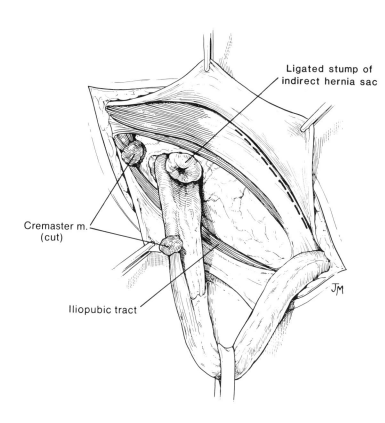

Ligated stump of indirect hernia sac

Cremaster m. (cut)

Iliopubic tract

6. HERNIAL SAC REDUCED OR SEVERED AND RELAXING INCISION

The indirect hernial sac is suture ligated and severed, which should permit the sac to retract up under the internal oblique muscle. A relaxing incision is made in the deep lamina of the rectus sheath just lateral to the fusion point of the external oblique aponeurosis. The incision must be carried inferiorly to the level of the pubic tubercle because this is the most inferior part of the incision and receives the most tension.

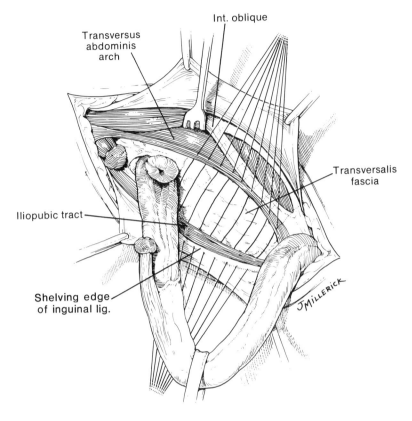

7. REPAIR FLOOR OF INGUINAL CANAL

▼

In the repair of an indirect hernia, a modified iliopubic tract approach is used. After the internal oblique muscle is retracted medially, the aponeurosis of the transversus abdominis muscle is identified as a separate structure from the transversalis fascia; this is actually the layer to be used for the medial suture. This may be fused to the internal oblique muscle as a conjoined tendon, which, if present, should be incorporated in the repair. Laterally, the iliopubic tract is identified again as a separate layer from the shelving edge of the inguinal ligament. Interrupted sutures of nylon are used, starting at the level of the pubic tubercle, to incorporate the transversus abdominis aponeurosis, the iliopubic tract, and the shelving edge of Poupart's ligament. The repair is most important at the internal ring, which must be reconstructed snugly to permit just a fingertip to be inserted next to the cord.

8. REPAIR OF COOPER'S LIGAMENT FOR DIRECT HERNIA

▼

For a direct hernia, the transversalis fascia is opened to permit visual identification and dissection of Cooper's ligament. This step must be accomplished by dividing the transversalis fascia to permit identification of an aberrant obturator artery that could cause excessive bleeding from the suture through Cooper's ligament.

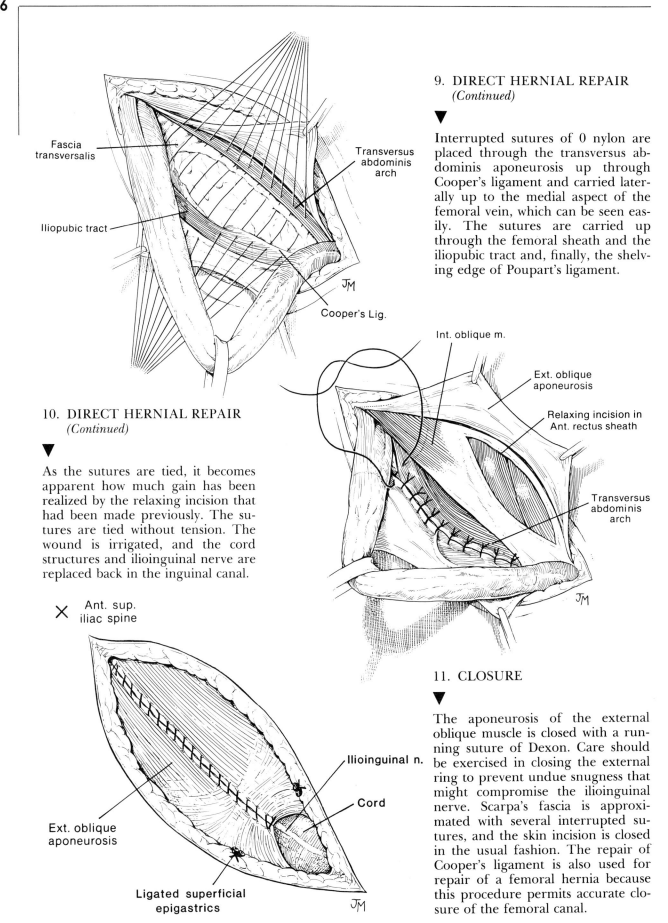

Fascia transversalis

Iliopubic tract

Transversus abdominis arch

Cooper's Lig.

9. DIRECT HERNIAL REPAIR
(Continued)

▼

Interrupted sutures of 0 nylon are placed through the transversus abdominis aponeurosis up through Cooper's ligament and carried laterally up to the medial aspect of the femoral vein, which can be seen easily. The sutures are carried up through the femoral sheath and the iliopubic tract and, finally, the shelving edge of Poupart's ligament.

Int. oblique m.

Ext. oblique aponeurosis

Relaxing incision in Ant. rectus sheath

Transversus abdominis arch

10. DIRECT HERNIAL REPAIR
(Continued)

▼

As the sutures are tied, it becomes apparent how much gain has been realized by the relaxing incision that had been made previously. The sutures are tied without tension. The wound is irrigated, and the cord structures and ilioinguinal nerve are replaced back in the inguinal canal.

✕ Ant. sup. iliac spine

Ilioinguinal n.

Cord

Ext. oblique aponeurosis

Ligated superficial epigastrics

11. CLOSURE

▼

The aponeurosis of the external oblique muscle is closed with a running suture of Dexon. Care should be exercised in closing the external ring to prevent undue snugness that might compromise the ilioinguinal nerve. Scarpa's fascia is approximated with several interrupted sutures, and the skin incision is closed in the usual fashion. The repair of Cooper's ligament is also used for repair of a femoral hernia because this procedure permits accurate closure of the femoral canal.

Ventral Herniorrhaphy with Marlex Mesh

58

J. LAWRENCE MUNSON, M.D.

▼ IMPORTANT FEATURES

Identification of Healthy Fascia and Resection of Attenuated Scarred
  Fascial Rim
Lysis of Adhesions Beneath the Fascial Edges to Permit Safe Closure
Interposition of Omentum Between Intestine and Marlex Mesh
Drainage of the Subcutaneous Space

▼ STEPS OR PLANS

Excision of Thinned-Out Skin Overlying the Hernia and Mobilization
  of Subcutaneous Fat Overlying Healthy Fascia
Dissection of the Hernia from the Fascial Rim
Excision of the Hernial Sac
Lysis of Adhesions Underlying the Fascial Rim
Excision of Attenuated and Scarred Fascia
Mobilization of Omentum over the Intestine Underlying the Wound
Sizing of the Prosthetic Mesh for the Repair and Placement of
  Mattress Sutures of Nylon
Placement of Subcutaneous Closed Suction Drains
Wound Closure

Double Marlex Mesh Technique

1. DISSECTION OF FASCIAL RIM

▼

The thinned-out skin overlying the hernia is excised in elliptical fashion back to healthy subcutaneous tissue. The healthy fascia is cleared of subcutaneous fat for several centimeters around the hernial defect. The hernial sac is opened and excised back to the fascial edge, lysing all adhesions of omentum or intestine to the hernial sac. Alternatively, the fascial rim can be freed circumferentially around the hernial sac, and the hernia can be reduced into the abdomen. The fascial rim of the hernia is usually attenuated and made up primarily of collagenous scar, which has poor suture-holding ability. The fascia therefore is excised back to healthy, thick, well-vascularized fascia circumferentially. The adhesions to this fascia are freed to permit safe closure. The omentum, if still present, is mobilized enough to permit it to be draped over the intestine that will be subjacent to the wound clo-

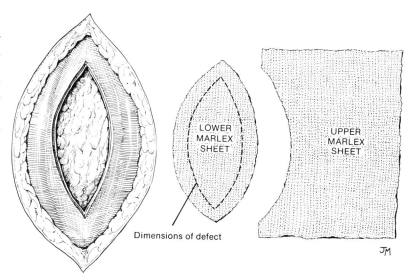

Dimensions of defect

sure. A Marlex sheet is fashioned in two sections for the upper and lower layers of the repair. The innermost or lower sheet approximates the dimensions of the hernial defect, allowing 2 cm on each edge for placement of sutures.

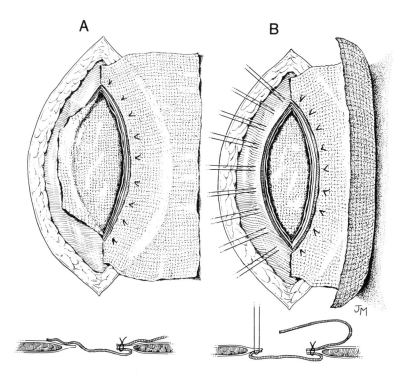

A   B

2. FIRST-STAGE PLACEMENT OF MARLEX SHEET

▼

A, The inner sheet is placed within the wound, and the lateral edge of the upper sheet is placed along the top of the fascia. Mattress sutures of 0 nylon are placed through both layers of the mesh and the healthy fascia and tied without undue tension. *B,* With one side of the hernial repair completed, the loose edge of the Marlex is approximated to the undersurface of the fascia with mattress sutures that are left untied. A needle is placed on the free end of the suture.

3. PLACEMENT OF OUTER MARLEX LAYER AND CLOSURE OF WOUND

A, The loose half of the upper sheet of Marlex is brought over the wound, and the mattress suture is brought up through the mesh where it is tied again. This procedure completes the sandwiching of Marlex to fascia and then to the upper Marlex. The rest of the Marlex sheet is excised, and the free edge is tacked to the underlying fascia with interrupted sutures. *B,* The subcutaneous tissue is mobilized off the underlying fascia only enough to permit closure of the skin without tension, although this technique creates a potential space that requires drainage. Two closed suction drains are placed through counterincisions and brought to overlie the mesh and drain the subcutaneous space. The wound is copiously irrigated and closed in layers.

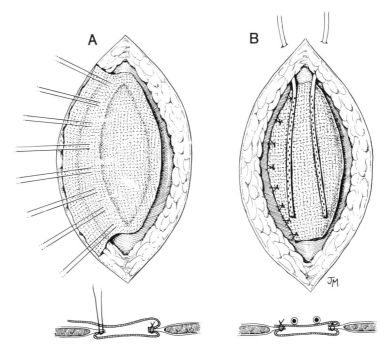

Binder Marlex Mesh Technique

4. PLACEMENT OF INTERNAL BINDER

A and *B,* The second type of repair of a ventral hernia involves the use of a binder technique first described using fascia lata but more conveniently now performed with Marlex mesh. The dimensions of the hernial defect are transcribed onto the center of a Marlex sheet, and strips 2 cm wide are fashioned, permitting 2 cm around the hernial defect. Each individual strip is twisted and threaded on a Gallie fascial needle, which is brought up through the healthy fascia approximately 3 cm from the fas-

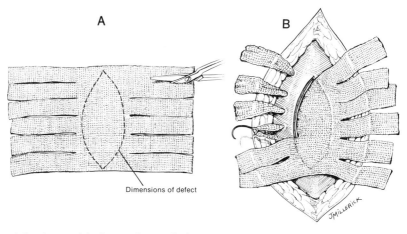

Dimensions of defect

cial edge. This is performed circumferentially so that the mesh is positioned underneath the fascia in a smooth fashion.

5. FIXATION OF BINDER AND CLOSURE OF INCISION

▼

A, All the strips are pulled anterior to draw the mesh securely up against the abdominal wall, with care being taken to avoid entrapment of omentum or intestine between the abdominal wall and mesh. Each strip is sutured to the fascia with a suture of 0 nylon, and the excess strip is excised. *B,* Closed suction drains are placed through counterincisions as the subcutaneous tissue has been mobilized to permit closure of the skin. The wound is irrigated and closed in layers without tension. After operation, the drains are left in place until drainage drops below 30 ml per 24 hours.

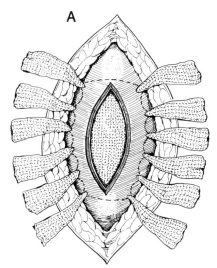

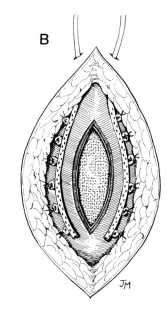

Repair of Umbilical Hernia

59

J. LAWRENCE MUNSON, M.D.

▼ IMPORTANT FEATURES
  Preservation of Umbilicus Unless the Hernia Is Exceedingly Large
  Inspection for Other Midline Defects
  Identification of Anterior Rectus Sheath
  Obliteration of Subcutaneous Dead Space

▼ STEPS OR PLANS
  Supraumbilical Incision; Elliptical Incision When the Hernia Is
      Excessively Large
  Dissection of Hernial Sac from Subcutaneous Tissue and
      Undersurface of the Umbilicus
  Circumferential Dissection of the Hernial Sac from the Fascial Edges
  Opening and Resection of the Hernial Sac and Lysis of Subjacent
      Adhesions
  Careful Inspection for Other Midline Defects That Will Require
      Repair
  Closure of the Peritoneum
  Repair of the Hernia Transversely with 0 Nylon After Accurate
      Identification of the Anterior Rectus Sheath
  Obliteration of Subcutaneous Dead Space
  Closure of Wound and Dressing

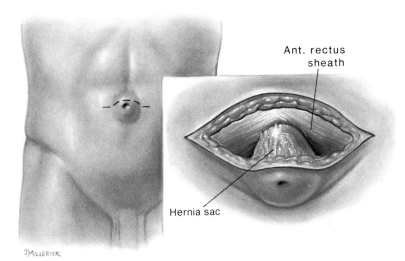

Ant. rectus sheath

Hernia sac

JMILLERICK

1. INCISION AND INITIAL DISSECTION

For the repair of a small umbilical hernia, a supraumbilical transversely aligned incision is used. Care must be exercised immediately adjacent to the umbilicus because the skin and dermis may be adherent to the hernial sac. It is often easier to begin the dissection at the two extremes of the incision, working toward the midline. This maneuver permits accurate identification of the hernial sac and prevents premature entrance into the sac immediately below the umbilicus.

2. DISSECTION OF HERNIAL SAC

A, The hernial sac is grasped with a traumatic forceps and sharply dissected from the undersurface of the umbilicus where the plane of dissection most often will be at the level of the dermis. Care must be taken to avoid devascularization of the skin of the umbilicus. The anterior rectus sheath and midline fascia are cleared completely around the hernial sac; notation should be made of the integrity of the linea alba above the umbilical hernia. As an umbilical hernia is commonly a congenital defect, other midline defects (most often superior to the umbilicus) that also require attention may be found. *B,* The hernial sac is dissected circumferentially around the fascial rim, often requiring extension of the defect laterally for accurate identification of the anterior rectus sheath and reduc-

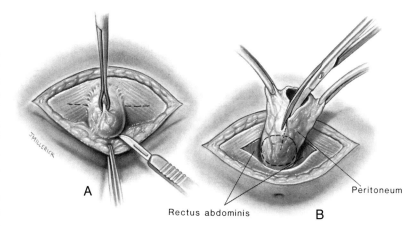

JMILLERICK

A

Rectus abdominis

Peritoneum

B

tion of the hernia. After full mobilization around the fascial rim, the hernial sac is opened, and any adhesions to the sac are divided. The redundant sac is excised, with care taken to obtain hemostasis in the peritoneal fat that often accompanies the sac.

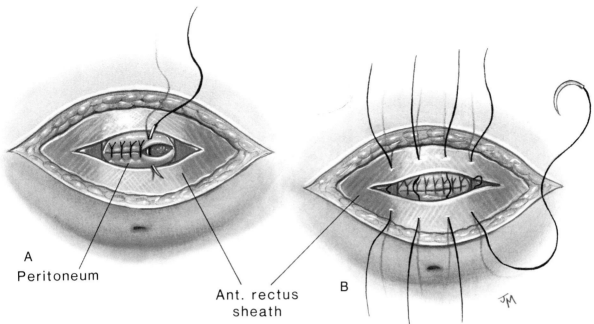

A
Peritoneum

Ant. rectus
sheath

B

3. REPAIR
▼

A, The peritoneum is closed with interrupted sutures of catgut, although this is not absolutely necessary and adds little to the functional repair. *B,* Interrupted sutures of 0 nylon are placed 1 cm back from the fascial edges, the length of the fascial defect, and brought up together by the assistant and tied sequentially. It is not necessary to overlap the fascial edges as is carried out in more classic repairs because direct fascia-to-fascia approximation enables greater wound strength on healing.

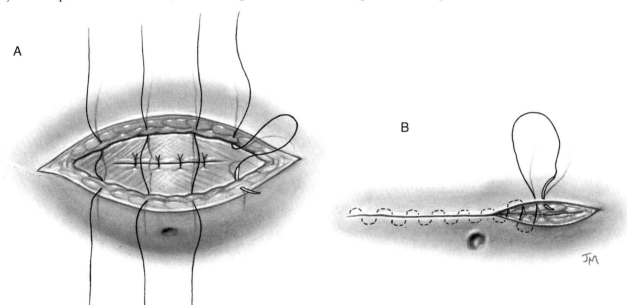

A

B

4. CLOSURE OF WOUND
▼

A, After the wound has been irrigated and hemostasis has been verified, the subcutaneous dead space is obliterated with interrupted sutures of plain catgut placed deep to the dermis. *B,* Closure of the wound is finished with a running subcuticular suture of Vicryl. The wound is dressed by placing surgical cotton within the umbilicus with a bulky compressive dressing to compress the subcutaneous tissue and permit the umbilicus to be fixed in its normal position to the fascia.

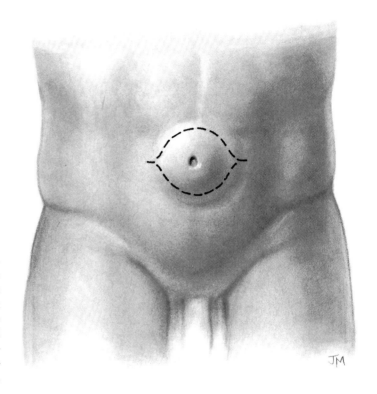

5. REPAIR OF LARGE UMBILICAL HERNIA

For a large umbilical hernia, an elliptical incision is planned to encompass the umbilicus and the subcutaneous tissue below it. The patient should be informed before the procedure that the umbilicus will be lost in performing the repair. The incision is carried laterally as an ellipse as far as necessary to identify the edges of the hernial sac and the rim of healthy fascia.

Hernia sac

Ant. rectus sheath

6. REPAIR OF LARGE UMBILICAL HERNIA
(Continued)

After an incision has been made through the subcutaneous tissue down to the anterior rectus sheath bilaterally, the dissection proceeds toward the midline to identify the edges of the hernial sac. The sac is dissected from the undersurface of the umbilicus or directly opened after the fascial rim has been dissected circumferentially. The distal sac is removed with an ellipse of skin and umbilicus as a specimen. The rest of the repair proceeds as for a smaller umbilical hernia. With a larger umbilical hernia, drainage of the subcutaneous dead space may be necessary, and drainage is best performed with closed suction drains brought through lateral counterincisions.

Appendix

Chapter 1

Figures 2, 4, and 7 through 11 are reproduced from Ellis FH Jr: Carcinoma of the distal esophagus and esophagogastric junction. *In* Cohn LH (ed): Modern Technics in Surgery. New York, Futura Publishing Co, 1979, with permission.

Chapter 3

Figures 1 and 2 are reproduced from Ellis FH Jr, Crozier RE, Shea JA: Paraesophageal hiatus hernia. Arch Surg 121:417 and 418, 1986, with permission. Copyright 1986, American Medical Association.

Chapter 8

Figures 1 and 2 are reproduced from Rossi RL, Braasch JW: Parietal cell vagotomy. Surg Clin North Am 60:248 and 251, 1980, with permission.

Chapter 9

Figures 1 through 5 and 7 through 14 are reproduced from Rossi RL, Braasch JW: Parietal cell vagotomy. Surg Clin North Am 60:248–255, 257, 1980, with permission.

Chapter 10

Figures 1, 3 through 9, and 11 are reproduced from Reiling RB: Staplers in gastrointestinal surgery. Surg Clin North Am 60:382, 385–389, 390, 392, 394, 1980, with permission.

Chapter 13

Figures 1 through 3 are reproduced from Cattell RB, Braasch JW: A technique for the exposure of the third and fourth portions of the duodenum. Surg Gynecol Obstet 111:378 and 379, 1960. By permission of Surgery, Gynecology & Obstetrics.

Chapter 19

Figures 1 through 13 and 16 through 24 are reproduced from Veidenheimer MC: Abdominoperineal excision of the rectum. *In* Rob C, Smith R: Operative Surgery: Fundamental International Techniques. Third ed, Section 3: Colon, Rectum and Anus (edited by I. P. Todd). London, Butterworth & Co (Publishers) Ltd, 1977, pp 133–142, with permission.

Chapter 20

Figures 3 through 11 are reproduced from Veidenheimer MC: Abdominoperineal excision of the rectum I. *In* Rob C, Smith R: Operative Surgery: Alimentary Tract and Abdominal Wall. Fourth ed, Section 3: Colon, Rectum and Anus (edited by I. P. Todd and L. P. Fielding). London, Butterworth & Co (Publishers) Ltd, 1983, pp 329–331, with permission.

Chapter 21

Figure 2 is reproduced from Reiling RB: Staplers in gastrointestinal surgery. Surg Clin North Am 60:391, 1980, with permission.

Chapter 22

Figure 8 is reproduced from Lahey FH: A discussion of the modified Mikulicz operation for carcinoma of the colon and its technic. Surg Clin North Am 26:615, 1946, with permission.

Chapter 23

Figure 2 is reproduced from Schoetz DJ Jr, Coller JA, Veidenheimer MC: Alternatives to conventional ileostomy in chronic ulcerative colitis. Surg Clin North Am 65:28, 1985, with permission.

Chapter 24

Figure 1 is reproduced from Schoetz DJ Jr: Rectal prolapse. A. Pathogenesis and

Chapter 23 *Continued*

clinical features. *In* Henry MM, Swash M (eds): Coloproctology and the Pelvic Floor: Pathophysiology and Management. London, Butterworth & Co (Publishers) Ltd, 1985, with permission.

Figures 2 and 3 are reproduced from Veidenheimer MC: Abdominoperineal excision of the rectum. *In* Rob C, Smith R: Operative Surgery: Fundamental International Techniques. Third ed, Section 3: Colon, Rectum and Anus (edited by I. P. Todd). London, Butterworth & Co (Publishers) Ltd, 1977, p 136, with permission.

Figures 13, 14, 16, and 17 are reproduced from Schoetz DJ Jr: Operative therapy for anal incontinence. Surg Clin North Am 65:44 and 45, 1985, with permission.

Figure 15 is reproduced from Horn HR, Schoetz DJ Jr, Coller JA, Veidenheimer MC: Sphincter repair with a Silastic sling for anal incontinence and rectal repair. Dis Colon Rectum 28:869, 1985, with permission.

Chapter 25

Figure 1 is reproduced from Corman ML: Anal sphincter reconstruction. Surg Clin North Am 60:459, 1980, with permission.

Figures 3 through 5 are reproduced from Schoetz DJ Jr: Operative therapy for anal incontinence. Surg Clin North Am 65:42 and 43, 1985, with permission.

Chapter 28

Figures 13 and 14 are reproduced from Corman ML: Rubber band ligation of hemorrhoids. Arch Surg 112:1258, 1979, with permission. Copyright 1979, American Medical Association.

Chapter 29

Figure 1 is reproduced from Seckel BR, Schoetz DJ Jr: Reconstruction of the perineum. Probl Gen Surg 2:565, 1985, with permission.

Figure 2 is reproduced from Corman ML, Veidenheimer MC, Coller JA: Anoplasty for anal stricture. Surg Clin North Am 56:728, 1976, with permission.

Figure 7 is reproduced from Seckel BR, Schoetz DJ Jr: Reconstruction of the perineum. Probl Gen Surg 2:567, 1985, with permission.

Figure 8 is reproduced from Seckel BR, Schoetz DJ Jr: Reconstruction of the perineum. Probl Gen Surg 2:568, 1985, with permission.

Figures 9 and 10 are reproduced from Schoetz DJ Jr: Operative therapy for anal incontinence. Surg Clin North Am 65:41, 1985, with permission.

Figures 11 through 14 are reproduced from Seckel BR, Schoetz DJ Jr, Coller JA: Skin grafts for circumferential coverage of perianal wounds. Surg Clin North Am 65:367–369, 1985, with permission.

Chapter 34

Figures 3 through 5 and 7 are reproduced from Linder RM, Cady B: Hepatic resection. Surg Clin North Am 60:352, 354, 357, and 361, 1980, with permission.

Chapter 35

Figures 2 and 16 are reproduced from Jenkins RL, Pinson CW, Stone MD: Liver transplantation. *In* McDermott WV Jr: Surgery of the Liver. Boston, Blackwell Scientific Publications, 1989, pp 481 and 482. By permission of Blackwell Scientific Publications, Inc.

Figures 1, 9, and 13 are reproduced with the permission of Roger L. Jenkins, M.D.

Figures 21 through 23 are reproduced with the permission of Roger L. Jenkins, M.D.

Figures 27 and 31 through 33 are reproduced from Jenkins RL, Pinson CW, Stone MD: Liver transplantation. *In* McDermott WV Jr: Surgery of the Liver. Boston, Blackwell Scientific Publications, 1989, pp 481, 484, and 485, with permission.

Figures 28 through 30 are reproduced with the permission of Roger L. Jenkins, M.D.

Chapter 40

Figure 2 is reproduced from Cattell RB, Braasch JW: Secondary operations on the biliary tract. Lahey Clin Bull 11:166, 1959, with permission.

Chapter 41

Figure 1 is reproduced from Cattell RB, Braasch JW: Secondary operation on the biliary tract. Lahey Clin Bull 11:166, 1959, with permission.

Chapter 43

Figure 2 is reproduced from Braasch JW: Secondary biliary tract procedures. Surg Clin North Am 40:709, 1960, with permission.

Figure 4*B* and *C* is reproduced from Bagley FH, Braasch JW, Taylor RH, Warren KW: Sphincterotomy or sphinctero-plasty in the treatment of pathologically mild chronic pancreatitis. Am J Surg 141:419, 1981, with permission.

Chapter 44

Figures 1, 5, and 7 are reproduced from Bolton JS, Braasch JW, Rossi RL: Management of benign biliary stricture. Surg Clin North Am 60:317, 323, and 325, 1980, with permission.

Figure 2 is reproduced from Cattell RB, Braasch JW: Strictures of the bile duct. Surg Clin North Am 38:651, 1958.

Figures 4, 8, and 10 are reproduced from Braasch JW: Current considerations in the repair of bile duct strictures. Surg Clin North Am 53:427 and 430, 1973.

Figures 6 and 9 are reproduced from Braasch JW: Postoperative strictures of the bile duct. *In* Schwartz SI, Ellis H (eds): Maingot's Abdominal Operations. 8th ed, Vol 2. Norwalk, CT, Appleton-Century-Crofts, 1985, pp 1967 and 1976, with permission.

Figure 12 is reproduced from Warren KW, Braasch JW: Repair of benign strictures of the bile ducts. Surg Clin North Am 45:625, 1965, with permission.

Figure 13 is reproduced from Braasch JW: Part II. Reconstruction of biliary tract. *In* Nora PF (ed): Operative Surgery: Principles and Techniques. 2nd ed. Philadelphia, Lea & Febiger, 1979, p 578, with permission.

Figure 14 is reproduced from Cattell RB, Braasch JW: Repair of benign strictures of the bile duct involving both or single hepatic ducts. Surg Gynecol Obstet 110:57, 1960. By permission of Surgery, Gynecology & Obstetrics.

Figure 17 is reproduced from Braasch JW, Rossi RL: Reoperations on the biliary tract. Probl Gen Surg 2:488, 1985, with permission.

Chapter 46

Figure 2 is reproduced from Linder RM, Cady B: Hepatic resection. Surg Clin North Am 60:355, 1980, with permission.

Figures 3 and 5 are reproduced from Pinson CW, Rossi RL: Extended right hepatic lobectomy, left hepatic lobectomy, and skeletonization resection for proximal bile duct cancer. World J Surg 12:56, 1988, with permission.

Figure 8 is reproduced from Rossi RL, Heiss FW, Beckmann CF, Braasch JW: Management of cancer of the bile duct. Surg Clin North Am 65:66, 1985, with permission.

Figure 9 is reproduced from Rossi RL, Gordon M, Braasch JW: Intubation techniques in biliary tract surgery. Surg Clin North Am 60:304, 1980, with permission.

Figures 15 and 16 are reproduced from Rossi RL, Braasch JW: Biliary cancer surgery: When to do what. Contemp Surg 20:16 and 17, 1982, with permission.

Chapter 51

Figure 4 is reproduced from Braasch JW, Gray BN: Technique of radical pancreatoduodenectomy with consideration of hepatic arterial relationships. Surg Clin North Am 56:644, 1976, with permission.

Figure 6 is reproduced from Braasch JW: Biliary tract. Probl Gen Surg 1:223, 1984, with permission.

Figures 7, 16, and 17 are reproduced from Braasch JW: Pancreaticoduodenal resection. Curr Probl Surg 25:344, 349, and 350, 1988, with permission.

Figures 8 and 12 are reproduced from Braasch JW: Surgical resection of cancer of the mid-duct and distal common bile duct: the Lahey Clinic experience. *In* Wanebo HY (ed): Hepatic and Biliary Cancer. New York, Marcel Dekker, Inc, 1987, pp 367 and 368, with permission.

Figures 9, 11, and 15 are reproduced from Braasch JW, Gray BN: Technique of radical pancreatoduodenectomy with consideration of hepatic arterial relationships. Surg Clin North Am 56:637, 638, and 640, 1976, with permission.

Figure 14 is reproduced from Braasch JW: Malignant disease of the distal bile duct. *In* Moody FG (ed): Advances in Diagnosis and Surgical Treatment of Biliary Tract Disease. New York, Masson Publishing USA, 1983, p 114, with permission.

Figure 18 is reproduced from Braasch JW: Current considerations in the repair of bile duct strictures. Surg Clin North Am 53:430, 1973, with permission.

Chapter 52

Figures 6 and 7 are reproduced from Warren KW, Braasch JW, Thum CW: Diagnosis and surgical treatment of carcinoma of the pancreas. Curr Probl Surg, pp 43 and 51, 1968, with permission.

Chapter 53

Figure 1 is reproduced from Cattell RB, Braasch JW: Secondary operations on the biliary tract. Lahey Clin Bull 11:166, 1959, with permission.

Figure 2 is reproduced from Braasch JW, Gray BN: Technique of radical pancreatoduodenectomy with consideration of

Chapter 53 *Continued*

hepatic arterial relationships. Surg Clin North Am 56:638, 1976, with permission.

Chapter 56

Figure 1 is reproduced from Libertino JA: Renal cell cancer with extension into vena cava. *In* Rob & Smith's Operative Surgery. 4th ed. Urology (edited by W. S. McDougal). London, Butterworth & Co (Publishers) Ltd, 1986, p 123, with permission.

Figure 20 is reproduced from Libertino JA: Surgery of adrenal disorders. Surg Clin North Am 68:1053, 1988, with permission.

Chapter 58

Figures 1, 2, and 4 are reproduced from Munson JL: Recurrent hernias of the abdominal wall. Probl Gen Surg 2:608, 609 and 611, 1985, with permission.

Index

439